WITHDRAWN FROM KENT STATE
UNIVERSITY LIBRARIES

BLOOD DISORDERS IN THE ELDERLY

By

J. H. THOMAS
M.R.C.P. (Lond.), D.C.H.

Consultant Physician (Geriatric Medicine), Bridgend General and Morgannwg Hospitals;
Formerly Federal Adviser, British Caribbean Territory

AND

D. E. B. POWELL
M.D. (Edin.), M.R.C.P. (Lond.), M.R.C.Path.

Consultant Pathologist, Bridgend General and Morgannwg Hospitals;
Formerly Senior Registrar, United Bristol Hospitals

With a Foreword by

W. FERGUSON ANDERSON
M.D., F.R.C.P. (Glas.), F.R.F.P.S., F.R.C.P. (Lond.), F.R.C.P. (Edin.)

Professor of Geriatric Medicine, University of Glasgow

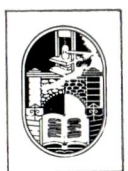

BRISTOL: JOHN WRIGHT & SONS LTD.
1971

COPYRIGHT NOTICE

© JOHN WRIGHT & SONS LTD., 1971

All Rights Reserved. No part of this publication may be reproduced, stored in a retrieval system, or transmitted in any form or by any means, electronic, mechanical, photocopying, recording, or otherwise, without the prior permission of the copyright owner.

Distribution by Sole Agents:
United States of America: The Williams & Wilkins Company, Baltimore
Canada: The Macmillan Company of Canada Ltd., Toronto

SBN 0 7236 0275 1

PRINTED IN GREAT BRITAIN BY JOHN WRIGHT & SONS LTD.,
AT THE STONEBRIDGE PRESS, BRISTOL BS4 5NU

PREFACE

THE number of elderly persons in the community is increasing, with the result that more attention is being given to prevention, rehabilitation, and to the social consequences of illness. Although the care of the elderly is a specialty in its own right, the boundaries between the specialties are artificial and increasingly difficult to maintain. This fact, together with the frequent association of diseases, made us consider the subject as part of general medicine. Blood disorders when present in the elderly are also best treated in this manner. However, the specialties of geriatrics and haematology are usually dealt with in separate departments and by different personnel, and because of this we decided to write a book that would, perhaps, help to bridge the gap.

The pattern of disease varies considerably with age, so that the medical practitioner, whether clinically or laboratory orientated, must take cognizance of this factor. We have found in the care of elderly patients the need for close co-operation between doctors and have endeavoured to incorporate this approach in the book. No attempt has been made to write a comprehensive textbook of haematology, but we hope that sufficient background is included to obviate the necessity for constant recourse to other sources. Both the subject-matter and bibliography are inevitably highly selective. Although conditions such as the haemoglobinopathies may be found in the elderly they are not discussed; other subjects, such as the congenital disorders, are not treated in any detail. Laboratory techniques are not described.

Case-history outlines have been included to illustrate or clarify certain features, although the majority are in no way exceptional. Several of them illustrate the more varied pattern of haematological disease seen in the elderly and underline the necessity of a multidisciplinary approach.

We hope that this basically practical rather than specialized treatment will make the book useful to senior students, membership candidates, and those dealing with sick elderly people, whether at home or in hospital. It could not have been written without the co-operation of colleagues, and we are particularly indebted to the following: Dr. A. G. Chappell, Dr. F. L. Dyson, Dr. R. Howell, Dr. F. W. Thomas, Dr. D. B. Richards, Mr. C. Havard, Mr. O. E. Owen, and Mr. A. W. Fowler. Dr. Alwyn Smith, the Senior Administrative Medical Officer of the Welsh Hospital Board, provided the South Wales cancer registration returns and Dr. Lewis Fanning the statistical evaluation. Dr. John Watkins and Dr. A. R. Mandal carried out surveys when registrars, and the nursing staff willingly co-operated. Mr. A. Dover, Mr. C. T. Dignam, Mr. D. H. Walters, and Mr. C. O. Rees did the bulk of the biochemical and haematological work, and Mr. W. T. Barr some

PREFACE

of the histological and photographic preparations. Mrs. Ann Robinson and Miss Glenys Philpotts were responsible for most of the typing. Finally, it is a pleasure to thank Professor Ferguson Anderson for the Foreword, and Mr. L. G. Owens, of the Publishers, for support and guidance.

J. H. T.
D. E. B. P.

CONTENTS

Preface	iii
Foreword	vii
1.—Introduction	1
2.—General Disease	18
3.—Iron Deficiency	58
4.—Megaloblastic Anaemias	86
5.—Folate Deficiency	110
6.—Other Deficiency States giving Rise to Macrocytic or Megaloblastic Anaemia	123
7.—Prevention of Anaemia	133
8.—Tumours of Lymphoid Tissues	142
9.—Leukaemia	164
10.—Protein Disorders	189
11.—Myeloproliferative Disorders	210
12.—Bleeding and Coagulation Disorders	224
13.—Haemolytic Anaemias	242
14.—Marrow Failure	256
Index	272

FOREWORD

By Professor W. Ferguson Anderson

WITH more older people in the population of the developed countries of the world and with the expectation of even longer life in the future, doctors and medical students need more knowledge about illness in the elderly. This book is a comprehensive account of blood disorders in the upper age range.

Diseases of the blood are not uncommon in older people, perhaps, as the authors state, because a long life gives opportunities for the body to acquire many diseases and for any defect that is present to be accentuated.

The normality of blood in old people is stressed and advancing age is found not to be associated with diminution of an erythrocyte life span or with compensatory failure.

Three aspects are noted to be of importance:—
1. Malabsorption—even of minor degree—especially when prolonged.
2. Antibody and enzyme level alterations and malignant change in cells.
3. Physiological recovery following illness which is incomplete, with diminished reserve power which may be further impaired by arterial disease.

Haemoglobin values, the present and main causes of anaemia, are described under the headings Blood Loss, Malabsorption, and Malnutrition. The importance of apathy, loneliness, impaired mobility, and financial stress is noted and attention is drawn to the compensatory mechanism whereby deficiency of a nutrient is associated with increased absorption. There is a most useful section on the investigation of anaemia with appropriate stress on clinical examination.

The chapter on general disease is complete, mentioning blood-pictures associated with tuberculosis, especially calling to mind the phenomenon of cryptic miliary tuberculosis. The completeness of the study is shown by reference to the anaemia in patients with bed-sores or trauma. Blood changes in rheumatoid arthritis are discussed in detail, while the effects of arterial disease are also considered.

As might be expected of the authors, an account of iron deficiency and metabolism with a practical and systematic approach to diagnosis is given. There is a most useful account of iron deficiency without anaemia, while the therapy of iron deficiency is fully discussed. The megaloblastic anaemias are considered in detail with a helpful account of the mental changes which may be found.

Deficiency of ordinary nutrients, prevention of anaemia, and a full account of other important blood diseases are given. This book thus contains a comprehensive and scholarly account of blood disorders with particular attention devoted to accurate diagnosis and adequate therapy. It is no bad thing that special attention is given to the elderly, where tiredness, depression, apathy, and weakness are so commonly ascribed to old age. This work will help innumerable old people as well as doctors and I commend it wholeheartedly. It is a combination of much study and research presented comprehensively by two well-informed physicians.

BLOOD DISORDERS IN THE ELDERLY

1

INTRODUCTION

BIOLOGICAL ageing must not be confused with the pathological ageing that results from disease—although both may occur together. The life span of cells is not uniform. When old they are desquamated and replaced by young cells. Eventually the process becomes defective and biological ageing supervenes, although man does not live long enough for this to be the cause of death. Most of the cells in an old person are young, except those of the central nervous system. These persist from birth, but even in the brain the changes due to biological ageing are usually overshadowed by those caused by arterial and other disease.

The cellular components of the blood follow the usual pattern. When old and effete they are destroyed and replaced by young cells formed in the marrow. Erythrocytes live 110–120 days, though their survival is not uniform; granulocytes survive approximately 3 weeks and lymphocytes a widely varied period from a few days to months in a complicated recirculating path involving the marrow, spleen, lymph-nodes, and peripheral blood.

In the healthy person, blood formation keeps pace with blood destruction and when necessary the rate varies. Reduction of red blood-cell survival to 20 or 30 days is compensated for by a sixfold increase of erythropoiesis, but beyond this the marrow fails. Advancing age is not normally associated with diminution of erythrocyte life span or with compensatory failure.

There are several studies on red-cell longevity, including that of Woodford-Williams, Webster, Dixon, and MacKenzie (1962). They compared the findings in 22 healthy subjects over the age of 80 (10 males and 12 females) with those obtained in 9 students between the ages of 18 and 25 years and concluded that no significant changes occurred with ageing.

The cells appear the same as they do at a younger age, although an increase in mean corpuscular volume was noted by Olbrich (1947) and in red-cell diameter by Spriggs and Sladden (1958).

The biological function of the red cells is similar at all ages, although there may be minor differences in the elderly as manifested perhaps in a decreased ability to transport potassium and to resist osmotic changes.

Studies on leucocyte counts by Allen and Alexander (1968) did not show any change with age in men, but women between 50 and 65 years had significantly lower total and polymorph leucocyte counts. This was present both in healthy blood donors and in hospital patients.

A long life gives opportunity for the body to acquire many diseases and for any defect that is present to be accentuated. The following three aspects are of considerable importance:—

1. Malabsorption of a minor degree has a cumulative effect and can cause a deficiency anaemia. When investigated, the extent of the failure may be less than one expects unless its prolonged nature is realized. Minor blood-loss has to be assessed similarly.

2. There is considerable opportunity for antibodies to develop and wane, for enzyme levels to alter, and for cells to become malignant.

3. Physiological recovery following illness may be incomplete and reserve power insufficient to withstand stress. Arterial disease reduces the reserve still further. Both factors combine to make the clinical features of anaemia more protean than in younger patients.

Many diseases in the elderly are degenerative and incurable, but symptoms can often be ameliorated by attending to associated treatable conditions. The anaemias come into this category; not only do they produce symptoms, but their clinical features are often superimposed on those of other diseases. Consequently a blood examination is mandatory in every elderly patient and even minimal anaemia must be treated.

The belief that a mild degree of anaemia is to be expected in the aged because of physiological reasons, such as diminution of marrow function, is erroneous. The haemoglobin level should be the adult normal, even in centenarians.

HAEMOGLOBIN VALUES: PREVALENCE OF ANAEMIA

The earlier surveys were designed to ascertain the normal haemoglobin level at different ages. Miller (1939) presented a haematological study of 160 fit men who were inmates of a home for the aged. The literature was summarized as follows: Leichtenstern (1878) found a drop in the haemoglobin from 55 to 60 years and a rise in old age; Nascher (1914) considered the normal haemoglobin level to be between 90 and 110 per cent, and the red-cell count from 3 million to $5\frac{1}{2}$ million; Williamson (1916) found the values to be fairly level between 16 and 60 years (16·9 g. per 100 ml. of blood in men), then a decline to 15·2 g. until the age of 75 years, and a rise to 15·6 g. beyond that age; Wintrobe (1930) concluded that there was no significant difference due to ageing. Miller's results averaged 14·3 g. per 100 ml.

The sex difference in haemoglobin levels was also studied. Olbrich (1947) found an average of 14·5 g. per 100 ml. in 23 males between 70 and 79 years and 13·4 g. in 20 women of the same age, but Hawkins (1954–6) stated that the sex difference in haemoglobin level diminished with advancing years.

Red-cell counts are slightly higher in males than in females. Olbrich (1947) indicated that 5·13 million red blood-cells per c.mm. was the normal in men at 70 years of age and 4·0 million in comparable women.

Kilpatrick (1961) reported the results of a survey carried out in a rural area of Yorkshire and compared them with those previously obtained in an industrial

INTRODUCTION

community in South Wales (Kilpatrick and Hardisty, 1961). There were 40 men and 54 women over 65 years of age in the Yorkshire survey, and of these 80 per cent of the men and 86 per cent of the women were assessed. Anaemia was defined as being 85 per cent or less (12·5 g. per 100 ml.) for men, and 81 per cent or less (12 g. per 100 ml.) for women. By these criteria 20 per cent of the women between 65 and 74 years (25 per cent over 75) and 21 per cent of the men were anaemic. In general the incidence was higher than in South Wales, but comparison in the elderly was not possible as too few had been investigated. Miall, Milner, Lovell, and Standard (1967) in Jamaica found a similar higher prevalence in a rural sample, particularly in males (14·5 per cent rural; 5 per cent suburban at ages 55–64 years). Fry (1961) in a study of 'anaemia' (haemoglobin below 80 per cent) in a London general practice of 5000 patients indicated that the most vulnerable ages were: in males, children under 10 years and men over 60 years, and in females, all age-groups over 30 years with a peak at 50–59. Iron deficiency accounted for 92 per cent of the anaemias. He recommended that full facilities for investigation be given to all family doctors in at least one hospital of each local hospital group.

There are several surveys dealing with the incidence in hospital patients. Lawson (1960) reported on a study of 319 patients over the age of 60 years. Twenty-six per cent were anaemic when first seen, and a further 11 per cent developed anaemia (the criterion being a haemoglobin level below 80 per cent, 11·9 g. per 100 ml.). Bedford and Wollner (1958) found a final incidence of 41 per cent. Our own figures are similar. In 333 consecutive admissions to the hospital a haemoglobin level below 80 per cent was present in 29 per cent. There was no difference in incidence between the sexes (Powell, Thomas, and Mills, 1968).

Read, Gough, Pardoe, and Nicholas (1965), while investigating folic-acid deficiency in 51 consecutive admissions to a welfare home, noted that 12 per cent had a haemoglobin level of 70 per cent or less when first seen.

Pincherle and Shanks (1967) gave the haemoglobin findings in 2000 business executives who included 262 males between 60 and 64 years and 44 males who were older. The level of 14·6 g. per 100 ml. did not drop with ageing and furthermore the incidence of even mild anaemia was negligible—0·32 per cent had a haemoglobin level between 80 and 85 per cent, and 0·1 per cent between 75 and 80 per cent. Lower levels were not found. They felt that the reason for this low incidence of anaemia compared with that in other surveys was the higher standard of nutrition and of medical care in the group studied.

Campbell and his colleagues (1968) gave the results of haemoglobin and plasma-urea concentration in a random sample of adults in Wales based on the electoral roll. Persons over 75 years of age were excluded as they probably needed a domiciliary visit. General practitioners co-operated by taking 2·5-ml. samples of venous blood. Patient refusal amounted to 6·5 per cent for males and 11·8 per cent for females. Four hundred and fifty-two blood samples were finally analysed. The mean haemoglobin level for men between 65 and 74 years of age was 15·2 g. per 100 ml., and for women 13·6 g. per 100 ml. No difference in haemoglobin concentration was noted in samples from different areas—whether rural or urban, agricultural or industrial. Ten per cent of the men had concentrations below 14·0 g. per 100 ml. and 11 per cent of the women below 12·0 g. per 100 ml. (14 per cent female in the age-group 65–75 years). They concluded that the haemoglobin level in men remained steady up to 74 years and that in women there was an increase from 25 to 65 years and then a fall of about 0·5 g. per 100 ml.

Hobson and Blackburn (1953) carried out a home survey of a 1 in 30 random sample selected from the food office register in Sheffield. Only those living alone or with a spouse were included. Anaemia (80 per cent haemoglobin—11·7 g. per 100 ml.—or less) occurred in 5·1 per cent of 177 males aged 66–85 years and in 6·5 per cent of 246 females aged 61–87 years. Eight out of 9 males had iron deficiency and 13 of 16 females. None was receiving treatment for anaemia. The main contributory factors were poor diet (44 per cent) and rheumatoid arthritis (28 per cent). The mean haemoglobin level among 46 males living alone was 13·9 g. per 100 ml. which was considerably lower than the mean level of 14·5 g. per 100 ml. obtained in those living with their wives. These authors put forward the interesting suggestion that there could be a selective removal by death with advancing age of those with low haemoglobin levels.

Parsons, Withey, and Kilpatrick (1965), while undertaking a social survey of a 2 per cent sample of the whole population of the County Borough of Swansea, investigated the haematological indices of 208 persons, 65 years of age or over. Anaemia was defined as a haemoglobin level of 85 per cent (12·5 g. per 100 ml.) or less for men, and 81 per cent (12·0 g. per 100 ml.) or less in women. By these criteria 10·8 per cent of the men and 15·7 per cent of the women were found to be anaemic. Subdivision at the age of 75 years supplied further information. There were 7·2 per cent anaemic men in the age-group 65–74 years and 20·8 per cent in the 75+ group, while in women the corresponding percentages were 11·1 and 23·3. Possible correlation with ingestion of aspirin was investigated but the result was negative. The anaemia was nearly always due to iron deficiency, only 3 having low serum vitamin-B_{12} levels.

From these and similar surveys it is apparent that the incidence of anaemia in the elderly is considerable and that its prevalence increases as age advances.

MORBIDITY AND MORTALITY

There are insufficient data on morbidity for worth-while comparisons to be made between those obtained in different countries. The incidence of pernicious anaemia and leukaemia varies, and iron-deficiency anaemia can be due to primary dietary deficiency in one country or to endemic hookworm disease in another. In this country the main cause of a macrocytic anaemia is vitamin-B_{12} deficiency whereas in India and the Far East it is folate deficiency. The age distribution of the population varies and in countries where the expectation of life is low the prevalence of pernicious anaemia, which is a disease of the elderly, is less than in those where the expectation of life is greater. Some anaemias are more easily treated than others, but the presence of concomitant disease—particularly in the very old—can still result in a high mortality. Moreover, anaemia can precipitate death when another disease is present, but death may not be attributed to it.

Response to therapy in iron-deficiency anaemia is satisfactory if the cause can be corrected, but the underlying disease, such as a carcinoma of the colon, may remain hidden or be inoperable. Diagnostic and therapeutic facilities differ within the same country and more so when several countries are compared. Nevertheless,

INTRODUCTION

despite all these variable factors, considerable information can be obtained from a study of mortality statistics.

The death-rate per million population for the years 1964–6 in the United Kingdom are given in *Table I*.

Table I.—DEATH-RATE PER MILLION POPULATION (W.H.O. REPORT)

TYPES OF ANAEMIA	50–59 Years	60–69 Years	70–79 Years	80+ Years
England and Wales				
Pernicious (other hyperchromic)	3·8	16·6	89·7	294·4
Iron deficiency	1·6	9·1	40·8	156·3
Other anaemia	8·4	23·1	51·7	93·6
Unspecified anaemia	1·4	9·0	30·9	99·7
Scotland				
Pernicious (other hyperchromic)	5·6	19·4	89·5	412·1
Iron deficiency	2·6	5·4	21·1	66·2
Other anaemia	8·7	26·1	62·1	139·8
Unspecified anaemia	5·6	14·0	79·5	179·9
N. Ireland				
Pernicious (other hyperchromic)	8·3	27·0	113·8	368·9
Iron deficiency	—	5·4	28·4	54·6
Other anaemia	10·3	24·3	66·4	68·3
Unspecified anaemia	2·1	21·6	71·1	327·9

The rate increases markedly beyond 60 years of age. The same trend occurs in other countries. Its incidence is similar in Australia and New Zealand, but is less evident elsewhere. Over the age of 70 the most common type is hyperchromic anaemia and this is more pronounced in those over 80, the percentage for England and Wales, Scotland, and Northern Ireland being 45·7, 52·1, and 45·0 respectively. Below the age of 70 death due to 'other anaemias' predominates.

The average death-rate for all types of anaemia rises from 5·8 per million persons in the 40–49 age-group to 409·4 in those aged 80 and over. Females predominate until the age of 70, and thereafter the mortality-rate is higher in males: 70–79 years: 146·6/135·9; 80+: 479/213·9.

The death-rate for hyperchromic and iron-deficiency anaemia remains higher in the female, the rate for hyperchromic anaemia at 80 and over being 130·5 per million in the female and 103·6 per million persons in the male, while for iron-deficiency anaemia the comparable rates are 37·2 and 20·4.

HAEMOPOIESIS AND AGEING

The various schemes of haemopoiesis have long been debated and are still subject to investigation, but we do not propose to recapitulate these arguments other than to summarize the important effects of ageing.

The anatomical effect can be seen in the extent and distribution of haemopoietic marrow. The normal adult has approximately 0·56 g. of marrow per gramme of blood, which constitutes 3·4–5·9 per cent of the body-weight (1600–3700 g.), i.e., it approximates to the weight of the liver. The classic observations of Custer and Ahlfeldt (1932) established that the functioning haemopoietic marrow recedes from the periphery with ageing (*Fig. 1*).

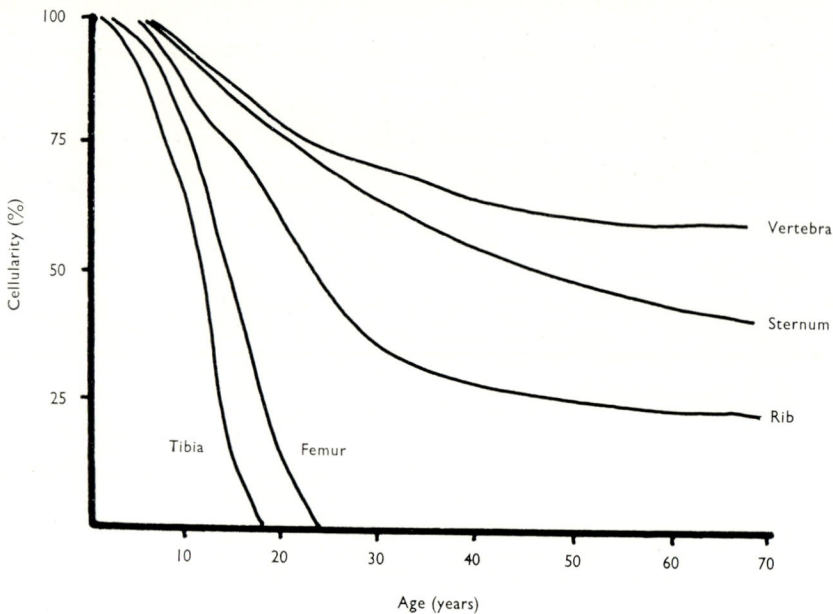

Fig. 1.—The cellularity of bone-marrow at different sites related to age.
(*After Custer and Ahlfedt*, 1932.)

Harstock, Smith, and Petty (1965) studied wedge biopsies of the iliac crest in 177 cases of sudden death where no disease likely to affect haemopoietic tissue had been found. They used a counting technique to assess the frequency of haemopoietic tissue in relation to fat and other structures. The mean percentage of haemopoietic tissue fell from 78·8 per cent under 10 years to 28·9 per cent at 70–79 years. There was a progressive decrease over the first three decades, followed by relative stability until a further decline took place after 60 years. The final stage could be related to an increase in fat subsequent to osteoporosis.

The physiological effects are difficult to evaluate because tests of haemopoietic function are either crude and imprecise or so artificial as to be of dubious relevance. Among the governing factors are erythropoietin, adrenocorticosteroids, thyroid and possibly other hormones, and many stimuli which provoke or depress haemopoiesis, such as oxygenation, body activity, fever, and toxins. There may be a considerable interplay of these factors.

Timaffy (1962) assessed the functional capacity of the leucopoietic system following stimulation by bacterial lipopolysaccharide (*Shigella sonnei*), and compared the responses of 25 healthy young adults (19–31 years) with those obtained in 25 elderly persons (70–83 years) the majority of whom were attending because of cataracts. The average rise in the leucocyte count was 108·07 per cent in the young

INTRODUCTION

and 29·09 per cent in the elderly. The greatest difference occurred in the neutrophils and young granulocytes which rose ×25 in the young and ×3 in the elderly. Cream (1968) measured the neutrophil granulocyte peak with prednisolone stimulation and found an impaired response in the elderly.

Little is known of the direct effect of ageing on erythropoiesis. Old people show a diminished capacity for regeneration after haemorrhage, but this is difficult to distinguish from that due to coexistent chronic disease and other factors, such as renal failure. The capacity of the elderly to produce optimal reticulocyte responses to vitamin-B_{12} therapy in pernicious anaemia may be impaired, but, on the other hand, response to haemorrhage and to vitamin B_{12} or iron therapy is sometimes as satisfactory as in the young. Extramedullary haemopoiesis is seldom seen, but this is hardly a normal index of reserve capacity. To summarize, there is no clear evidence linking the morphological hypoplasia of erythropoietic marrow with functional impairment.

CAUSES OF ANAEMIA

The *main causes* of anaemia are:—

>Blood-loss
>Malabsorption
>Malnutrition

Specific causes are considered separately in subsequent chapters.

BLOOD-LOSS

This is generally accepted as the most important single factor in the production of iron-deficiency anaemia. The mean daily blood-loss in the stools is about 3 ml., but Holt, Mayet, Warner, Callender, and Gunning (1968) found that the average blood-loss in 19 anaemic patients with a gastric hernia was 15 ml. Nearly half were losing the equivalent of 500 ml. a month (250 mg. elemental iron). In all, except 2, there was a fourfold compensatory increase of iron absorption, and the response to iron therapy was good. Many were free from gastric symptoms and 14 had negative occult blood tests.

The cause of gastro-intestinal bleeding is sometimes obscure although haemorrhoids, peptic ulceration, gastric herniation, and neoplastic lesions are fairly common. The diagnoses in 77 consecutive anaemic patients with gastro-intestinal blood-loss, other than from haemorrhoids, are given below:—

Carcinoma:	Colon, 8; Stomach, 9; Rectum, 8; Oesophagus, 1; Jejunum, 1
Hiatus hernia:	6
Ulceration:	Gastric, 10—2 giant; Duodenal, 6; Anastomotic, 1; Oesophageal, 1; Gastric and duodenal, 1; Gastric erosion, 2
Diverticula:	Colon, 5; Duodenal, 4; Oesophageal, 1; Jejunal, 1; Gastric, 1
Ulcerative colitis:	2
Thrombocytopenic purpura:	1
Uraemia:	1
Aspirin ingestion:	2
Unknown cause:	5

Occult blood testing is not an accurate method of detecting gastro-intestinal bleeding because the loss is often intermittent. Nevertheless, it is valuable in view of its simplicity and sensitivity, being positive when the loss is 5 ml. a day. However, undue reliance should not be placed on negative results. Bedford and Wollner (1958) found the Gregersen test positive in 55 per cent of admissions and in 78 per cent of those who were anaemic. Agate (1963) considered that hiatus hernia was probably the most commonly missed cause.

Those in whom no reason for the bleeding is found form an interesting group. They amounted to 14 per cent of patients with iron-deficiency anaemia described by Bannerman, Beveridge, and Witts (1964). The follow-up was negative in 75 per cent and they concluded that although gastric erosions perhaps accounted for some, in the majority the cause remained obscure. Anaemia tended to recur but responded to therapy. In the elderly, more so perhaps than in the young, it is difficult to decide how thoroughly one should pursue the investigation when radiological examination of the gastro-intestinal tract is negative. Intestinal polypi, erosions, ischaemic colitis, and vascular anomalies may remain undetected. Laparotomy is not justified, but in view of the frequency of neoplastic lesions at this age barium studies should be repeated in 3–4 months. Despite these precautions it is not unusual for a neoplasm to be obvious a year or two later.

Other sources of bleeding, such as haematuria, vaginal bleeding, and epistaxis, are fairly common reasons for admission to hospital. Obvious loss may be intermittent, with less in between. This may not be noted, with the result that the anaemia may seem excessive. Bleeding from the urogenital tract, as in carcinoma of the prostate, bladder, and kidney, is a common cause of this phenomenon, as the urine may contain excess red blood-cells when haematuria is not evident. The amount of iron normally lost in the urine is about 0·5 mg. a day, but this is probably exceeded in many elderly persons, especially males. Oesophageal varices have occasionally to be considered because cirrhosis of the liver is not unusual. McKeown (1965) gave an incidence of 1·5 per cent in necropsy material.

MALABSORPTION

Iron and folates are absorbed in the upper part of the small intestine, and vitamin B_{12} in the lower ileum. The incidence of atrophic gastritis increases as age advances, with the result that the production of 'intrinsic factor' may diminish and consequently fail to participate in the absorption of the dietary vitamin B_{12}. Normal gastric function also has a complex role in iron metabolism. Jejunal diverticula sometimes develop and interfere with the normal absorption of folate. Steatorrhoea is not an uncommon finding, although gluten enteropathy is rare. Patients who have undergone surgery of the gastro-intestinal tract may present several years later with anaemia due to malabsorption. Of 85 consecutive patients who were anaemic from a gastro-intestinal cause 5 had had a previous partial gastrectomy.

MALNUTRITION

The normal diet contains 10–12 mg. of iron, 10 μg. vitamin B_{12}, and 100 μg. folate per day, which is sufficient to supply the 1 mg. of iron, 2 μg. vitamin B_{12}, and 50 μg. folate that are necessary to maintain erythropoiesis. A diet devoid of all meat, fish, fowl, dairy produce, and grain products still contains about 0·4 μg.

INTRODUCTION

vitamin B_{12} per day and would have to be taken continuously for about 2 years before vitamin-B_{12} deficiency developed, provided absorption was satisfactory and the stores full when the diet commenced. Such limitation of food intake is unlikely to be encountered except in vegans and even in them few symptoms develop. Smith (1962) investigated 12 such subjects and found that apart from 2 who had subacute combined degeneration of the cord, they were healthy. Four were over 50 years of age, and 1, a female of 71, had been a vegan for 30 years. Her haemoglobin was 83 per cent, serum vitamin B_{12} 80 pg. per ml., and serum iron 25 μg. per 100 ml. None had a haemoglobin below 80 per cent and in 7 it was 90 per cent or above. The serum vitamin-B_{12} level was below 150 pg. per ml. in 8, and in 5 it was 90 pg. per ml. or less, the lowest being 48 pg. per ml. This was in a female aged 48, who had been a vegan for 18 years. He contrasted their lack of physical signs, despite the low serum vitamin-B_{12} levels, from that seen in patients with tobacco amblyopia, where the levels of serum vitamin B_{12} could be normal, and yet the condition responds to cytamen injections. However, as the amblyopia is probably due to failure of cyanide detoxication by vitamin B_{12} it is more likely to develop when vitamin B_{12} is deficient than when dietary intake and absorption are satisfactory. The oldest patient among the 65 reported on by Foulds, Chisholm, Bronte-Stewart, and Wilson (1969) was aged 84 years.

Despite the adequacy of haematinic factors in normal diets malnutrition still occurs. Apathy, loneliness, impaired mobility, and financial stress are potent causes. Moreover, the body stores may already be low and when combined with occult blood-loss and decreased absorption, deficiency may become severe.

The body normally compensates for a deficiency by increasing absorption so that when this mechanism is defective or the dietary intake insufficient, anaemia results.

ERYTHROCYTE SEDIMENTATION RATE (E.S.R.)

Although Westergren (1957) indicated that the upper limit of normality was 5 mm. in the first hour in men, and 10–15 mm. in women, higher values are frequently obtained in 'healthy' elderly persons.

The rate of red-cell sedimentation is governed by factors affecting both cell and plasma. Increased viscosity retards sedimentation, while a decrease in red-cell volume accelerates it. When these factors are allowed for, the rate is mainly dependent on the concentration in the plasma of fibrinogen, alpha-2, and gamma-globulin, the most important being fibrinogen. Elevation of this fraction, as may occur with ageing (Steinman, 1964), perhaps accounts for the unexpected high values that are sometimes obtained. An increased serum lipid concentration is another possibility.

Women have higher normal values than men, but the explanation is obscure because the greater incidence of anaemia that occurs among women in the younger age-group is not a feature in the elderly. Perhaps hormonal influences are in some way responsible.

Bottiger and Svedberg (1967) analysed the E.S.R. in 1457 men and 1021 women between the ages of 20 and 70. They were all physically healthy. Those whose parents suffered from, or had died from, ischaemic heart disease or cerebrovascular accidents were excluded. The results indicated that above the age of 50 the upper normal limit for men was 20 mm. and for women 30 mm. in the first hour.

Boyd and Hoffbrand (1966) studied the E.S.R. in 303 patients admitted to a geriatric unit, and concluded that in nearly a third there was no apparent cause for values above 20 mm. in the first hour, and that in some instances this was so when the value was as high as 40 mm. They decided that occult urinary tract infection was not the explanation.

The presence of such a wide range in the E.S.R. of healthy elderly persons diminishes the value of the test as a diagnostic aid. In exceptional circumstances similar values may be obtained, for example, in a patient with early myelomatosis or temporal arteritis as in another who is healthy. Serial readings help clinically, but they are seldom available.

The enormous variety of pathological states associated with a raised E.S.R. is not surprising, as most infections, whether acute or chronic, can produce an altered serum protein pattern. When a grossly elevated reading is obtained, collagen disease, arteritis, and myelomatosis have to be considered although the elderly are also subject to the same diseases as affect younger people. Their presentation, however, is often different so that well-recognized entities such as pyometra, bacterial endocarditis, septicaemia, abscesses, and purulent arthritis may be overlooked. Occasionally a high E.S.R. is obtained for which there is no apparent explanation.

PLASMA PROTEINS

There is wide variation in the levels of protein fractions. Reduction of albumin and elevation of gamma-globulin are often noted, but this could be physiological.

Haferkamp, Schlettwein-Gsell, Schwick, and Störiko (1966) measured the protein fractions of 145 inhabitants of a village in Switzerland, ranging in age from 15 to 91 years (55 over 61 years). There was no significant difference in the total protein content between the different age-groups, but electrophoresis and quantitative immunological tests showed an increase in gamma-globulin and a decrease of albumin as age advanced. This change appeared in the fifties and was maintained.

Other authors have been less definite. Some have shown that protein patterns are unchanged with ageing in healthy individuals, while others regard a fall in serum albumin and high values of gamma-globulin to be normal in the elderly. The difficulty in differentiating between health and disease in these persons is often semantic, owing to the frequent occurrence of occult disorders in the apparently healthy. The distinction is largely theoretical because for practical purposes it is only in ill people that serum proteins need be assessed.

Chesrow, Turner, Shaffner, and Musci (1957) showed that gamma-globulins increased and ascribed it to intercurrent infection and malnutrition. Eckerström (1958) investigated 30 persons between 70 and 90 years of age. They had normal blood-pictures, erythrocyte sedimentation rate, renal and hepatic function, and were all well nourished. There was an elevation of gamma-globulin and this was considered to be primarily due to infection or tumour. Woodford-Williams, Alvarez, Webster, Landless, and Dixon (1964) concluded that the changes seen were probably the result of numerous factors, with underlying disease, immobility, and malnutrition being the most important. Chronological ageing as a cause

INTRODUCTION

seemed less significant. Very ill patients, whatever their illness, had markedly abnormal protein patterns. After the age of 60 the mean level for albumin was 3·56 g. per 100 ml. compared with 4·19 g. in young normals, and the globulin fractions had mean levels of 0·27 g. for alpha-1, 0·91 g. for alpha-2, 0·89 g. for beta, and 1·41 g. for gamma (compared with 0·23, 0·76, 0·80, and 1·21 in the young). The lower albumin was not statistically related to either dietary intake or nutritional state, but was influenced by chronic infection, particularly of the renal tract.

We measured the total protein in 293 consecutive admissions over the age of 60 years (173 females, 120 males) and obtained comparable results. Although moribund patients were excluded the majority were seriously ill. No difference relating to sex was demonstrated.

The level was between 6·1 and 8·0 g. per 100 ml. in 82 per cent of the males and in 83 per cent of the females.

Albumin

The mean level was 3·0 g. per 100 ml. No further reduction occurred beyond the age of 60 years in either sex except that a slightly lower level was obtained in men in the 81–90 age-group. The association with disease categories is shown in Table II.

Table II.—Association of Albumin and Disease Categories

Clinical Diagnosis	Albumin Values (g. per 100 ml.)						
	<1·5	1·6–2·0	2·1–2·5	2·6–3·0	3·1–3·5	3·6–4·0	4·1+
Blood-loss and gastro-intestinal disease	0	0	8	10	10	3	0
Infection and rheumatoid disease	1	5	11	20	20	6	2
Neoplasm	0	0	5	9	3	0	1
Cardiovascular	0	1	18	25	23	1	5
Complex anaemia	0	1	1	2	1	1	1
Miscellaneous	0	0	5	16	14	4	3
Total No. of patients	1	7	48	82	71	15	12.

In the infection group, 6 had levels below 2·0 g. per 100 ml. compared with 1 in the vascular disease group and none in the others. Only 12 of 236 had an albumin above 4·0 g. per 100 ml., none of whom were in the alimentary disease group, so possibly deficient dietary intake and absorption may have contributed, although infection seemed a much more important cause.

We correlated the albumin level with that of haemoglobin, defining anaemia as a haemoglobin below 80 per cent (11·6 g. per 100 ml.). Among 59 anaemic patients an albumin below 2·5 g. per 100 ml. was obtained in 25 per cent, while in 148 non-anaemic patients the corresponding number was 29 (19 per cent).

There was no relationship with serum vitamin B_{12}.

It is evident that infection is associated with hypoalbuminaemia, but iron-deficiency anaemia, which is common in the elderly, may also have a contributory role. Other factors such as immobility, deficient protein intake, disease of liver and kidneys, together with carcinoma, must also be included.

Globulin

A high level of globulin is common in elderly hospital patients. *Table III* shows the results obtained from an analysis at different ages.

Table III.—Analysis of Serum Proteins at Different Ages

	Serum Proteins (mean levels)					
	61–70 Years		71–80 Years		81–90 Years	
	Male	*Female*	*Male*	*Female*	*Male*	*Female*
Albumin	2·9±0·6	3·0±0·6	3·1±0·6	3·0±0·6	2·8±0·5	3·2±0·6
Alpha-1 globulin	0·35±0·18	0·36±0·29	0·38±0·13	0·35±0·13	0·42±0·13	0·35±0·17
Alpha-2 globulin	0·88±0·39	0·89±0·41	0·90±0·31	0·91±0·30	0·88±0·25	0·93±0·33
Beta-globulin	0·81±0·50	0·99±0·41	0·82±0·51	0·84±0·34	0·90±0·67	0·77±0·28
Gamma-globulin	1·54±0·37	1·64±0·53	1·55±0·61	1·47±0·50	1·56±0·73	1·34±0·64

Table IV.—Gamma-globulin in Disease Categories

Clinical Diagnosis	Gamma-globulin Values (g. per 100 ml.)						
	<0·5	0·51–1·00	1·01–1·50	1·51–2·00	2·01–2·50	2·51–3·00	3·01+
Blood-loss and gastro-intestinal disease	0	6	9	11	4	1	0
Infection and rheumatoid disease	0	17	14	23	9	11	1
Neoplasm	0	3	7	8	1	0	0
Cardiovascular	1	19	24	23	13	3	0
Complex anaemia	1	3	1	1	0	2	0
Miscellaneous	1	6	17	12	5	0	0
Total No. of patients	3	54	72	78	32	17	1

Gamma-globulin has received more attention than the other fractions, but alpha-1, alpha-2, and beta-globulins may be higher than the corresponding levels in younger patients.

Although the mean levels are not significantly elevated, there is a considerable standard deviation. Even in the absence of an established cause high levels may still be obtained. This is shown in *Table IV*.

INTRODUCTION

A level above 2·0 g. per 100 ml. was present in 12 per cent of the miscellaneous group, 17 per cent of the gastro-intestinal and infection groups, in 20 per cent of those with vascular disease (hemiplegia and cardiac infarction), but in only 5 per cent of the neoplastic group. When levels below 1·0 g. per 100 ml. were considered again there was no association with a particular disease category. As the mean level was 1·5 g. per 100 ml. it is possible that in the presence of illness a level below 1·0 g. per 100 ml. signifies gamma-globulin deficiency. Whether this has clinical implications, either in the disease process itself or in its prognosis, is debatable. The percentage with this level of gamma-globulin increased from 9 per cent (3/32) in the age-group 61–70 years to 19 per cent (20/103) between 71 and 80 years, and to 32 per cent (19/60) in those aged 81–90 years.

We compared the gamma-globulin levels obtained in 59 anaemic with those of 149 non-anaemic patients and noted that 58 per cent had a level above 1·5 g. per 100 ml. as against 44 per cent. A similar finding occurred when the serum iron was below 70 μg. per 100 ml. These results are the same as those obtained in patients with low measurements of serum albumin, but they are not due to specific diseases because they are present in all the disease categories.

Woodford-Williams and others (1964) concluded that immobility itself was an important cause. In their series a group with osteoarthritis had the lowest albumin and the highest gamma-globulin levels.

It is evident that routine fractionation of serum proteins, as usually performed, is of little, if any, value in the elderly other than in the detection of paraproteins. Identical results are obtained in a variety of diseases.

There is possibly an unknown factor associated with ageing and illness that stimulates the plasma cells to form more gamma-globulin, and it has been suggested (Martin, 1961) that very high levels may be forme fruste of myelomatosis. Likewise, low levels of gamma-globulin may indicate displacement by a closely related paraprotein.

Studies of antibody components have shown a decrease, despite elevation of the gamma-globulin. Haferkamp and others (1966) stated that antistreptolysin O, staphylolysin, staphylococcal coagulase, and mixed coli antigens diminished with age. The immunoglobulins IgG and IgA increased while no change occurred in the level of IgM globulin. They suggested that tissue changes could be responsible. The cells producing immunoglobulins are of lymphoid origin. Although minute quantities are probably lost in the urine and via the gastro-intestinal tract, much more is destroyed by catabolism, the site of which is not known.

Whether an increase in IgG is a general finding in the elderly remains to be seen. The wide scatter around the mean gamma-globulin level suggests that the quantity of immunoglobulins is unlikely to be constant. Low levels are not rare.

Many elderly people are surprisingly resistant to infection, but others succumb readily and become progressively more susceptible.

TYPES OF ANAEMIA

Iron deficiency is the most common cause of anaemia in the elderly, but depletion of vitamin B_{12} and folate is commoner than at other ages. Indeed, pernicious anaemia is primarily a disease of persons over the age of 60 years, and in our experience is seen about three times as often as anaemia due to folate deficiency.

A characteristic of the deficiency anaemias at this age is that frequently more than one haematinic factor is at fault, despite the fact that the blood-picture may be typical of a lone deficiency. Lack of iron for instance, associated with hypochromia, does not exclude a deficiency of vitamin B_{12} or of folate. Iron therapy can be successful even when there is such a deficiency, but there is always a possibility that the deficiency will become more pronounced with increased erythropoiesis. In many instances there is initial improvement and then a relapse. A similar state of affairs can exist with pernicious anaemia. A typical macrocytic blood-picture does not exclude the presence of iron deficiency. Evans, Pathy, Sanerkin, and Deeble (1968) found that in 90 cases of megaloblastic anaemia, vitamin B_{12} was deficient in 48, folic acid in 36, and both factors in 6, while more than half had associated iron deficiency. Similarly, when they studied those over 65 years who had iron deficiency, no less than 47 per cent had evidence of other haematinic factor deficiencies.

The tendency to multiple pathology complicates the issue. Wilkinson (1949) reported that of 301 patients with pernicious anaemia who had died, 28 did so because of a carcinoma of the stomach and 42 because of a non-gastric cancer. Involvement of the gastro-intestinal tract can lead to blood-loss, but carcinoma elsewhere in the body can also affect haemopoiesis. Other diseases, such as rheumatoid arthritis and chronic infection, can cause anaemia because of a failure of iron utilization, although in the elderly the overall picture is modified by the frequency of iron deficiency.

A low serum level of pyridoxine may be part of a wider deficiency and can cause a hypochromic anaemia resistant to iron therapy. Lack of vitamin C can be associated with a macrocytic anaemia. A low protein intake, as for instance after gastrectomy, may lead to a normocytic normochromic anaemia, possibly due to inadequate globin synthesis. Malabsorption and malnutrition in general can cause a complex blood-picture, particularly when other diseases are also present. Moreover, haematinic factors may be deficient in persons who have not yet become anaemic.

Hypoplastic anaemia and marrow infiltration with neoplastic or fibrous tissue are seen more often in the elderly than in the middle aged, but nevertheless are much rarer than the deficiency anaemias. The reticuloses, leukaemia, erythraemia, and myelomatosis are also commoner at this age.

Certain blood disorders, such as congenital spherocytic anaemia and idiopathic thrombocytopenic purpura, are rarer than in younger life, though typical examples occur.

The relative frequency of disorders is seen from the accompanying analysis of 100 consecutive patients with a haemoglobin level of 60 per cent (8·6 g. per 100 ml.) or less:—

Pure iron deficiency	45
Lone vitamin-B_{12} deficiency	18
Lone folate deficiency	7
Iron and folate deficiency	10
Iron and vitamin-B_{12} deficiency	11
Iron, vitamin-B_{12}, and folate deficiency	6
Acute leukaemia	1
Leuco-erythroblastic anaemia	1
Aplastic anaemia	1

INTRODUCTION

INVESTIGATION

Tests requested in anaemic patients obviously depend a great deal on the available facilities, but when several departments use the same laboratory different approaches are still evident. They can be divided into three broad groups:—

1. The routine system: A series of investigations are carried out in every case.
2. The clinical approach: The investigations instigated are governed by the clinical findings.
3. The combined approach: After initial routine assessment investigations are performed as required.

The differences can be illustrated in the management of a patient with hypochromic anaemia. By the routine system, serum levels of iron, vitamin B_{12}, and folate, reticulocyte count, and the result of a sternal puncture are obtained; while the clinical approach is satisfied if a hypochromic anaemia responds to iron therapy. The combined method desires information on serum iron, vitamin B_{12}, and folate, and then continues with further requests only if specifically indicated. Investigation involves assessment of marrow function, blood-loss, and red-cell destruction.

Marrow Function

Disturbance is usually due to a deficiency of haematinic factors, but sometimes the marrow is hypoplastic or infiltrated with leukaemic, neoplastic, or myeloma cells. Fibrosis may be prominent. Increased reticulocyte counts in the peripheral blood indicate hyperactivity of the marrow as with chronic blood-loss, haemolysis, or response to haematinics.

Microscopic study of marrow smears, or of marrow biopsy material, is essential when anaemia persists.

Blood-loss

Occult-blood testing of the stools should always be performed when iron deficiency is suspected. The test is also required when response to adequate iron therapy is unsatisfactory.

Haemolysis

Evidence of increased haemolysis should be sought when there is unexplained reticulocytosis or persistent anaemia.

Clinical Examination

Clinical examination is imperative. A sore tongue and angular stomatitis indicate the presence of multiple deficiencies. Enlarged lymph-nodes suggest leukaemia, lymphosarcoma, or Hodgkin's disease. Splenomegaly can be due to infiltration with leukaemic or myeloid tissue, with extramedullary erythropoiesis in myelofibrosis, or increased blood destruction in haemolytic states. Petechiae occur in thrombocytopenia, whether primary or secondary, and in bacterial endocarditis which can present as anaemia. No system of the body can be excluded because anaemia is usually a secondary phenomenon and investigation is not complete until the cause has been ascertained. Previous surgery, particularly of the gastrointestinal tract, must be considered.

If a deficiency anaemia is present, then dietary intake, absorption, and blood-loss must be assessed. Measurement of the faecal fat and radiological study of the gastro-intestinal tract are necessary when malabsorption is suspected.

More sophisticated investigations are sometimes required. Measurement of vitamin-B_{12} absorption, with and without intrinsic factor, may be the only means whereby the presence of pernicious anaemia can be demonstrated. Iron or folate absorption can also be ascertained.

Guiding Principles

When investigating anaemia particular attention should be paid to the most common cause. In the elderly this is iron deficiency due to blood-loss, but multiple deficiencies are often seen. Consequently, estimation of serum iron, vitamin-B_{12}, and folate levels is frequently necessary unless another cause, such as leukaemia, is present—and even then the information is useful. A patient with iron-deficiency anaemia often has low serum levels of the other main haematinic factors, and treatment with iron alone is only partially successful. After initial improvement anaemia recurs, though its character may change from hypochromic to macrocytic. Close supervision is often impossible so that early relapse is difficult to detect. In view of this, prevention is preferable. Despite the complexity of the inter-relationship between the three main haematinics we believe that their serum levels should ideally be ascertained whatever type of deficiency the blood-picture suggests.

Measurement of the haemoglobin and haematocrit levels are the only reliable means of detecting anaemia, and a blood-film should always be studied. Hypochromia, even of a mild degree, usually shows the need for iron therapy. There are exceptional states, however, such as pyridoxine deficiency and sometimes chronic infection, when the utilization of iron is faulty, rather than its quantity. A normocytic normochromic anaemia occurs after acute blood-loss, but in the elderly it is much more likely to be due to a combined deficiency.

Reticulocyte counts supply valuable diagnostic and therapeutic information. A persistently low count suggests marrow hypoplasia, particularly when the serum level of the main haematinics is satisfactory. Conversely, reticulocytosis indicates marrow hyperfunction and is an accepted means of measuring response to therapy.

Examination of marrow smears should perhaps be carried out more often, but aspiration is sometimes difficult and the procedure disturbing to the patient. In general it is necessary when the cause of the anaemia is obscure or response to therapy unsatisfactory. The type of erythropoiesis and its extent can be judged, and abnormal cells observed. The detection of macrocytic anaemia should be followed by examination of the marrow. Perls's staining for iron is an integral part of the investigation. Myelofibrosis cannot be diagnosed unless the architecture of the marrow is assessed, but this is not possible with sternal puncture material. Biopsy, usually of the iliac crest, is then necessary.

In those with a low serum B_{12} gastric analysis should be carried out, as pernicious anaemia does not occur unless histamine-fast achlorhydria is present. A search for paraproteins is worth while when the E.S.R. is unaccountably elevated, particularly if there is bleeding. Elevation of the blood-urea often accounts for a refractory anaemia.

Whenever the clinical features are unusual, periodic reassessment is necessary.

INTRODUCTION
REFERENCES

AGATE, J. (1963), *The Practice of Geriatrics*, p. 338. London: Heinemann.
ALLEN, R. N., and ALEXANDER, M. K. (1968), *J. clin. Path.*, **21**, 691.
BANNERMAN, R. M., BEVERIDGE, B. R., and WITTS, L. J. (1964), *Br. med. J.*, **1**, 1417.
BEDFORD, P. D., and WOLLNER, L. (1958), *Lancet*, **1**, 1144.
BOTTIGER, L. E., and SVEDBERG, C. A. (1967), *Br. med. J.*, **1**, 85.
BOYD, R. V., and HOFFBRAND, B. I. (1966), *Ibid.*, **1**, 901.
CAMPBELL, H., GREENE, W. J. W., KEYSER, J. W., WATERS, W. E., WEDDELL, J. M., and WITHEY, J. L. (1968), *Br. J. prev. soc. Med.*, **22**, 41.
CHESROW, E. J., TURNER, C. C., SHAFFNER, F., and MUSCI, J. (1957), *Geriatrics*, **12**, 642.
CREAM, J. J. (1968), *Br. J. Haemat.*, **15**, 259.
CUSTER, R. P., and AHLFELDT, F. E. (1932), *J. Lab. clin. Med.*, **17**, 960.
ECKERSTRÖM, STEN (1958), *Geriatrics*, **13**, 744.
EVANS, D. M. D., PATHY, M. S., SANERKIN, N. G., and DEEBLE, T. J. (1968), *Geront. clin.*, **10**, 228.
FOULDS, W. S., CHISHOLM, I. A., BRONTE-STEWART, J., and WILSON, T. M. (1969), *Br. J. Ophthalm.*, **53**, 393.
FRY, J. (1961), *Br. med. J.*, **2**, 1732.
HAFERKAMP, O., SCHLETTWEIN-GSELL, D., SCHWICK, H. G., and STÖRIKO, K. (1966), *Gerontologia*, **12**, 1, 30.
HARSTOCK, R. J., SMITH, E. B., and PETTY, C. S. (1965), *Am. J. clin. Path.*, **43**, 326.
HAWKINS, W. W. (1956), *Am. Geriat. Soc.*, **4**, 24.
— — SPECK, E., and LEONARD, V. G. (1954), *Blood*, **9**, 999.
HOBSON, W., and BLACKBURN, E. K. (1953), *Br. med. J.*, **1**, 647.
HOLT, J. M., MAYET, F. G. H., WARNER, G. T., CALLENDER, S. T., and GUNNING, A. J. (1968), *Ibid.*, **3**, 22.
KILPATRICK, G. S. (1961), *Ibid.*, **2**, 1736.
— — and HARDISTY, R. M. (1961), *Ibid.*, **1**, 778.
LAWSON, I. R. (1960), *Geront. clin.*, **2**, 87.
LEICHTENSTERN (1878), quoted by WILLIAMSON, C. S. (1916), *Archs intern. Med.*, **18**, 505.
MCKEOWN, F. (1965), *Pathology of the Aged*. London: Butterworths.
MARTIN, N. H. (1961), *Lancet*, **1**, 237.
MIALL, W. E., MILNER, P. F., LOVELL, H. G., and STANDARD, K. L. (1967), *Br. J. prev. soc. Med.*, **21**, 45.
MILLER, I. (1939), *J. Lab. clin. Med.*, **24**, 1172.
NASCHER, I. L. (1914), *Geriatrics. The Diseases of Old Age and their Treatment*. Philadelphia: Blakiston.
OLBRICH, O. (1947), *Edin. med. J.*, **54**, 306.
PARSONS, P. L., WITHEY, J. L., and KILPATRICK, G. S. (1965), *The Practitioner*, **195**, 656.
PINCHERLE, G., and SHANKS, J. (1967), *Br. J. prev. soc. Med.*, **21**, 40.
POWELL, D. E. B., THOMAS, J. H., and MILLS, P. (1968), *Geront. clin.*, **10**, 21.
READ, A. E., GOUGH, K. R., PARDOE, J. L., and NICHOLAS, A. (1965), *Br. med. J.*, **2**, 843.
SMITH, A. D. M. (1962), *Ibid.*, **1**, 1655.
SPRIGGS, A. I., and SLADDEN, R. A. (1958), *J. clin. Path.*, **11**, 53.
STEINMAN, B. (1964), *Gerontologia*, **10**, 100.
TIMAFFY, M. (1962), *Geront. clin.*, **4**, 13.
WESTERGREN, A. (1957), *Triangle (En)*, **3**, 20.
WILKINSON, J. F. (1949), *Lancet*, **1**, 336.
WILLIAMSON, C. S. (1916), *Archs intern. Med.*, **18**, 505.
WINTROBE, M. M. (1930), *Medicine*, **9**, 195.
WOODFORD-WILLIAMS, E., ALVAREZ, A. S., WEBSTER, D., LANDLESS, B., and DIXON, M. P. (1964), *Geront. clin.*, **10**, 86.
— — WEBSTER, D., DIXON, M. P., and MACKENZIE, W. (1962), *Ibid.*, **4**, 183.
WORLD HEALTH ORGANIZATION (1969), 'Anaemias, 1926–66, Mortality Statistics', *Wld Hlth Org. Stat. Rep.*, **22**, 409.

2
GENERAL DISEASE

GENERAL disease is frequently associated with changes in the blood, and this is particularly so in the elderly. A patient with cerebral thrombosis or cardiac infarction, for example, may be anaemic due to blood-loss from a carcinoma of the colon or as a result of chronic pyelonephritis, and consequently the practice of requesting routine investigation of the haemoglobin, blood-film, and urea assumes considerable importance. Not only may the result explain the presence of congestive failure or mental confusion but appropriate treatment facilitates rehabilitation and the whole future management is simplified.

The association between the disease and the blood disorder can be straightforward as in anaemia from blood-loss due to peptic ulceration, or complex and ill understood as in the anaemia of chronic infection.

All diseases that interfere with mastication, ingestion, digestion, and absorption are important in the development of anaemia, as are those associated with blood-loss. They are numerous but not specific to the elderly, although edentulous states, badly fitting dentures, pseudobulbar palsy, oesophageal strictures, gastric hernias, jejunal diverticula, and neoplasms of the gastro-intestinal tract are commoner at this age than at any other. Whenever mobility is limited from whatever cause, malnutrition leading to anaemia may follow. Diseases causing mental disturbances and social upheaval often result in a disinterest in food.

It is unnecessary to expand on the clinical features of many of these diseases, but there are some that warrant further consideration owing to their special role in the production of blood changes.

INFECTION

A neutrophilia with a shift to the left in the Arneth count is not sufficiently prominent or characteristic to be relied upon when the diagnosis of infection is in doubt.

In 50 consecutive patients with bronchopneumonia, the total white-cell count varied from 4600 to 16,200 per c.mm. with the majority lying between 9000 and 12,000 per c.mm. This was elevated compared with the normal count of 4000–8000 per c.mm. The polymorph proportion was between 60 and 90 per cent. A shift to the left was commonly noted, even when there was no leucocytosis. Overlap with that obtained in persons with no apparent infection was considerable. A similar range occurred in those with carcinoma of the lung, acute exacerbation of chronic bronchitis, asthma, and pulmonary infarction.

Even an abscess or empyema may be associated with a normal white-cell count, although occasionally the leucocytosis may reach 20,000–30,000 per c.mm.

Similar counts may also be produced by multiple secondaries, particularly when the liver is involved, so that the presence of a subphrenic abscess may be suspected.

The lymphocyte, eosinophil, and monocyte counts have the same significance in the elderly as in younger persons except that the disease pattern may be different and certain conditions, such as infectious mononucleosis, rarer.

In general, the marrow is slower to respond than in the young or middle aged, and the degree of response may be less. Similarly with lymphoid tissue. Adenitis in the drainage area of a superficial infection may not develop as expected, although lymph-node participation in reticulosis and neoplasm is unaffected.

The erythrocyte sedimentation rate is usually raised by the time the patient is admitted to hospital, but the time taken to produce this elevation is not known. Experience with long-term hospital patients suggests that the rate is raised within 24 hours, but these are ill people and their plasma proteins often abnormal, so that comparison between them and healthy persons developing acute infection is probably misleading. The level to which the rate rises is not of diagnostic or prognostic significance, but levels above 100 mm. in the first hour are unlikely in uncomplicated bacterial or viral disease. The rate of reduction is sometimes rapid and parallels clinical improvement, although usually there is delay of 2–3 weeks after apparent complete recovery before a normal fixed level is reached. Should a raised sedimentation rate persist then the presence of another disease, such as arteritis or myelomatosis, or the possibility of a complication has to be considered.

Anaemia is often seen but its incidence in patients with acute infection is probably not increased unless haemolysis results or the infection is prolonged. There may be a deficiency of haematinic factors from unrelated causes, and coincidental disease may affect the blood-picture.

Case 1.—A man, aged 83, was admitted with bronchopneumonia of the right base. He had been ill for 2 days and was delirious. The diagnosis was confirmed and it was noted that he had slight tenderness below the right costal margin. The Hb was 54 per cent and the white-cell count 11,000 with 80 per cent polymorphs. The red cells were hypochromic. Serum iron was 45 μg. per 100 ml., serum folate 1·1 ng. per ml. and vitamin B_{12} 90 pg. per ml. Blood-urea was 30 mg. per 100 ml. Marrow puncture showed normoblasts with a few megaloblasts. Despite antibiotic and haematinic therapy he died on the sixth day.

Post-mortem: Bronchopneumonia of right base; suppurative cholecystitis with gangrene of gall-bladder; spleen enlarged; gastric polyp; cysts of colon; aneurysm of descending aorta; cerebral atherosclerosis.

Bacterial Endocarditis

This disease is often peculiarly difficult to diagnose in the elderly and the significance of certain physical signs may not be appreciated—petechiae and ecchymoses may be confused with senile purpura, mild clubbing may be missed, an apical murmur may be ignored, mild pallor can be ascribed to the many causes that are frequently present, and low-grade fever may be thought to be due to bronchopneumonia or urinary infection. Symptoms can be minimal and the only finding a mild hypochromic anaemia resistant to iron therapy. The erythrocyte sedimentation rate and the white-cell count are usually raised, but are sometimes normal. A cardiac lesion need not be present. Wedgwood (1955) reported on 65 cases of subacute bacterial endocarditis, 13 (20 per cent) of whom were 60 or over, and in 1961 he described these elderly patients in greater detail. The oldest was 81 years of age, and duration of symptoms varied from 2 to 23 weeks. He suggested that the disease ran a quieter and more insidious course than in the young. The haemoglobin concentration was within normal limits in 3, between 60 and 80 per cent (Haldane) in 7 cases, and low (39 per cent) in 1. Occasionally there is haemolysis, due either to the infecting organisms or to penicillin, in which case penicillin antibody may be found.

The disease is frequently preceded by dental sepsis, urinary infection, pneumonia, bladder instrumentation, or surgery of the prostate or colon. Vague joint pains, mental disturbance, embolic lesions, lassitude, loss of weight, pallor, clubbing, haematuria, and splenomegaly are a few of the presenting features. Whenever anaemia persists in a patient, or the cause is obscure, it is essential that a blood-culture is carried out.

Sometimes the patient has received inadequate or incorrect antibiotic therapy because of an erroneous diagnosis, with the result that further management is difficult. Combined antibiotic therapy may then have to be given even when repeated blood-cultures are sterile. *Streptococcus faecalis*, coliforms, and other enterococci are the usual organisms in this type of case.

Fulminating Septicaemia

Fulminating septicaemia may produce widespread petechiae and sometimes haemorrhage from rupture of a vessel with infective arteritis. A deficiency of clotting factors can develop, perhaps secondary to disseminated intravascular coagulation. Haemolysis and toxic vacuolation of the neutrophils can occur, while the presence of hypotension and of anuria makes the prognosis grave.

Tuberculosis

Tuberculosis may be associated with bizarre blood-pictures, and sometimes the blood disorder is the most prominent feature of the disease. Polycythaemia, eosinophilia, monocytosis, hypochromic anaemia, macrocytic anaemia, pancytopenia, and leukaemoid reactions have been observed. The diagnosis is often difficult as symptoms may be minimal. Pyrexia is seldom noteworthy and may be absent, but in others there is cachexia, fever, and obvious pulmonary involvement.

The presence of tuberculosis may not be suspected because of the similarity of the clinical features with those seen in patients with leukaemia, Hodgkin's disease, or aplastic anaemia. Corticosteroid therapy may be given and aggravate or disseminate the tuberculous lesion. Even when there is no activity of a tuberculous focus, reactivation can occur following steroid therapy and it is sometimes difficult to decide whether the tuberculosis is primary and the cause of the blood disorder, or secondary to treatment. The complication may not be recognized until necropsy is carried out.

Miliary tuberculosis can be particularly difficult to diagnose, especially in the very old. There may be no recognizable evidence of dissemination—either clinically or radiologically—and the abnormal blood-picture, usually leukaemoid, can be the sole manifestation. When the presence of leukaemia cannot be confirmed in a marrow smear, and there is no evidence of a causative disease, it is justifiable to institute therapeutic trial with antituberculous drugs on the assumption that a response confirms the diagnosis. Proudfoot, Akhtar, Douglas, and Horne (1969) indicated that in patients over the age of 60 years the cryptic type was as common as the overt type, and that the peak incidence was in the eighth decade.

Leukaemoid blood reactions are produced when there is an unusual response to infection, intoxication, or malignancy, and is recognized by a leucocytosis with some primitive cells, and an anaemia with nucleated red blood-cells. In tuberculosis the blood-picture may resemble that of acute myeloid leukaemia, aleukaemic leukaemia, and occasionally lymphatic or monocytic leukaemia. The significance of the reaction is not known.

'Sideroblastic' anaemia is not uncommon in tuberculous patients treated with isoniazid in conjunction with P.A.S., cycloserine, or pyrazinamide. This was confirmed by Roberts, Hoffbrand, and Mollin (1966). When treatment with isoniazid and P.A.S. continued for longer than 6 months, 57 per cent of the marrows they examined contained excess sideroblasts. Their study, which was concerned with 68 randomly selected tuberculous patients, ranging from 17 to 72 years of age, also showed that folate deficiency was common.

Chronic Infection

This term refers to persistent or recurrent infection and does not implicate any particular organism, although there is a tendency to regard infection with certain organisms, such as the tubercle bacillus, as chronic, and that due to others, such as the pneumococcus, as acute. The blood-picture produced depends more on the duration of the infection than on the organism involved.

Loss of weight, malnutrition, anorexia, and cachexia may be marked, while persistent infection of some organs, as for example the kidney, may be symptomless or associated with minimal disturbance. Nevertheless, blood changes may be produced, but as these are due more to the altered renal function than to the infection, they are discussed separately.

Chronic bronchitis is commonly associated with secondary polycythaemia, but its degree can be limited by iron deficiency. A haemoglobin level of 120 per cent does not exclude sideropenia. The blood viscosity may be greatly increased. There is no alteration of the white-cell count in the uncomplicated case. Underlying bronchiectasis with retention of pus may be associated with polymorpholeucocytosis, and the polycythaemia resulting from hypoxia can be overshadowed by anaemia from defective iron utilization—even when there is no overt iron deficiency.

Another difficulty is that acute infection is often an exacerbation of chronic infection, or a complication of chronic disease. In a patient with bronchopneumonia, for instance, there is often underlying chronic bronchitis or bronchiectasis.

Classically, chronic infection produces a resistant normocytic normochromic anaemia. There is reduction of the serum iron values possibly due to increased uptake or failure of release from the reticulo-endothelial system, and a lowering of the iron-binding capacity with consequent maintenance of a normal saturation. Marrow smears contain abundant haemosiderin. This is unlike the typical picture of iron deficiency, where the lowered serum iron is associated with absence of marrow haemosiderin and elevation of the iron-binding capacity. It is postulated that the changes are due to a failure of iron utilization by the red blood-cells. The condition can be referred to as 'pseudo-iron deficiency' and the anaemia as 'secondary refractory anaemia'. There is less impairment of haemoglobin synthesis in infection than in iron deficiency despite the low plasma iron in both conditions (Bothwell and Finch, 1962). Diversion of iron to the stores is an accepted factor (Cartwright and Wintrobe, 1949) and elevation of the erythrocyte protoporphyrin is often observed.

Nixon and Olsen (1968) stated that the impaired erythropoiesis was paralleled by an increase of iron stores, and of marrow haemosiderin which displayed particles of larger size than were seen when there was an increase of plasma iron turnover, as occurred following haemorrhage or haemolysis. Rath and Finch (1948) maintained that a clear-cut differentiation could usually be made between the anaemia of infection and that of iron deficiency by examining the marrow smear. Absence of haemosiderin indicated iron deficiency. When the patient recovered iron values returned to normal. In the elderly, however, the presence of true iron deficiency modifies the picture. This is illustrated in *Table V* in a comparison of the haemoglobin and serum iron values obtained in two groups of elderly patients—one with infection and the other with vascular disease.

Table V.—Comparison of Haemoglobin and Serum Iron Values in Patients with Infection and Others with Vascular Disease

	Hb <80 per cent 11·6 g. per 100 ml.	M.C.H.C. (per cent) <33	Serum Iron (μg. per 100 ml.)		T.I.B.C. (μg. per 100 ml.)			
			<35	<50	<300	301–400	401–500	501+
Infection (including rheumatic disease)	(35/106) 32 per cent	18/95 19 per cent	26/107 24 per cent	44/107 42 per cent	13/83 16 per cent	29/83 35 per cent	28/83 34 per cent	13/83 15 per cent
Vascular disease (cerebral infarction, cardiac infarction)	(30/135) 22 per cent	44/126 35 per cent	28/139 20 per cent	54/139 39 per cent	14/99 14 per cent	38/99 38 per cent	26/99 26 per cent	21/99 21 per cent

There is no significant difference between the two in their serum iron values. Sideropenia is common in both, as is a raised binding capacity. Similarly with the result of sternal punctures. Marrow haemosiderin is absent in patients with chronic infection not only when there is concomitant iron deficiency, but sometimes when iron deficiency does not appear to be present. Perhaps the easiest way of recognizing an anaemia of infection is to evaluate the effect of iron therapy after confirming that there is no increased loss of iron, no haemolysis, no hypoplasia of the marrow, and no diminution of any other haematinic factor. When there is no response it is justifiable to assume that the cause may be the chronic infection, but follow-up is still necessary lest another abnormality, such as a neoplasm, becomes evident.

Although the red-cell life span may be slightly reduced, this is not such that a normal marrow would not be able to compensate, so that fundamentally there is impaired marrow activity. This explains the slow response to iron therapy or to vitamin B_{12} when patients with chronic infection have iron-deficiency anaemia or pernicious anaemia. Failure of the anaemia to stimulate the production of more erythropoietin is a possibility, but does not explain the altered iron metabolism—the reduced transferrin and the avidity of the reticulo-endothelial system for iron. Diminished absorption of iron may occur, but cannot be important in the classic case, because there is no shortage of tissue iron.

Changes in serum protein are well documented. There may be reduction of albumin and elevation of globulin, particularly of the gamma fraction. Again the changes are not distinctive in the elderly, as can be seen from *Table VI* in which the albumin and gamma-globulin levels of 65 patients with infection are compared with the levels of 83 with vascular disease.

Table VI.—Comparison of Serum Albumin and Gamma-globulin in Patients with Infection and Others with Vascular Disease

	Albumin (g. per 100 ml.)			Gamma-globulin (g. per 100 ml.)		
	<2·0	<2·5	<3·0	<1·0	1·01–1·5	1·51+
Infection	6/65 9 per cent	17/65 26 per cent	37/65 57 per cent	17/65 26 per cent	37/65 57 per cent	11/65 17 per cent
Vascular diseases	1/83 1·2 per cent	19/83 23 per cent	44/83 53 per cent	19/83 23 per cent	48/83 58 per cent	16/83 19 per cent

Lower levels of albumin were present in those with infection, but the gamma-globulin levels were similar in the two groups. It was mentioned in the section on plasma proteins that most diseases affected the globulins and that there was some evidence to suggest that ageing itself was a factor.

Paraproteins may be found. Although in rare instances an immune body response may be the cause it is much more likely that the patient has monoclonal gammopathy or myelomatosis.

Amyloidosis can develop and produce a blood disorder from involvement of marrow, spleen, kidney, or liver.

Bed-sores

Anaemia in patients with bed-sores or pressure sores is due to: the effect of the underlying disease, the presence of septicaemia or of chronic infection, and sometimes to protein deficiency. Usually there is hypochromia with sideropenia. Improvement in the blood-picture is often slow or absent, until the bed-sore heals. It then becomes satisfactory unless another cause persists. Where there is deficiency of iron, vitamin B_{12}, or folate, they should always be given, in order to improve cell metabolism and to replenish iron-dependent skin enzymes. As healing sometimes coincides with their introduction it is possible that they have a curative effect. Extra protein, in an easily assimilable form, is always indicated.

CARCINOMA

Several types of blood changes can occur, depending on the presence of haemorrhage, secondaries in the marrow or liver, the organ concerned, or whether there is chronic infection. Hypochromic anaemia is associated with blood-loss, and a leuco-erythroblastic picture is sometimes found if there are secondaries. Increased haemolysis may be present. Thrombocytosis is fairly common and its degree may be such that the serum acid phosphatase is elevated.

The incidence of anaemia depends a great deal on which organ is involved, but changes due to the carcinoma itself are important, because normocytic normochromic anaemia is often present when there is no other apparent cause. Sometimes it is an early manifestation, but occasionally does not become evident until a late or terminal stage has been reached. It is then difficult to be certain that the carcinoma has not spread (*Fig.* 2).

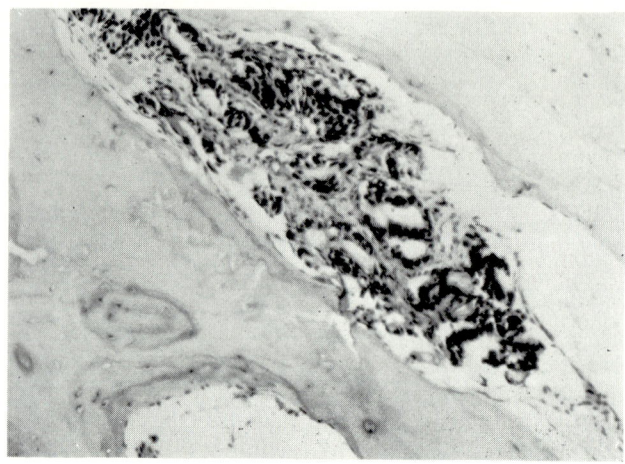

Fig. 2.—Iliac crest biopsy from male, aged 53 years, containing secondary adenocarcinoma from prostate. The patient had been investigated extensively and treated with haematinics before a marrow smear suggested the diagnosis, supported by a raised acid phosphatase level. ($\times$ 150.)

Sideropenia may develop and become more pronounced as the carcinoma advances, but the patient need not necessarily be anaemic. There is no correlation between the serum-iron value and the prognosis. Kinetic studies suggest that the lowered level is associated with impaired release of iron from the reticulo-endothelial cells.

The iron-binding capacity is also reduced, but as the serum iron is affected to a greater extent there is a tendency for the saturation to be low. Marrow haemosiderin is present unless there is iron deficiency.

Miller, Chodos, Emerson, and Ross (1956) investigated 38 patients with carcinoma—breast, prostate, kidney, lung, stomach, sigmoid, and testes were the primary sites. Metastases were present in all but 4. Blood-loss, infection, and overt haemolytic anaemia were excluded. Twenty-two were anaemic and in 19 the anaemia was normochromic. Depressed serum-iron levels were found in 17. More than half the patients studied had increased red-cell destruction, but no evidence of any antibody mechanism was found. Storage iron in liver, spleen, and marrow was normal or slightly increased. There was hypercellularity of the marrow with increased erythropoiesis, but the authors believed that its degree was insufficient to combat the anaemia. In their words, there was a 'functional inadequacy of the marrow'.

Another reason for the anaemia is decreased red-cell production. This is usual when there is widespread metastasis in the marrow, but sometimes it occurs when the marrow is not obviously involved.

A flattening of the mucosa in the upper small intestine may occur. Loehry and Creamer (1966) found from necropsy material that flattening of the mucosal folds in the duodenum and to a lesser extent in the jejunum, similar to that seen in coeliac disease, was present in 18 per cent of patients with malignancy. A similar abnormality of the intestine was noted in some patients with uraemia or cirrhosis of the liver. These changes suggest that malabsorption may occur.

In the patients we have studied the changes in serum iron and iron-binding capacity are not remarkable when compared with those obtained in other diseases. In 27 consecutive cases the serum iron was found to be below 35 μg. per 100 ml. in 7, below 50 μg. per 100 ml. in 15, between 50 and 70 μg. per 100 ml. in 7, and between 71 and 100 μg. per 100 ml. in 5. In no instance was a level above 100 μg. obtained. The iron-binding capacity ranged from 201 μg. per 100 ml. to 750 μg. per 100 ml. and the majority had a level of over 400 μg. per 100 ml.

Changes in the serum proteins are often observed: the albumin value may be low and that of the gamma-globulin high. In a series of 20 patients the albumin level was below 3·0 g. per 100 ml. in 14 and less than 2·6 g. per 100 ml. in 5; while the gamma-globulin measurement was above 1·50 g. per 100 ml. in 9 (the highest being 2·4 g. per 100 ml.) but in 3 a value below 1·0 g. per 100 ml. was obtained. Again the changes are comparable with those seen in other disease categories. In rare instances paraproteins are found, and they have been known to diminish or disappear when treatment of the carcinoma is successful. Usually, however, they persist, in which case their presence is unlikely to be due to the carcinoma. Fibrinolytic effects are rarely encountered, but should be considered if there is bleeding or purpura, particularly when the prostate or lung is involved.

Polycythaemia can occur when the carcinoma arises in the kidney, ovary, adrenal, or liver.

Haemolytic anaemia of some degree is common in all types of carcinoma, particularly when advanced, and an auto-immune haemolytic state, as revealed by a positive Coombs's test, may be present. Green, Wakefield, and Littlewood (1957) found an antibody of the 'cold' incomplete non-gamma-globulin type in many of those with a positive test. Anaemia was not invariable because it can be combated by increased erythropoiesis—unless the marrow function is depressed. They stated their view as follows: '... in terms of the immunological theory the cancer cell is an aggressive parasite in the sense that it is capable of invading, and perhaps damaging host tissue because it is, immunologically speaking, a new race of cells. It may possibly prove that not only the anaemia, but the general emaciation of cancer is in part due to this immune aggressive reaction of the tumour to the host.'

SURGERY

Persons who have been operated upon are often anaemic. This is not surprising, as approximately 30 per cent of patients admitted to medical wards are anaemic, irrespective of the underlying disease, but nevertheless the pathogenesis can be complex.

Rapid onset following surgery may be due to haemorrhage or haemolysis from drug sensitivity, blood transfusion, or septicaemia, and the first manifestation can be a disturbance of consciousness rather than pyrexia or pallor. Septicaemia can be particularly deceptive and characterized solely by lassitude with mild anaemia. In others, mental confusion is prominent. It may take several months before septicaemia is even suspected.

An abscess need not cause leucocytosis. The only abnormality in the peripheral blood may be a normochromic anaemia due to failure of iron utilization. If true iron deficiency predominates hypochromia may be present, but response to therapy can still be unsatisfactory owing to the infection.

Deficiency of haematinic factors has always to be considered. Low serum levels of iron, vitamin B_{12}, and folate can occur even in the non-anaemic, so that when metabolism is altered by trauma or inadequate diet true deficiency anaemia can be precipitated or accentuated.

The serum iron and the iron-binding capacity are both reduced in the postoperative phase, so that a fairly normal saturation is maintained. These changes develop irrespective of the presence or absence of anaemia. Marrow haemosiderin is unaltered.

A marked increase in the platelet count can occur with trauma, asphyxia, and acute blood-loss. The maximal increase, which may range from 30 to 100 per cent, is usually seen from the seventh to the twentieth postoperative day. Although it may develop after any operation it is more constant and pronounced after splenectomy. The increase may persist for weeks, or possibly months.

Protein malnutrition can probably affect erythropoiesis. Neale, Anteliff, Welbourn, Mollin, and Booth (1967) reported on 5 patients who had a normocytic normochromic anaemia following partial gastrectomy. There was no response to therapy with iron, vitamin B_{12}, folate, and other vitamins, but there was rapid improvement when protein deficiency was corrected. The lowest serum-protein measurement in these patients was 3·7 g. per 100 ml., and the lowest albumin value was 1·7 g. per 100 ml. A negative protein balance normally follows surgery and this could reduce the production of globin and possibly of erythropoietin. Features suggestive of mild kwashiorkor may be seen.

When anaemia develops several years later it is nearly always due to occult bleeding or malabsorption. Investigation of patients after partial gastrectomy or small-bowel resection, particularly when the jejunum or lower ileum is removed, shows that the incidence of anaemia increases with the length of follow-up. This is well recognized in those who have had a partial gastrectomy, and is related more to the presence of gastritis than to the amount of stomach removed. Anaemia in these patients can be due to several factors, such as continued bleeding, inadequacy of the stores prior to operation, restricted diet, rapid gastric emptying, and, according to Turnberg (1967), a mucosal enzyme that facilitates iron absorption may be deficient. Although inorganic iron is absorbed normally, there is no augmentation when the patient becomes anaemic. The same applies to organic iron, with the result that iron-deficiency anaemia persists and may develop within a year of operation. Sideropenia, without anaemia, is seen more often and probably indicates an earlier stage. Vitamin-B_{12} deficiency is less common, but tends to develop in those who have become iron deficient. Its incidence increases progressively for about 3–6 years, and then evens off. The level of serum vitamin B_{12} is seldom as low as in pernicious anaemia, although the degree of anaemia may be equally severe. Subacute combined degeneration of the cord or myelopathy can develop and is not directly related to the level of serum vitamin B_{12} or the anaemia (Williams and others, 1969). Evidence of malabsorption may be obtained within a few months of the operation, but only a proportion develop anaemia. Steatorrhoea is a late complication and these patients are often folate deficient. Loss of weight is often prominent. According to Hines, Hoffbrand, and Mollin (1967) vitamin-B_{12} deficiency is more common following partial gastrectomy for gastric ulcer than for duodenal ulcer, regardless of the type of operation, the relative proportions being 30 per cent and 9 per cent.

Deller and Witts (1962) stated that 'the incidence of anaemia in different series has varied from 4 per cent to 63 per cent depending on the criterion of anaemia which has been adopted, the proportion of men and women in the series, the indication for operation, the type of gastro-intestinal anastomosis, the interval of time between operation and blood examination, and the thoroughness with which anaemia is searched for'. They studied 265 patients 1–12 years after surgery; 187 were male and 78 female. The total incidence of anaemia was 20·4 per cent (54 patients), anaemia being defined as a haemoglobin level of less than 13·6 g. per 100 ml. in men and 11·6 g. per 100 ml. in women. Thirty-eight had lone iron-deficiency anaemia, 12 had combined deficiency of iron and vitamin B_{12}, and in 4 vitamin-B_{12} deficiency alone was diagnosed. Subnormal serum vitamin-B_{12} values were commoner with the Polya type of operation than with the Billroth I, and when the operation was for a gastric rather than a duodenal ulcer, but age and sex did not appear to influence the results. 'Dumping' syndrome, bilious vomiting, diarrhoea, and loss of weight were not related to the anaemia.

Gastro-enterostomy and vagotomy may also produce late effects. Wheldon, Venables, and Johnston (1970) reviewed 255 patients (ages 37–80 years) more than 15 years after this operation, and found weight-loss of more than 6 kg. in 32·5 per cent of men and in 60 per cent of women. Iron-deficiency anaemia was present in 43·5 per cent of men and in 84 per cent of women. The incidence of sideropenia may well have been considerably higher because the serum iron was estimated only in those found to be anaemic. Serum vitamin-B_{12} levels were within the normal range, although 14 were below 150 pg. per ml. This again was done in the anaemic patients only. Another important finding was that 7 per cent developed pulmonary tuberculosis.

The incidence of anaemia after gastro-intestinal surgery increases with time, and this is related to the preponderance of hypochlorhydria in these patients. The speed of gastric emptying and intestinal transit may also be important, because Wastell (1969) found a lower incidence of anaemia after pyloroplasty than after gastroenterostomy. Cox, Bond, Podmore, and Rose (1964) had shown a reduction in serum-iron levels after vagotomy and gastro-enterostomy, but did not find as much anaemia and their patients gained rather than lost weight. However, these findings were based on a 4-year follow-up.

Intestinal anastomoses, resections, and by-pass operations can cause an anaemia similar to that produced by other abnormalities of the small intestine, such as strictures, diverticula, and fistulae. There are several reasons for this development, among which are: removal of the absorptive area for vitamin B_{12}, folate, vitamin C, and pyridoxine; shortening of transit time; and abnormal proliferation of intestinal bacteria which block vitamin B_{12} or folate absorption—possibly by diverting them from the host or interfering in their relationship with 'intrinsic' factor or some other enzyme. Abdominal distension, loss of weight, flatulence, diarrhoea, and glossitis may precede or accompany the anaemia. Steatorrhoea is not unusual. The intestinal bacterial proliferation can sometimes be controlled by oral antibiotic therapy.

Although patients with malabsorption or small-bowel resection may have delayed excretion of ingested ascorbic acid, Williamson, Goldberg, and Moore (1967) found the leucocyte ascorbic acid levels to be low. Similar results were obtained in patients after gastric surgery. They considered the most likely cause to be malabsorption of the vitamin, although demand could have increased because of the role of vitamin C in wound healing. Five of their 26 patients had evidence of increased capillary fragility, and 3 had purpura.

When a hypochromic type of anaemia develops which is refractory to iron therapy the possibility of pyridoxine deficiency has to be considered.

TRAUMA

Some traumatic lesions, such as fractures of the femoral neck, are seen more often in the elderly than in the young, and, as in other conditions in this age-group, underlying or unrelated disease may be present. Osteoporosis, osteomalacia, neoplastic secondaries, rheumatoid arthritis, and myelomatosis are obvious examples, but there may be latent disease or occult neoplasm, and occasionally a blood disorder, for example, chronic lymphatic leukaemia or pernicious anaemia, is detected.

The effect of trauma on iron metabolism is similar to that produced by chronic infection. There is sideropenia with maintenance of a fairly normal transferrin saturation—unless iron deficiency is also a feature. Serum-iron values below 70 μg. per 100 ml. are usually obtained.

In general there are three broad groups of blood disorders to be considered, namely: anaemia, bleeding, and thrombosis, but as they are discussed elsewhere only brief comments are included in this section.

Anaemia

Various degrees of a normochromic or a hypochromic type of anaemia are often present. The haemoglobin level may lie between 60 and 70 per cent, but sometimes it is lower, depending on the amount of bleeding. When they cannot be correlated it is reasonable to assume that the patient was anaemic before the injury occurred, that blood has been redistributed, or that both factors are operating simultaneously. The haemoglobin value on admission may be falsely low or high and it is only when there is a progressive fall, after allowing for haemodilution or haemoconcentration, that the presence of persistent oozing can be inferred. If the blood is visible its quantity can be assessed, but when it leaks into the thigh, pelvis, or abdomen, clinical judgement can be very inaccurate although the amount lost may be considerable.

The haemoglobin values, together with those of iron, vitamin B_{12}, and folate, obtained in 50 consecutive female patients with a fracture of the femoral neck are given in *Tables VII* and *VIII*. No reason, other than inadequacy of the blood

GENERAL DISEASE

sample, affected the number tested. The haemoglobin was measured in each case, the serum iron in 43, and vitamin B_{12} and folate in 47. Values obtained at a later date were excluded.

Table VII.—HAEMOGLOBIN AND SERUM IRON VALUES

AGE AND TOTAL	HAEMOGLOBIN PERCENTAGE			SERUM IRON (μg. per 100 ml.)				IRON SATURATION PERCENTAGE			T.I.B.C. (μg. per 100 ml.)		
	1–60	61–80	81–100	1–35	36–50	51–70	71+	1–10	11–15	16+	200–300	301–400	401+
60–69 (2)	0	1	1	1	0	1	0	1	1	0	0	1	1
70–79 (28)	2	12	14	12	8	0	3	12	6	5	5	8	10
80–89 (16)	3	8	5	4	8	1	1	5	6	3	2	7	5
90+ (4)	0	4	0	2	0	1	1	2	0	2	0	3	1
50	5	25	20	19	16	3	5	20	13	10	7	19	17
		50			43				43			43	

Table VIII.—SERUM VITAMIN-B_{12} AND FOLATE VALUES

AGE AND TOTAL	VITAMIN B_{12} (pg. per ml.)				SERUM FOLATE (μg. per ml.)				
	1–80	81–110	111–150	151+	0·1–1·0	1·1–2·0	2·1–3·0	3·1–5·0	5·1+
60–69 (2)	1	0	0	1	0	0	0	1	1
70–79 (28)	3	2	4	17	1	8	5	6	6
80–89 (16)	2	1	4	8	0	1	3	8	3
90+ (4)	0	3	1	0	0	0	1	2	1
50	6	6	9	26	1	9	9	17	11
		47					47		

The haemoglobin level was less than 81 per cent in 30 and below 61 per cent in 5, the lowest being 41 per cent. This was in a patient aged 81 years whose vitamin-B_{12} value was 50 pg. per ml. Of the 30 anaemic patients (i.e., Hb below 81 per cent) the serum iron was below 51 μg. per 100 ml. in 22, the iron saturation less than

16 per cent in 20, the serum vitamin B_{12} under 110 pg. per ml. in 9, and folate below 2·5 ng. per ml. in 7 (although iron values were not obtained in 3, vitamin-B_{12} value in 1, and folate in 2). The results indicate the frequency with which combined low serum levels of the main haematinic factors occur in these patients, despite the presence of trauma. There was a fall in haemoglobin of over 10 per cent following surgery in 16, of 20 per cent or more in 11, and of over 30 per cent in 3. The largest was in a female of 86 years whose haemoglobin fell from 88 per cent to 52 per cent.

Serum-iron values were below 51 μg. per 100 ml. in 35 of 43 patients (81 per cent) and below 36 μg. per 100 ml. in 19 (44 per cent) compared with 42 per cent and 24 per cent in those with infection, and 39 per cent and 20 per cent in patients with vascular disease. Sideropenia was profound in 6, values below 25 μg. per 100 ml. being obtained. Faecal occult blood was present in 6 of the 25 tested.

The T.I.B.C. was above 400 μg. per 100 ml. in 20 (46 per cent), but in general the reduction in serum iron was greater than the elevation of the binding capacity when compared with patients suffering from acute vascular disease. The saturation was less than 16 per cent in 33 of 43 patients, and less than 11 per cent in 20 (46 per cent).

Serum vitamin-B_{12} values below 111 pg. per ml. were found in 12 of 47 patients, and a folate below 2·1 ng. per ml. in 10.

Multiple low levels were often present. For instance, a female of 78 years with a haemoglobin of 55 per cent had a serum-iron value of 30 μg. per 100 ml. (saturation 13 per cent), a serum vitamin B_{12} of 60 pg. per ml., and a serum folate of 1·5 ng. per ml. She also had myxoedema and congestive cardiac failure.

It is evident that attention has to be given to the general medical picture if the best results are to be obtained, because social difficulties, malnutrition, malabsorption, and occult blood-loss are as common in these patients as in those admitted to medical wards.

Bleeding

When a blood-vessel is torn, intravascular, vascular, and extravascular factors combine to limit the bleeding. Laxity of tissues and diminution of muscle tone reduce the effectiveness of the extravascular component in the elderly, while thickening of the wall and loss of elasticity diminish that of the vessels. Vasoconstriction and retraction are less prompt, so that initiation of clotting and local deposition of platelets and fibrin may be delayed. Haematomas are often extensive, and the amount of bruising excessive for the degree of injury—owing to the added effect of increased capillary fragility, combined sometimes with vitamin C and other deficiencies.

Despite these complications the management of bleeding and of haematomas is usually straightforward. In rare instances, however, there may be an unrelated bleeding or clotting disorder which may not be suspected until unsatisfactory results are obtained following repeated blood transfusion. The present frequency of accidents is such that the possibility of these conditions occurring by chance cannot be ignored. Temporary elevation of the haemoglobin level and then a fall may wrongly suggest that traumatic bleeding is continuing.

Liver disease, renal disease, infection, haemolysis, and thrombocytopenia should be excluded, but clotting-factor deficiencies or the presence of anticoagulants may have to be considered. Blood transfusion can sometimes supply the missing or deficient factor, but when antibodies or anticoagulants are present transfusions merely replace lost blood temporarily, and are otherwise valueless or harmful, as they may increase the antibody titre. These circulating anticoagulants are mainly anti-factor VIII and antithromboplastin. Full haematological investigation is time consuming and complex, and, moreover, these patients are usually critically ill. The prognosis is grave though spontaneous recovery may occur. Corticosteroid therapy can be beneficial.

Another possibility is that fibrinolytic mechanisms are hyperactive, particularly when the patient is shocked. Not only may this be primary, but it can also be secondary to disseminated intravascular coagulation. These conditions are considered in greater detail in Chapter 12.

The platelet count continues to fall for 1–3 days after injury, and if this is associated with bleeding and a poor marrow response homeostasis can be impaired.

Case 2.—Mrs. C. L., aged 65 years, was admitted to hospital after falling and injuring her left hip. Prior to this she had been in bed for 5 weeks complaining of back and leg pains. A fractured neck of the left femur was found. The Hb fell repeatedly to 40 per cent despite the transfusion of 15 pints of blood over a 3-week period. All tests for haemolysis or external haemorrhage were negative. The only positive findings were a one-stage prothrombin ratio of 1·5 and a platelet count of 20,000 per c.mm.

At autopsy severe generalized purpura was found and the serous surfaces and cavities contained fresh blood.

Thrombosis

The elderly are prone to thrombotic lesions, and when treatment necessitates immobilizing a limb or prolonging bed-rest the tendency is increased, particularly when the circulation is slowed from congestive cardiac failure or limb pressure. Other factors contribute, for instance, Geill (1960) found that serum thromboplastin activity was increased when the trauma was associated with tissue injury or a haematoma, and Sevitt (1960) believed that these serum changes were highly significant because thrombi in leg veins were usually bilateral. Quick (1960), on the other hand, considered that local liberation of thromboplastin from the damaged vessel wall was primarily responsible. Platelets are usually increased a week or so after trauma, and counts may reach 400,000 per c.mm. or more. This thrombocytosis can persist for prolonged periods in the severely injured.

Physiotherapy and early mobilization, with or without anticoagulation, are the accepted means whereby the hazard is prevented or minimized, and when commencing thrombosis is detected reliance is usually placed on anticoagulants alone, as discussed in Chapter 12. Management would be simplified if individual predisposition to thrombosis could be detected. In an effort to clarify the problem den Ottolander, Schreuder, and Hoorweg (1963) investigated the clotting and lysis activity of the serum in 140 healthy persons over the age of 70, and then followed them up in order to identify which blood characteristic indicated a likelihood to thrombosis. They found that a tendency to hypercoagulability existed in 13 per cent, but it was not related to the serum fibrinogen content, the clotting time, or the composition of the prothrombin complex. In 12 per cent, nearly all men, increased fibrinolytic activity was demonstrated. Six persons died of thrombosis within a year, but in none had hypercoagulability been detected. They concluded that hypercoagulability was more common in the elderly as a group than in younger persons, but that, unlike enhanced fibrinolysis, the finding was not constant in the individual. It appears that there is no reliable haematological means at present whereby a tendency to thrombosis can be detected.

According to Innes and Sevitt (1964) there is a rapid increase in fibrinolytic activity after trauma, followed within a few hours by a marked reduction which persists for 4–11 days before returning to normal. This reduction could be a contributory factor in the development of thrombosis. Chakrabarti, Hocking, and Fearnley (1969) obtained similar results following electroplexy, surgery, and myocardial infarction.

LIVER DISORDERS

Several factors operate. Gastro-intestinal symptoms, such as anorexia, can cause nutritional defects resulting in iron and folate deficiency; blood-loss from oesophageal varices can account for the iron-deficiency anaemia that is often present; liver secondaries may cause a variety of blood disorders; abscesses are associated with leucocytosis; and splenomegaly when present can give rise to hypersplenism with reduction of red cells, white cells, and platelets, or any combination of the three. In addition, jaundice and parenchymatous disease have their own special blood characteristics.

Hepatic involvement in the elderly is usually due to congestive cardiac failure, secondary neoplastic infiltration, or cirrhosis. Obstructive jaundice from gallstone impaction or carcinoma of the head of the pancreas is seen fairly often and so is cholestasis following drug therapy. Hepatitis and acute necrosis are relatively rare.

OBSTRUCTIVE JAUNDICE

An increase in the diameter of the red cells with diffuse flattening and diminished osmotic fragility is often present. Although the explanation is obscure, it is likely that a substance such as bile-salts circulating in the blood-stream is implicated. Target cells—which are red blood-cells with a pigmented centre and periphery—are probably manifestations of this altered shape. According to Jandl (1955), there is no correlation between these changes and the degree of anaemia. Moreover, the characteristic is not basic to red-cell destruction, because when haemolysis is present the red cells may be spherocytic and fragmented (*Fig. 3*).

HEPATOCELLULAR NECROSIS

High serum vitamin-B_{12} values are usually obtained in the early stages of acute hepatitis, but the level cannot be correlated with the intensity of the jaundice, nor the biochemical changes (Rachmilewitz, Aronovitch, and Grossowicz, 1956), and may return to normal long before the liver-function tests.

The raised level is probably due to liver vitamin B_{12} being released into the circulation, and there is evidence to suggest that the binding is increased. The explanation is obscure, but presumably an alteration in serum proteins is implicated, though the alpha-globulin fraction to which the vitamin B_{12} is chiefly bound is not always increased when the level is high. Reduced excretion of vitamin B_{12} by the kidney is unlikely to be the cause, because this would elevate the free and not the bound form. The serum folate level is reduced and urinary folate increased (Retief and Huskisson, 1969).

Serum-iron values are raised when necrosis is severe, probably due to cellular release.

Macrocytosis may be present, the degree of which is roughly proportional to the liver dysfunction (Hall, 1956). Marrow hypoplasia has been observed.

Haemolysis and coagulation defects may develop, and there is failure to synthesize prothrombin, factor V, and Christmas factor (Sherlock, 1968).

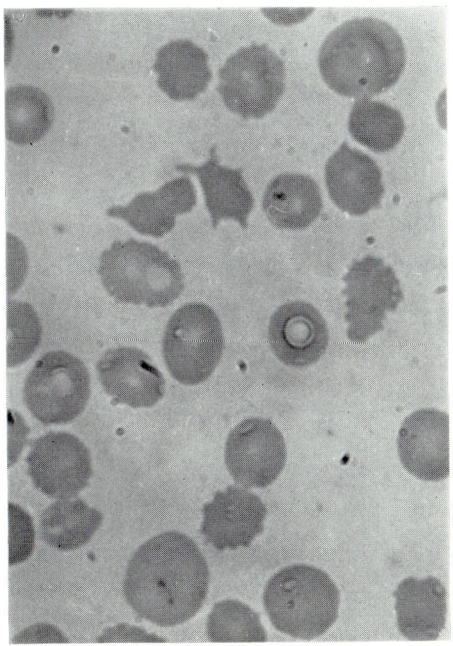

Fig. 3.—Peripheral blood showing bizarre erythrocytes in jaundice. ($\times$ 1100.)

Cirrhosis

Moderately severe anaemia is usually present, but its degree cannot be correlated with the duration of the illness or the severity of the hepatic lesion, but there is a tendency for the anaemia to remit when function improves.

An accelerated red-cell turnover occurs, probably due to diminished red-cell survival, so that when a border-line nutritional defect exists the combination may produce a deficiency anaemia.

The blood-film in anaemic patients usually shows macrocytosis of a moderate or mild degree, but a similar picture may be seen when there is no anaemia. Stippling can be a feature and target cells may be found. Therapy with vitamin B_{12} and folate does not influence either the anaemia or the red-cell characteristics. In view of this it has been postulated that a specific factor (or factors) is produced by the diseased liver which acts uniformly on all cells, either during erythropoiesis or after the cells have left the marrow, but so far such a factor has not been isolated.

Berman and others (1949) reviewing 25 cases ranging in age from 31 to 71 years stated that 21 were anaemic, and in approximately 75 per cent of them macrocytosis was present with normal or elevated mean corpuscular haemoglobin values.

The white-cell count is often lowered. Lymphopenia is sometimes found. The response of the granulocytes to infection is unimpaired. Platelets are reduced to a level below 100,000 per c.mm. in approximately half the patients, and bleeding may occur.

Acute haemolytic episodes are sometimes seen and the direct Coombs's test may be positive, but a diminished red-cell life span was present in 5 cases reported by Chaplin and Mollison (1953) when the test was negative. These patients were below 60 years of age. Jandl (1955) suggested that the spleen was the major site of red-cell destruction when cirrhosis was associated with anaemia, and he found that haemoglobin synthesis in these patients was increased to about three times the normal rate. Consequently a mild degree of reticulocytosis may be present.

Raised serum vitamin-B_{12} levels are sometimes found. In 3 of the 6 cases of portal cirrhosis investigated by Rachmilewitz and others (1956) values of 1175, 1250, and 1350 were obtained, and in 5 of their 6 cases with biliary cirrhosis a similar range was observed. The common factor in these cases appeared to be hepatocellular damage. The serum-folate level is reduced and urinary loss increased in portal and cardiac cirrhosis.

Sweinseid, Hvolboll, Schick, and Halsted (1957) analysed the vitamin-B_{12} content of liver tissue obtained at autopsy from 132 males and found greatly reduced values in those with cirrhosis, but these values could not be correlated with the degree of anaemia prior to death.

The level of iron in the serum is unpredictable. Cell necrosis and haemolysis cause elevation while nutritional deficiencies and blood-loss result in a lowering. Simultaneously intestinal absorption may be increased and this can occur even when there is no anaemia or sideropenia. It was noted in 38 per cent of the non-anaemic patients investigated by Williams and others (1967), and the serum-iron saturation values were sometimes considerably raised due mainly to a reduction in iron-binding capacity. The increased absorption could not be correlated with the clinical state of the patient, the serum-iron values, the haematological and biochemical findings, the presence of collateral circulation, the type of cirrhosis that was present, or the degree of hepatocellular failure.

Liver damage *per se* can cause increased iron absorption, but the possible presence of associated pancreatic insufficiency has always to be considered.

Excess absorption may be particularly evident when alcohol is the cause of the cirrhosis, because alcohol enhances iron absorption and can cause pancreatitis, which has a similar effect. Moreover, many alcoholic beverages have a high iron content.

Bothwell and Finch (1962) stated that the plasma iron was usually normal unless there was also liver-cell necrosis or megaloblastic anaemia, and they found that transferrin saturation was increased. This they considered to be due to diminished circulating protein.

Other findings are: expansion of the plasma volume and the rare occurrence of an L.E. phenomenon. The immunological system can be severely disturbed (Caroli and Salmon, 1969).

Marrow

According to Berman and others (1949) there is an increase of functioning marrow and a tendency to hypercellularity—macronormoblastic in type—even when there is no anaemia. Megaloblasts are not usually found. In elderly patients the picture is variable, because of deficiencies of haematinic factors and the presence of other disease. There may be increased haemosiderin deposits, and this, combined with a lowering of the serum-iron and binding-capacity values, resembles that classically seen in patients with chronic infection. According to Nixon and Olsen (1968) the haemosiderin particles are of the large pattern type (greater than 4–5 μ) which in their opinion indicates decreased utilization.

There are no characteristic changes in the white-cell series, but the plasma cells may be slightly increased.

Coagulation Defects

There is failure to absorb vitamin K, which is necessary for the synthesis of prothrombin and of factor VII. The defect is more pronounced when jaundice is present.

Functional impairment of the parenchymatous cells is associated with a complex pattern of deficiencies in which factor V, factor VII, and sometimes prothrombin and Christmas factor are markedly diminished.

Cowling (1956) noted that a gross reduction of plasma-coagulation factors was not always associated with bleeding. Their level fluctuated rapidly and paralleled the clinical state of the patient. Although thrombocytopenia and oesophageal varices were the main causes of bleeding, he concluded that a reduction of Christmas factor sometimes contributed.

Fibrinolytic activity can occasionally be sufficient to impair haemostasis (Fearnley, 1956). Fibrinogen may be reduced because of defective synthesis or excessive destruction by an enzyme, such as plasmin.

Haemochromatosis

In this disease multilobular hepatic cirrhosis is associated with iron overloading. It primarily affects the middle aged and elderly. Of 58 patients reported on by Williams and others (1969) 11 were over 60 when the disease presented. This was the average age at which death occurred in 57 cases followed up at the Boston City Hospital (Macdonald and Mallory, 1960).

The aetiology is obscure. It may be a variant of alcoholic cirrhosis (Macdonald 1964), but the general view in this country appears to be that the fundamental abnormality is an inborn error of iron metabolism, manifested by excess absorption only partially controlled by the state of the stores. The mechanism is not understood, but there may be more than one genetic pattern. It has been claimed that excessive iron absorption was due to deficiency of an iron-binding protein 'gastroferrin', which normally inhibited absorption (Davies, Luke, and Deller, 1966). About 70 per cent of symptom-free relatives have excess liver iron and absorption was abnormally high in 55 per cent of those studied by Williams, Manenti, Williams, and Pitcher (1966). Familial cases have occasionally been described. The preponderance of males which is evident in younger life is not apparent in the elderly, presumably due to the absence of menstruation.

The patients have a slaty pigmentation of the exposed parts and sometimes buccal pigmentation. Hepatomegaly and diabetes mellitus are usually present. Other features include testicular atrophy and progressive polyarthritis. This occurred in half the patients reported on by Hamilton, Williams, Barlow, and Smith (1968). Most of them had chondrocalcinosis. These authors indicated that joint abnormalities were particularly common in patients over the age of 50.

The level of serum iron is usually raised, but may be normal in 20 per cent (Dreyfus and Schapira, 1964). According to Bothwell and Finch (1962) diurnal fluctuation is absent. The iron-binding capacity is normal or reduced and the saturation abnormally high—in the region of 80–100 per cent. The raised serum iron may persist despite repeated venesection, and iron absorption can be increased by treatment (Williams and others, 1966). Excess iron is present in marrow, spleen, kidney, liver, skin, pancreas, adrenals, heart, endocrine glands, and aortic lymph-nodes. In advanced cases it may amount to 30–40 g. compared with the normal of approximately 4 g. Variation is considerable.

Anaemia is unlikely to develop in the uncomplicated case unless there is superadded vitamin-B_{12} or folate deficiency. In alcoholic cirrhosis, on the other hand, iron deficiency is common.

Liver biopsy shows the iron to be located not only in the cells of the reticuloendothelial system, as is usual in other kinds of iron overloading, but also within the parenchymatous cells. This difference, however, may not be significant, because with excessive iron overloading from any cause, such as repeated blood transfusion or prolonged iron therapy, an appearance similar to that seen in haemochromatosis can sometimes be produced.

When the total chelatable body store is assessed by the differential ferrioxamine test high values are obtained in untreated or partially treated haemochromatosis, thus distinguishing it from cirrhosis with secondary siderosis where normal or slightly raised values are obtained (Smith, Studley, and Williams, 1967).

The patients may present with diabetes mellitus, hepatic derangement, skin pigmentation, or anaemia, but often there is no evidence of altered liver function, or indeed of haemochromatosis. This was so in a man of 72 who had folic-acid-deficiency anaemia. It was only when a high transferrin saturation persisted that the possibility of haemochromatosis was considered. Pyridoxine responsive anaemia can also occur.

The diabetes mellitus is not usually different from that normally seen, although sometimes it may be insulin resistant, and it is possible that retinal changes are less likely to develop when the pituitary is involved. Oesophageal varices develop in about a third. Cardiac manifestations are not unduly rare. There may be congestive failure, precordial pain, or dysrhythmia and the heart is often dilated. Increased melanin in the lower layers of the skin is a far more common finding than is the presence of haemosiderin. Iron may be present in the distal renal tubules. Deposition in the brain, particularly cerebellum and basal ganglia, can cause neurological features. Carcinoma of the liver develops in 5–6 per cent.

Treatment is directed towards both the cirrhosis and the diabetes. Regular venesection in order to remove excess iron is valuable (Williams, 1969) and can be assessed by means of the ferrioxamine test.

When death occurs it is usually from liver failure, haematemesis, carcinoma of the liver, heart failure, diabetic complications, infection, or incidental disease.

GENERAL DISEASE

RENAL DISEASE

Nephrosclerosis and chronic pyelonephritis are the most common renal diseases in the elderly, although calculi, cysts, adenomata, and carcinoma are sometimes seen. Acute glomerulonephritis is rare, but the chronic stage is found fairly often.

POLYCYTHAEMIA

This may occur when the underlying lesion is cystic or neoplastic. Among the 28 published cases reviewed by Forsell (1958) 22 had a hypernephroma, 4 polycystic disease, 1 a fibromyxoma, and 1 hydronephrosis. Nephrectomy relieved the polycythaemia in all but 1. It is a rare association, occurring in 2–3 per cent of patients with hypernephroma. Splenomegaly may be present. Drivsholm (1960) described a man of 60 with hypernephroma and splenomegaly, in whom polycythaemia responded to nephrectomy despite the presence of a pulmonary secondary.

It is generally accepted that there is increased production of erythropoietin by the kidney—possibly in the juxtaglomerular cells—and that this leads to overstimulation of the red-cell series, but the mechanism concerned and the exact role of the kidney have not been determined. Erythropoietin is a glycoprotein with a rapid turnover. It has been isolated from tumours, urine, and plasma. Extrarenal production can occur. One of these sites is the liver and increased amounts can sometimes be detected in the plasma when the patient has a hepatoma with polycythaemia (Cannon and Penington, 1967). Its role in normal erythropoiesis is not known. Perhaps it only serves as an emergency mechanism when, for instance, there is blood-loss, and that otherwise any alteration is pathological.

ANAEMIA

Probably every patient with progressive renal insufficiency develops some degree of anaemia during the course of the illness, irrespective of the pathology, but it may not be present for many years. Usually it is of the normocytic, normochromic type unless there is iron deficiency. Three factors operate, namely, blood-loss, decreased erythropoiesis, and accumulation of toxic products in the plasma.

1. BLOOD-LOSS

Bruising, gingival bleeding, epistaxis, haemoptysis, and haemorrhage from the gastro-intestinal tract are occasional complications of uraemia, but a bleeding tendency and defective haemostasis can be present when there is no overt blood-loss.

Thrombocytopenia may be found and the bleeding time prolonged, but qualitative changes in the platelets have been demonstrated even when the count is normal. Platelet adhesiveness can be diminished, and clot retraction and platelet aggregation impaired. Castaldi, Rosenberg, and Stewart (1966) showed that the abnormality seemed to be related to the level of the blood-urea and could be corrected by dialysis. They suggested that release of platelet factor 3 was inhibited. Abnormal capillary fragility may also occur.

Haemolysis is often present in the terminal stages, but it is not usually detected when the disease is stationary (Chaplin and Mollison, 1953). A male, aged 70, with a stable blood-picture was investigated twice by Loge, Lange, and Moore

(1958), the last being a few days before death, and on neither occasion was red-cell survival impaired. The anaemia, seemingly, has to be progressive. Slight reticulocytosis is sometimes seen and urobilinogen excretion may be a little increased, but usually haemolysis is mild. No reduction in red-cell life span is detected when blood from an affected patient is transfused into a healthy person, indicating that the defect is not intracorpuscular—although a reduction has been noted in isolated instances. There is no alteration of the mechanical or osmotic fragility. When blood from a healthy donor on the other hand is transfused into the patient, the life of the donor's red cell is shortened, showing that the cause of the haemolysis is extracorpuscular, and as the Coombs's test is negative it is almost certainly due to toxic or biochemical factors. Red-cell survival measured 36–76 days in the 5 patients reported by Loge and others, while survival in normal persons varied from 90 to 130 days. The degree of haemolysis is seldom sufficient to cause anaemia, but in combination with other abnormalities its effect is considerable. The blood-urea in these patients is invariably high. Decreased fibrinolysis has been reported in patients with chronic renal disease, and elevation when a carcinoma is present. Erythrocyte protoporphyrin was increased in 38 per cent of the patients investigated by Loge and his colleagues.

Table IX.—LEVEL OF BLOOD-UREA IN DISEASE CATEGORIES IN 363 PATIENTS

BLOOD-UREA (mg. per 100 ml.)	GASTRO-INTESTINAL DISEASE	INFECTION	NEOPLASM	CARDIO-VASCULAR DISEASE	COMPLEX ANAEMIA	MISCEL-LANEOUS
151+	0	5	1	2	0	0
101–150	3	4	0	4	1	4
61–100	2	13	3	15	1	7
41–60	8	27	7	49	3	16
21–40	23	45	11	55	3	36
0–20	2	3	1	5	0	4
Total	38	97	23	130	8	67

Table X.—HAEMOGLOBIN AND BLOOD-UREA IN 298 PATIENTS

HAEMOGLOBIN (g. per 100 ml.)	BLOOD-UREA (mg. per 100 ml.)					
	0–20	21–40	41–60	61–100	101–150	151+
<11·6	5	39	18	11	4	6
>11·6	7	108	69	22	7	2
Total	12	147	87	33	11	8

The normal range for the blood-urea is not affected by ageing, so that a raised value indicates gross anaemia, dehydration, or renal failure. Among 363 consecutive hospital admissions the level was as follows: below 20 mg. per 100 ml. in 15, from 21 to 40 mg. per 100 ml. in 173, 41–60 mg. per 100 ml. in 110, 61–100 mg. per

100 ml. in 41, 101–150 mg. per 100 ml. in 16, and above 151 mg. per 100 ml. in 8. The value obtained in different disease categories is indicated in *Table IX*.

Comparison of the haemoglobin and blood-urea values showed that a haemoglobin value below 80 per cent (11·6 g. per 100 ml.) was likely when the blood-urea was above 150 mg. per 100 ml. Further information is given in *Table X*.

The serum iron was low. Only 1 of 19 patients had a level of 70 μg. per 100 ml. or more when the blood-urea was above 100 mg. per 100 ml. This can be seen from *Table XI*.

Table XI.—SERUM IRON AND BLOOD-UREA IN 298 PATIENTS

SERUM IRON (μg. per ml.)	BLOOD-UREA (mg. per 100 ml.)					
	0–20	21–40	41–60	61–100	101–150	151+
<70	7	89	54	28	10	8
>70	5	58	33	5	1	0
Total	12	147	87	33	11	8

Table XII.—T.I.B.C. AND BLOOD-UREA

BLOOD-UREA (mg. per 100 ml.)	T.I.B.C. (mg. per 100 ml.)						
	200	201–300	301–400	401–600	601–700	701+	Total
0–20	0	2	3	3	0	0	8
21–40	1	14	39	44	3	3	104
41–60	0	11	24	18	3	0	56
61–100	0	3	9	8	0	0	20
101–150	0	0	3	5	0	0	8
151+	0	0	1	4	1	0	6
Total	1	30	79	82	7	3	202

An increased incidence of sideropenia seemed to be evident when the blood-urea was more than 60 mg. per 100 ml.

Measurement of the T.I.B.C. in 202 patients showed that a level above 500 μg. per 100 ml. was common and that in 3 of the 6 with a blood-urea above 150 μg. per cent the value was 501–700 μg. per 100 ml. Detail is presented in *Table XII*.

2. DECREASED ERYTHROPOIESIS

There is diminution of red-cell precursors in the marrow, and increasing aplasia is seen as renal failure progresses. Callen and Limarzi (1950), however, noted hypoplasia only in those whose non-protein nitrogen value was above 150 mg. per 100 ml. In 80 per cent of their patients there was hyperplasia.

The marrow appearance is not constant and depends on the clinical features, such as the presence or absence of bleeding, haemolysis, iron deficiency, gross elevation of the blood-urea, and whether blood transfusion or iron therapy have been given. The haemopoietic state of the marrow as judged microscopically is of little if any prognostic significance.

More precise information obtained by radioactive iron uptake indicates that iron utilization by the marrow is decreased when the patient is uraemic. Diminished uptake occurs even when haemolysis is not releasing excess iron into the plasma. It is now generally accepted that this reduced erythropoiesis is the most important single factor in producing the anaemia. Incorporation of iron into the developing erythron is faulty, but according to Carter, Hawkins, and Robinson (1969) the uptake improved temporarily when iron dextran was given intravenously.

The serum-iron level is usually low although it may be within normal limits when haemolysis is present. The iron-binding capacity can be normal, but according to Bothwell and Finch (1962) it is reduced in uraemic patients or where there is gross albuminuria, probably due to loss of transferrin in the urine. Marrow haemosiderin is present unless there is iron deficiency. When multiple blood transfusions are given, tissue iron is increased.

Two reasons are being postulated for the reduced erythropoiesis, namely: diminution of erythropoietin and accumulation of toxic products.

a. Reduced Erythropoietin.—The discovery of an erythropoietic factor in patients with erythrocytosis and certain types of renal disease gave rise to the theory that the anaemia of renal failure was due to a reduction of the factor. When it was found that an increase sometimes occurred with extrarenal disease, the possibility of more than one factor was recognized, and also that perhaps a precursor found elsewhere could be modified by the kidney. This theory received a setback when van Dyke, Keighley, and Lawrence (1963) failed to stimulate erythropoiesis in an anaemic nephritic patient by giving erythropoietin. It was later shown (Nathan, Schupak, and Merrill, 1963) that normal erythropoiesis could be maintained after bilateral nephrectomy had been performed. Moreover, post-dialysis improvement of the blood-picture is not associated with increase of erythropoietin, although inhibitory factors may be removed. Most workers have found absent or reduced serum levels of the enzyme, but in 2 of the patients investigated by Eschbach and others (1967) the level was raised.

b. Presence of Biochemical Abnormality.—If azotaemia and biochemical changes are treated by dialysis, the haemoglobin level rises, although it usually stops short of normal. The higher levels are maintained until uraemia recurs. Iron deficiency may develop with repeated dialysis. It is possible that removal of inhibitory factors allows the marrow to respond to the anaemia, but that later a substance essential for erythropoiesis is lost.

Carter and others (1969) administered parenteral iron until the serum iron was raised to normal levels and a further rise of haemoglobin not observed. The expected fall in haemoglobin level after cessation of iron therapy did not occur in dialysed patients. Their studies with ^{59}Fe showed that the iron was well utilized in the formation of haemoglobin.

It is evident that abnormal blood chemistry has an inhibitory effect on erythropoiesis, but the mechanism has not been elucidated.

3. SERUM FOLATE AND VITAMIN-B_{12} LEVELS

Sevitt and Hoffbrand (1969) found that the serum folate level may be raised in acute renal failure but reduced in the chronic stage. Peritoneal dialysis reduced the folate level. The serum vitamin B_{12} was raised in both acute and chronic renal failure and was not affected by dialysis. Hypersegmented polymorphs were a common feature, but their presence was not related to the level of blood-urea, serum folate, or serum vitamin B_{12}.

Other aspects of the haematological effects are considered in the context of the hypoplastic anaemias (Chapter 14).

GASTRO-INTESTINAL DISEASE

Occult blood-loss from the gastro-intestinal tract is so common that it has to be accepted as one of the main causes of anaemia. Atrophic gastritis, malabsorption, and the consequence of surgery, such as partial gastrectomy, have also to be considered. But this section confines discussion to acute blood-loss, and the effect this has on an elderly person.

Approximately 5–8 per cent of emergency geriatric admissions are due to acute blood-loss. Although haematuria, epistaxis, and vaginal bleeding occur fairly often the most common seems to be haematemesis and/or melaena. In a survey at Swansea, Thomas and Rees (1954) found that of 435 admissions for gastro-intestinal bleeding due to peptic ulceration, 106 (24·3 per cent) were in the age-group 60–90 years, the mortality being 11·3 per cent. Among the total of 483 with acute gastro-intestinal bleeding there were 25 in whom the cause was a carcinoma of the stomach. A higher proportion of elderly subjects has been reported in other surveys—for instance, Avery Jones (1947), 33 per cent; Fergusson and Wyman (1951), 46·5 per cent; and Banning and others (1965), 39 per cent.

Diverticula, oesophageal varices, polypi, blood disorders, and uraemia may also cause acute bleeding. Avery Jones (1969) emphasized hiatus hernia as a cause. In his series 65 per cent were over 60 years of age and 20 per cent over 80. Strange (1963) analysed 116 patients with a giant innocent gastric ulcer and indicated that acute haemorrhage was the commonest reason for admission. The peak age incidence in males was between 60 and 70, and in females between 70 and 80.

The earliest blood change after acute haemorrhage is an increase in the platelet count and shortening of the coagulation time. Within 2–5 hours a moderate neutrophilia occurs with a left nuclear shift and an occasional myelocyte and myeloblast may be seen.

The red-cell count, haemoglobin, and haematocrit are unchanged immediately after haemorrhage, but then fall progressively as haemodilution takes place. This is soon followed by the regenerative phase when a reticulocytosis, maximal between 3–7 days after a single bleed, can be shown. The mean corpuscular volume increases slightly, and many of the macrocytes appear polychromatic. After a brisk haemorrhage nucleated red blood-cells appear in the peripheral blood.

The serum iron is usually low, but the iron-binding capacity may be normal or raised, and adequate stores may be present in the marrow even though the patient is actively bleeding. Presumably mobilization of iron is not sufficiently rapid to meet the need of the body when acute (Beutler, Robson, and Buttenwieser, 1958). At a later stage marrow haemosiderin disappears. According to Bothwell and Finch (1962) an increase in the saturation of transferrin can sometimes occur owing to iron being released from the tissues in excess of what can be used by the erythroid marrow.

The clinical picture depends largely on the rate and quantity of bleeding, but there is always a danger of irreversible progressive uraemia. Hypotension often causes confusion, and sometimes cardiac infarction. The elderly are particularly prone to recurrent bleeding with the result that surgical intervention is required more often than in the young. Whether the cause is an acute or chronic ulcer is of no particular significance, in so far as the immediate management is concerned. Routine investigation on admission should include examination of a blood-film, grouping and cross-matching of blood, and the estimation of serum electrolytes and blood-urea. Whether further investigation is justified during the first 24 hours is debatable. It is generally accepted that there is a higher mortality when bleeding is from a gastric ulcer than from a duodenal ulcer, and that surgery is more likely to be required.

Mailer and others (1965) stated that any of the following features suggested a loss of blood exceeding 1 litre: pallor of the skin, tachycardia of over a 100 per minute, systolic blood-pressure of under 100 mm. Hg, and a haemoglobin level of less than 75 per cent (11 g. per 100 ml.).

Measurements of blood-volume have shown that reliance should not be placed on the haemoglobin level obtained immediately on admission, as the effect of haemoconcentration can be considerable. Of 11 patients who had lost over 3 litres of blood the haemoglobin was 75 per cent or over in 3 (Mailer and others, 1965). Repeat estimation of the haemoglobin a few hours after the first is necessary, particularly when transfusion has not been carried out, but a fall in value does not in itself indicate that bleeding has recurred or continued. Similarly with the blood-pressure—readings above 100 mm. Hg do not exclude severe blood-loss, as the normal blood-pressure reading tends to be higher in the elderly.

Dehydration, electrolytic imbalance, and hypotension are often difficult to combat, but nevertheless adequate blood transfusion is the most important single measure. In an analysis of 73 consecutive elderly patients who had been transfused, Gibbins (1966) noted that in 37 the underlying reason was gastro-intestinal bleeding.

Mortality is so high in the elderly that a combined medical and surgical approach is essential.

RHEUMATOID ARTHRITIS

This is a common affliction in the elderly and is a frequent reason for hospital admission. Sometimes the disease develops at this age but usually it is the aftermath of acute disease—the distorted joints, impaired mobility, and the social consequences—that ultimately leads to hospitalization, although in many instances there are acute exacerbations. In a survey of patients in geriatric and chronic sick wards it was found (MacCarthy and Thomas, 1963) that over a period of 18 months 66 had been admitted with severe disabilities from a population of approximately half a million.

A summary of the findings is presented in *Table XIII*. Blood examination was not carried out in all the patients. Joint deformities were sometimes extreme and a few had been admitted in a terminal state with bed-sores and unrelated general medical diseases, such as bronchopneumonia and cerebral thrombosis. In the 60–69 age-group 50 per cent had suffered from the disease for over 20 years and 14 were totally incapacitated; 60 per cent of those aged 70–79 had had the disease for over 20 years and half were bedridden; while all the 10 patients over 80 years had been afflicted for longer than 15 years and 5 were severely incapacitated.

Seventeen had an erythrocyte sedimentation rate above 70 mm. in the first hour (Westergren), and 7 had a level above 100 mm.—the highest being 130 mm. This patient had a haemoglobin level of 88 per cent. Only 4 in this group had a haemoglobin percentage below 75. One patient had an abscess of the buttock, 3 had severe infection of the urinary tract, and 1 a carcinoma of the lung, but in 10 patients the reason for the high sedimentation rate could not be ascertained. Their arthritis did not appear to differ clinically, either in activity or in extent, from that present in those with a lower rate.

Table XIII.—Advanced Rheumatoid Arthritis in 66 Patients

Age	Sex		E.S.R. (Westergren) mm. in first hour					Deformities		Haemoglobin Percentage					
	M.	F.	<19	20–29	30–39	40–49	50+	Severe	Moderate	80+	70–79	60–69	50–59	40–49	30–39
60–69	14	15	3	1	4	3	15	4	25	15	7	5	1	1	0
70–79	6	21	1	0	3	4	11	14	13	12	4	2	2	0	0
80–89	1	9	1	1	2	1	0	5	5	4	1	2	0	0	1
Total	21	45	24				26	23	43	31	12	9	3	1	1

The chance occurrence of other diseases was well exemplified. Five had diabetes mellitus, 2 Parkinson's disease, 2 Paget's disease, 1 a large aneurysm of the abdominal aorta, 1 myxoedema, and 1 cirrhosis of the liver. Definite urinary infection was noted in 10 cases and chest infection in 8. Death occurred in 17 patients—2 from cardiac infarction, 3 from congestive failure, 3 from a cerebrovascular accident, 3 from pyelonephritis, 4 from bronchopneumonia, 1 from gangrene of a leg, and 1 from follicular lymphoma.

In this survey the anaemia was usually of the iron-deficiency type although in many instances other haematinic factors were also deficient. In only 1 case was the anaemia caused by lack of vitamin B_{12} and folate. This patient had steatorrhoea. Among the 92 rheumatoid patients described by Carter and others (1968) nearly half had anaemia of less than 12·0 g. per 100 ml., and this was either due to iron deficiency or was the anaemia of chronic disease. Only 2 had a megaloblastic anaemia, 1 being due to folate deficiency and the other, a female of 71, had pernicious anaemia.

For the sake of convenience and clarity it is proposed to discuss the blood changes in relation to the haematinic factor involved.

Iron Deficiency

At this age anaemia is present in approximately 30 per cent of hospital admissions and sideropenia in about 50 per cent, irrespective of the underlying disease, so that a high incidence of anaemia in patients with rheumatoid arthritis is not surprising. Some surveys, however, indicate that the deficiency is greater than can be accounted for by chance. Jeffrey (1952) found that in 136 cases the M.C.H.C. was above 32 per cent in only 5. Values below 30 per cent were obtained in 97 (71 per cent). The mean haemoglobin level in males with active disease was 10·9 g. per 100 ml. and the corresponding level in females 9·6 g. per 100 ml. There was no direct relationship with age or with the duration of the disease. The mean corpuscular volume was within normal limits in 75 per cent of the cases so that the anaemia was usually of the normocytic hypochromic type.

The serum-iron level is nearly always low. Values of 40–45 μg. per 100 ml. are commonly obtained. This does not necessarily indicate iron deficiency as the iron-binding capacity may also be low. It has been suggested that there may be a delay in the release of iron from senescent red blood-cells.

Examination of marrow smears revealed the presence of haemosiderin in almost 70 per cent of the 64 cases investigated by Richmond, Gardner, Roy, and Duthie (1956), but they could not establish any correlation between the presence or absence of stainable iron in the marrow with the haemoglobin level, the mean corpuscular haemoglobin concentration, the erythrocyte-sedimentation rate, or the serum-iron concentration. Thirty-eight of the patients were between 40 and 49 years of age, and 19 between 60 and 79. They concluded that the anaemia bore a significant relationship to the activity of the disease and was associated with, but not directly due to, a disturbance of iron metabolism. There was a tendency for a higher proportion to have absent marrow iron when the disease was of long duration. This was the case in 41 per cent of those in whom the rheumatoid arthritis had been present for 10 years or longer.

Studies on iron absorption have given conflicting results. Roy, Alexander, and Duthie (1955) found that absorption of iron from the gut was unimpaired, but Jeffrey (1952) thought that this was not so in 8 of his 50 cases following an oral dose of 9 g. of ferrous sulphate when one accepted that absorption is normally increased in the presence of anaemia. In 2 of his cases plasma iron rose by only 2 and 5 μg. despite a haemoglobin value of 10·8 and 10·3 g. per 100 ml. respectively. On the other hand, there is strong evidence to suggest that iron turnover is increased, so that technical difficulties are encountered when absorption is assessed by this method.

Iron administered parenterally may be shunted rapidly to the tissues, resulting in only temporary elevation of the serum-iron value, but Lovgren (1959) stated that this was not so in over half his cases.

The iron content of liver, spleen, lungs, lymph-nodes, and adrenals is the same as in control cases, but a large spleen may contain a greater amount than expected (Gardner and Roy, 1961). Synovial tissue may also contain excess iron in the form of ferritin.

Splenomegaly in association with chronic arthritis of the rheumatoid type, anaemia, leucopenia, and often lymphadenopathy is known as Felty's syndrome. Pengelly (1966) described such a case in a man of 68 years. Studies indicated a mild haemolytic process, a normal red-cell volume, and a greatly increased plasma volume. The haemoglobin level was 37 per cent. Corticosteroid therapy elevated the haemoglobin to 72 per cent in 3 weeks, and the spleen was not palpable 2 months after treatment commenced. The plasma volume also returned to normal. It was thought that reticulo-endothelial hyperplasia had been controlled. Some authors consider the splenomegaly to be a chance occurrence, or due to systemic lupus erythematosus (*Fig.* 4). Ruderman, Miller, and Pinals (1968) found that splenomegaly could be present without leucopenia, and vice versa. Of the 27 cases they described 14 were aged 60 and over, the eldest being 79, and the longest interval between the diagnosis of rheumatoid arthritis and the development of Felty's syndrome was 38 years. These elderly patients were nearly all females and all except 1 had severe joint deformities, but in only 4 was adenopathy detected. The lowest haematocrit percentage was 19, and the lowest W.B.C. was 500 per c.mm. Immunoglobulins were increased in 7 and in general their level was higher than in uncomplicated rheumatoid arthritis. Gamma-G and gamma-A were raised in

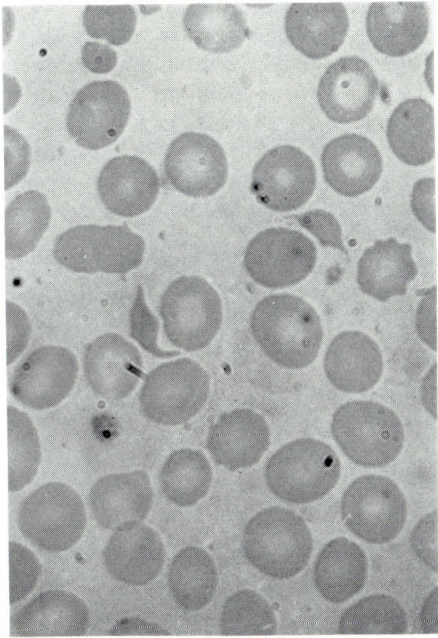

Fig. 4.—Distorted erythrocytes with haemolysis in disseminated lupus erythematosus and rheumatoid arthritis. ($\times 1100$.)

6 and gamma-M in 3. The total haemolytic complement was normal in 5, and lowered in 2 (as in S.L.E.). Antinuclear antibody was present in 6. Four patients had splenectomy performed, but in only 1 was the granulocyte count markedly affected. According to Blendis and others (1970) anaemia in Felty's syndrome can be due to alteration in iron or folate metabolism (as in rheumatoid arthritis), to gastro-intestinal bleeding from salicylate therapy, to haemolysis because of hyperplenism, or to haemodilution due to an increase in plasma volume.

Clinical response to iron therapy in rheumatoid arthritis is variable. Anaemia improves in the majority when iron salts are given orally and presumably these patients have simple iron deficiency with normal absorption. A few require administration by the intravenous or intramuscular route but then respond satisfactorily, and it is perhaps legitimate to assume that they also have iron deficiency although gut absorption may be inadequate. Occasionally the anaemia is refractory to medication with iron, but responsive to cortisone preparations. The explanation remains obscure although it is possible that the turnover of plasma iron is reduced so that more becomes available for erythropoiesis, or perhaps iron is released from synovial tissue when activity diminishes. An anaemia of chronic infection sometimes occurs. Care is always necessary to exclude blood-loss and the presence of other diseases or complications.

FOLATE METABOLISM

Gough and others (1964) reported that 65 per cent of 46 patients had subnormal serum-folate levels and that in 33 per cent the range was such that megaloblastic anaemia could have been expected, but in only 6 was it encountered. Some authors have regarded the deficiency as being coincidental while others have been unable to confirm its existence. Inadequate diet is common in these patients and can cause a lowering of the serum level which would not in itself be indicative of a reduced body folate, but nevertheless one would be suspicious if the level was below 2·0 ng. per ml.

Omer and Mowat (1968) investigated folate metabolism in 37 patients, 17 of whom were over 60 years of age. Their finding in these older patients is indicated in *Table XIV*.

Table XIV.—CHARACTERISTICS OF 17 PATIENTS WITH RHEUMATOID ARTHRITIS (OMER AND MOWAT, 1968)

AGE	SEX	GRADE	DURATION	Hb. (g. per 100 ml.)	E.S.R. (mm. in 1 hour)	FILM	MARROW	PLASMA FOLATE (ng. per ml.)	ERYTHROCYTE FOLATE (ng. per ml.)	FOLIC ACID ABSORPTION
64	F.	II	6 mth	12·7	32	Normal	Normo.	1·4	183	Normal
62	F.	II	30 yr.	11·5	48	Normal	Normo.	1·5	103	Normal
78	F.	II	1 yr.	8·7	52	Normal	Normo.	4·4	209	Normal
65	F.	II	14 yr.	10·5	30	Normal	Normo.	2·0	88	Normal
73	F.	II	2 yr.	7·3	107	Normal	Normo.	3·6	194	Normal
71	M.	II	4 mth	9·8	58	Hypo.	Normo.	2·4	290	Normal
64	M.	III	7 mth	12·4	43	Normal	Normo.	6·1	251	—
70	M.	II	8 yr.	14·6	22	Normal	Early megalo.	2·3	189	—
74	F.	II	3 yr.	8·4	53	Normal	Normo.	2·9	175	—
64	F.	III	15 mth	8·2	112	Normal	Early megalo.	1·4	153	—
69	F.	III	3 mth	10·6	112	Normal	Early megalo.	2·0	126	—
63	M.	I	7 yr.	12·8	22	Normal	Early megalo.	2·8	208	—
62	M.	I	6 yr.	12·1	22	Normal	Normo.	2·2	205	Normal
73	F.	II	3 yr.	8·4	40	Hypo.	Normo.	1·7	111	Normal
63	M.	II	8 yr.	9·4	36	Occ. mac.	Early megalo.	1·5	55	Normal
62	M.	II	22 yr.	7·8	26	Hypo.	Normo.	2·9	232	Normal
73	F.	II	18 mth	8·4	40	Hypo.	Normo.	1·8	215	Normal

In Grade I the disease was clinically inactive, in Grade II moderately active, and in Grade III greatly so. The normal erythrocyte folate value was considered to be above 130 ng. per ml. of packed red cells.

From the table it is seen that 5 patients had abnormally low erythrocyte folate level and that 2 of them had evidence of early megaloblastic erythropoiesis. The serum folate was 2·0 ng. per ml. or below. It is also evident that megaloblastosis can be present when both folate values are normal and that the picture can be normoblastic when both are low. Moreover, the association between the serum and red-cell folate levels is inconstant.

The megaloblastosis in the 'non-folate-deficient patients' was not accounted for by vitamin-B_{12} deficiency. This was measured in every patient and no definitely subnormal values were obtained although in 1 it was intermediate—132 pg. per ml.

Megaloblastic marrow changes were found in 22 per cent of the total series, and a subnormal plasma folate in 65 per cent and a subnormal red-cell folate in 37 per cent. FIGLU urinary excretion was increased in 66 per cent of cases, but in many instances could not be ascribed to folate deficiency. According to the authors no relationship existed between FIGLU excretion and folate values. Deller and others (1966) reported the findings in 80 patients—21 treated rheumatoid arthritis, 20 untreated, and a group of 39 with various bone diseases. Thirteen (32 per cent) of those with rheumatoid arthritis had a serum level below 2·1 ng. per ml., but normal levels were obtained in the others. There was no statistical difference between the treated and untreated groups, suggesting that drug therapy had not influenced the results. Low serum folate levels were not related to duration or severity of the arthritis and, in their opinion, folic-acid deficiency was unimportant in the mechanism of anaemia in this disease.

Urocanic acid, which may be present in the urine of folate-deficient patients, is also increased in many with rheumatoid arthritis, but it is possible that this is due to alteration in protein metabolism rather than to folate deficiency. A similar increase can occur in patients with a low serum albumin, which is fairly common in the elderly.

An increased utilization during cellular proliferation in the joints has been suggested as a possible cause by Gough and others (1964), but there does not appear to be a relationship between the folate values and the apparent activity or duration of the disease.

Low values are often obtained in patients admitted to geriatric units, and bearing in mind dietary difficulties the incidence in those with rheumatoid arthritis does not appear to be unduly high.

Vitamin B_{12}

Partridge and Duthie (1963) found the incidence of megaloblastic anaemia to be 1·38 per cent in patients with rheumatoid arthritis, as opposed to 0·27 per cent in a control group. In 77 per cent of these cases pernicious anaemia was considered likely. On the other hand, Carter and others (1968) investigated the incidence of anaemia, parietal cell antibody, intrinsic factor antibody, and serum vitamin B_{12} and folate levels in 92 patients with rheumatoid arthritis and in a matched control group, and concluded that no significant difference could be demonstrated. The mean age of their rheumatoid patients was 57·7 years (range 19–85) and the mean duration of the disease 10 years. Three of the patients had low serum vitamin-B_{12} levels, but only 1 had pernicious anaemia. Parietal cell antibody was present in 8 per cent but none had intrinsic factor antibody.

Marrow Cytology

Moderate depression of the red-cell series has been described with an increase in normoblasts, which, according to Jeffrey (1952) was directly proportional to the degree of anaemia, especially in cases of more than 2 years' duration.

An increase in reticulum cells with mild plasmacytosis is often observed. Hayhoe and Smith (1951) stated that the plasma cells exceeded 2 per cent in most patients and that it was often associated with hyperglobulinaemia, but Richmond and others (1956) did not find any definite abnormality in their 60 cases. There was a slight increase of the plasma cells in 35 per cent, but this was no greater than in any other disease associated with the production of antibodies.

OTHER FACTORS

Complications, such as pyoarthrosis, vasculitis, and amyloidosis can affect the blood-picture.

Protein and porphyrin metabolism may be profoundly altered and could result in impaired haemoglobin synthesis.

Hypo-albuminaemia and hyperglobulinaemia are often present, but many diseases in the elderly affect the serum proteins. Occasionally a paraprotein may be produced. Waldenström (1964) described 3 such cases. An unusually rapid rate of destruction of circulating red blood-cells may be a factor in producing the anaemia (Alexander, Richmond, Roy, and Duthie, 1956). Abnormalities of tryptophan metabolism and a relative deficiency of pyridoxine were suggested by Bett (1966). Increase of the plasma volume with dilution of the erythrocytes was considered important by Dixon, Rachmaran, and Ropes (1955).

Ekelünd (1962), summarizing the position, stated that the anaemia had been variously ascribed to depressed erythropoiesis, haemolysis, dilution by increased plasma volume, or to an unknown factor interfering with the absorption and utilization of iron.

OSTEO-ARTHRITIS

Degenerative joint disease is common in the elderly and minor degrees may be physiological, but sometimes it is so advanced that it becomes pathological. The dividing line between the two is vague and recognition depends to a considerable

Table XV.—ANALYSIS OF 39 PATIENTS ADMITTED BECAUSE OF ADVANCED OSTEO-ARTHRITIS

Age	No.	M.	F.	Sedimentation Rate (mm. in first hour)					Deformities		Haemoglobin (percentage)				
				<19	20–29	30–39	40–49	50+	Severe	Moderate	80+	70–79	60–69	50–59	40–49
60–69	6	1	5	1	2	1	0	2	1	5	3	1	2	0	0
70–79	15	3	12	7	1	2	1	4	2	13	10	2	2	1	0
80–89	18	6	12	8	2	2	4	2	11	7	10	5	2	0	1
Total	39	10	29	16	5	5	5	8	14	25	23	16			

extent on the personality of the patient. If the complaint is of pain or limited movement a clinical diagnosis is made, whereas in their absence the condition is overlooked. The severity of the symptoms is not related to the radiological appearance. Frequently underlying rheumatoid or traumatic changes exist and the presence of osteoporosis or osteomalacia may be observed.

Although there are no specific blood changes in the uncomplicated disease there are many that are non-specific. A reduction of serum albumin and elevation of gamma-globulin may be due to immobility or to the ageing process itself.

Furthermore, in many of those admitted with severe or moderate deformities anaemia is present. Almost invariably the cause lies outside the skeletal system, but it is as well to realize that when an elderly person is seen with advanced osteo-arthritis the blood-picture is unlikely to be entirely normal. This is illustrated in *Table XV*.

As was noted with rheumatoid arthritis a variety of other diseases were present. Anaemia was nearly always due to iron deficiency and in most instances responded to oral iron medication. One patient had a haemoglobin level of 42 per cent and a serum iron of 25 µg. per 100 ml. due to bleeding haemorrhoids.

ARTERIAL DISEASE

ATHEROSCLEROSIS

This occurs so often in the elderly that it is difficult to assess its direct impact on haemopoiesis, although its indirect effect is considerable. Vascular disease diminishes the reserve power of an organ and may precipitate failure when further stress due to anaemia is added.

Renal involvement can lead to azotaemia and anaemia. It is also possible that other organs can influence haemopoiesis when their blood-supply is reduced. Woodford-Williams and others (1964) noted a reduction in albumin and elevation of globulin in patients with diffuse cerebral arteriosclerosis which was more marked in those with atherosclerosis and hemiplegia. The role of the nervous system in regulating haemopoiesis may be important, as the hypothalamus may be sensitive to oxygen tension and concerned with erythropoietin production.

Necrotic tissue, as in cardiac infarction, is usually associated with a varying degree of neutrophilia and elevation of the erythrocyte sedimentation rate. There is often no precordial pain, and the presenting feature may be confusion, dyspnoea, congestive failure, uraemia, or gangrene, and consequently any blood changes that are present may be ascribed to a condition other than that of the heart.

Atherosclerosis of the mesenteric vessels can probably cause malabsorption. Although intermittent abdominal pain and loss of weight are common the condition can be silent and manifested solely by the development of a mixed type of anaemia. Mild steatorrhoea may be present.

The role of platelet adhesiveness and of fibrin deposition in the pathogenesis of atherosclerosis is well recognized, and the common occurrence of thromboses during old age has drawn attention to possible disturbances in the clotting mechanism of the blood or in fibrinolytic activity. Although atheromatous roughening of the intima, endothelial damage due to hypertension, inflammatory changes associated with arteritis, and a slowing of the circulation rate are important in the development of thrombosis, it is possible that there are occasions when there is a 'latent preparedness for coagulation, characterized by an increase in one or more factors that promote coagulation, or a decrease of factors which inhibit coagulation' (Geill, 1960). In his study, however, using a modified thrombin generation test, Geill was unable to detect any such abnormality in patients with arteriosclerosis who had no local damage, although there was clearly a hypercoagulable state, reflected by increased thromboplastin activity, when a haematoma had developed following tissue injury.

Giant-cell Arteritis
(Temporal Arteritis)

This disease is seldom found in persons below the age of 60. Seventy-one of the 76 cases reported on by Paulley and Hughes (1960) were over 60 years of age, 42 were over 70, and 12 over 80. The modes of presentation include head pains, facial neuralgia, psychotic states, visual disturbances, cardiac ischaemia, anarthritic rheumatism, pain in the ear, vertigo, deafness, strokes, vomiting, cachexia, meningeal irritation, pyrexia of unknown origin, polyarthritis, and aortic arch syndrome.

The erythrocyte sedimentation rate is elevated within the 60–100 mm. range, although *rarely* it is below 30 mm. in 1 hour. The elevation may last for weeks, months, or even years in some instances.

A normocytic normochromic or a hypochromic anaemia is often present and there may also be a mild neutrophilia. An increase in the globulin fraction, especially alpha-2 and beta, may be demonstrated on electrophoresis.

The diagnosis can be confirmed by temporal artery biopsy. An obliterative giant-cell reaction is usually seen, but treatment should not be delayed pending the result if arteritis is likely.

Steroid therapy is effective, provided sufficient is given to lower the sedimentation rate to normal. If discontinued prematurely the elevation returns, as cortisone has a 'damping down' rather than a curative effect. Although the disease is self-limiting it should never be allowed to run its natural course because blindness or some other permanent damage may develop. Therapy has to be continued until the sedimentation rate remains normal after a trial period of cessation lasting 2–3 weeks. It is usually possible to discontinue treatment permanently after 6–9 months, but in some instances small doses of steroids have to be given for periods of up to 3 years.

Polyarteritis Nodosa

This is associated with a moderate leucocytosis and a high erythrocyte sedimentation rate. There may be a relative or an absolute increase of eosinophils. Evidence of haemolysis may be obtained. Anaemia is nearly always present and it may be severe. According to Dollery (1969) the gamma-globulin fraction of the plasma proteins is not usually elevated.

Giant-cell Granuloma
(Wegener's Granulomatosis)

Although rare, this disease can occur. Three of the 10 cases described by Walton (1958) were aged 62, 73, and 75, and we have seen the condition in a female aged 84. It should be suspected when there is a persistent destructive lesion of the upper or lower respiratory tract, together with evidence of widespread disease, such as haematuria, uraemia, polyarthritis, or peripheral neuritis.

There is usually a normocytic or a hypochromic anaemia which becomes profound in the terminal stages, probably due to uraemia, although sometimes there is haemolysis. The erythrocyte sedimentation rate is raised, and there may be leucocytosis, with or without eosinophilia. The serum globulin level is increased, but as this is observed so often in the elderly its significance is doubtful.

Systemic Lupus Erythematosus

The condition is rare in the elderly. There may be a normocytic, normochromic, or a hypochromic anaemia which is usually resistant to haematinics but may respond to steroid therapy. Hypoplasia of the marrow sometimes occurs.

Red-cell survival may be diminished in the acute phases, and frank haemolytic anaemia can be a presenting feature.

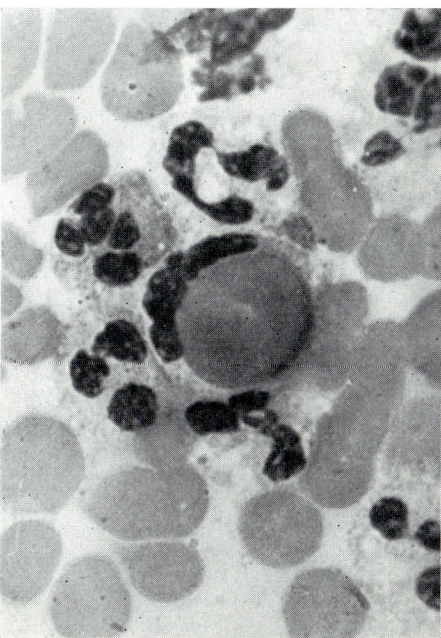

Fig. 5.—*Case* 3. Age 61 years. L.E. cell present 2 weeks before death. ($\times 1100$.)

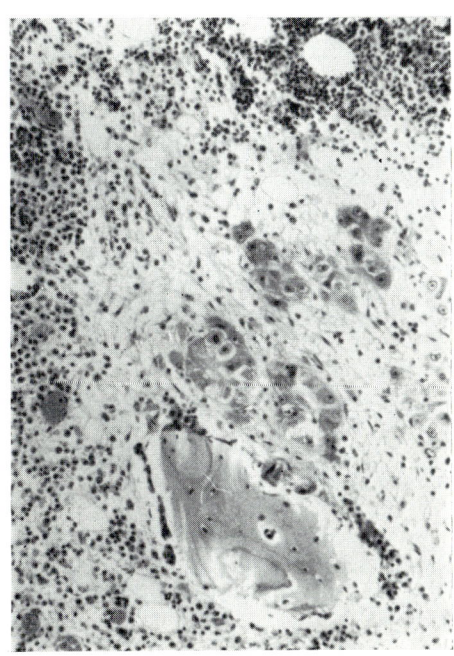

Fig. 6.—*Case* 3. Marrow infiltrated by carcinoma. ($\times 150$.)

Leucopenia is often present, but a normal or a raised count does not exclude the diagnosis. A mild or a severe degree of thrombocytopenia may occur leading to haemorrhages, and this can be the initial manifestation.

The erythrocyte sedimentation rate is raised and may persist during remissions.

Electrophoresis usually shows a reduction of albumin and a marked elevation of gamma-globulin. Cold agglutinins, cryoglobulins, and other paraproteins may be found. Owing to the production of abnormal antibodies these patients may show false-positive serological tests for syphilis and develop reactions when given blood transfusions.

The L.E. cell phenomenon has been widely used as a diagnostic test and may be positive in about 90 per cent of cases. False-positive results are rare, although they may occur in patients with severe drug reactions, but Wilkinson and Sacker (1957) were unable to find L.E. cells in 20 patients with reactions to chlorpromazine, mersalyl, carbimazole, penicillin, phenylbutazone, streptomycin, and serum. Collagen diseases, other than systemic lupus erythematosus in which a positive L.E. test may be found, are rheumatoid arthritis, polyarteritis nodosa, dermatomyositis, and scleroderma. In rare instances a positive result may be obtained in hepatitis and cirrhosis.

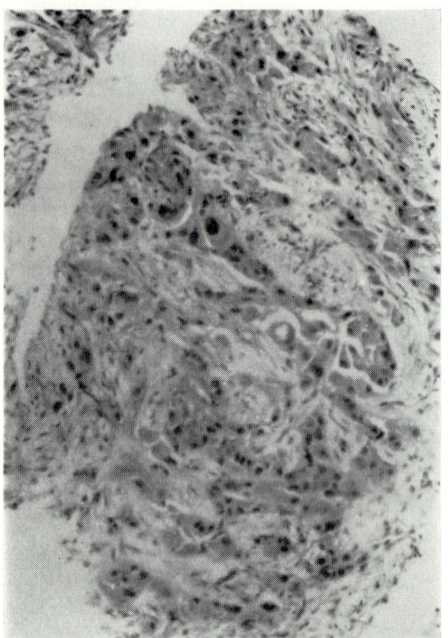

Fig. 7.—Case 3. Pleural biopsy showing carcinoma. ($\times$150.)

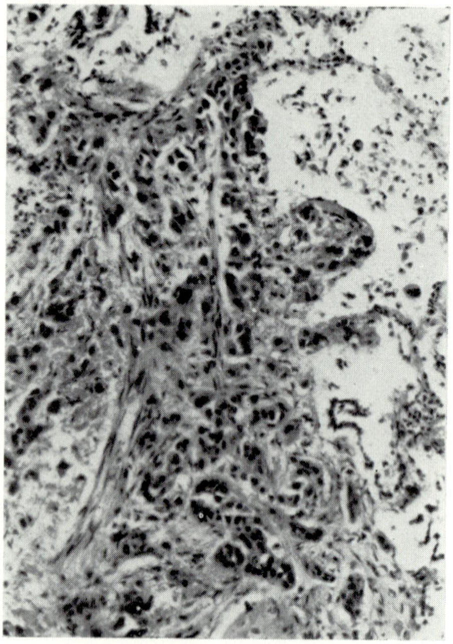

Fig. 8.—Case 3. Lung—bronchogenic carcinoma. ($\times$150.)

Case 3.—Female, aged 61 years. This lady developed arthritic features and psoriasis at the age of 36 years. Five years later rheumatoid arthritis was diagnosed (D.A.T. 1 in 2048). At age 54 L.E. cells were found. She was given repeated courses of steroids and developed septic arthritis with discharging sinuses. When 61 years old she was admitted with dyspnoea, anorexia, vomiting, severe back pain, and cough. X-ray showed wedging of the lower dorsal vertebrae. Hb, 87 per cent, P.C.V., 41 per cent, W.B.C., 7900 per c.mm., E.S.R., 40 mm. The L.E. latex fixation test was positive, L.E. cells were found, and the A.N.F. positive. A pleural biopsy showed a poorly differentiated carcinoma.

At autopsy the principal findings were: an encircling peribronchial tumour of the right lower lobe bronchus; right lung collapse; secondary carcinomatosis of the right pleura; secondary nodules in the skull, liver, and spine. The histological appearance was that of an anaplastic carcinoma. The kidneys and adrenals showed vascular fibrinoid degeneration, microthrombi, and wire-looping of glomerular tufts.

This patient showed typical clinical and laboratory features of rheumatoid arthritis and disseminated lupus erythematosus. However, her terminal picture, which initially was attributed to steroid therapy, was in fact due to bronchogenic carcinoma (*Figs.* 5-9).

The latex agglutination test provides a useful screening procedure and confirmation is obtained by using fluorescence to demonstrate an antinuclear factor. The latter is more sensitive than the L.E. cell test.

Nephropathy is a common complication and can effect haemopoiesis, particularly in the terminal stages.

Other Forms of Angiitis

Terminal obstruction of peripheral vessels may be due to cryoglobulinaemia, cold agglutination, polyarteritis nodosa, Buerger's disease, giant-cell arteritis,

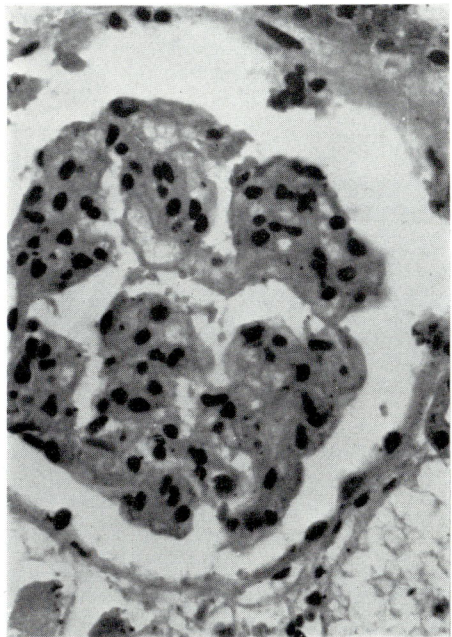

Fig. 9.—Case 3. Kidney glomerulus showing fibrinoid deposition and wire-looping. ($\times 540$.)

syphilis, multiple emboli, scleroderma, vasospasm, crutch arteritis, or thrombosis in association with atherosclerosis or diabetes.

In patients with rheumatoid arthritis or systemic lupus erythematosus there may be minor acute vascular lesions in the digital pulp, severe lesions leading to bone absorption, and others with gangrene (Dubois and Arterberry, 1962). This type of arteritis shows intimal proliferation of fibroblasts, accumulation of mucoid material, secondary changes in the elastic lamina, and sometimes fibrin clots. It seems distinct from polyarteritis nodosa which occurs occasionally in patients with rheumatoid arthritis and from the minor pathological vessel changes that are often present in this disease (Bywaters, 1957).

The erythrocyte sedimentation rate is elevated, and there may be a normochromic or a hypochromic anaemia with a mild degree of leucocytosis. Whether these changes are partly due to the angiitis or entirely to the underlying collagen disease has not been ascertained.

ENDOCRINE DISEASE

THYROID

HYPERTHYROIDISM

There are no characteristic blood changes, although an increase in lymphocytes and in eosinophils may occasionally occur. There is a higher incidence of overt and latent pernicious anaemia than in the general population, and from the findings of Schiller, Spray, Wangel, and Wright (1968) it appears that this varies from 5 to 12 per cent.

HYPOTHYROIDISM

Pallor is nearly always present and about 60–70 per cent are anaemic, but it is only when there is iron or vitamin-B_{12} deficiency that it is prominent. According to Simpson (1959) three kinds may occur, namely, iron deficiency, vitamin-B_{12} deficiency, and a type thought to be due to a deficiency of thyroid. Bomford (1938) described it thus: 'this simple hyperchromic anaemia is never severe, the colour index is normal or a little above 1. There is some macrocytosis, but no poikilocytosis and no excessive anisocytosis. The reticulocyte count may be normal and there may be achlorhydria. The administration of liver or iron has no effect on the anaemia, but the anaemia does respond slowly to treatment with thyroid alone, in such doses as are found to keep the patient free from symptoms of myxoedema or overdosage. The rate of response is very slow, the blood-count attaining normal levels in from 3 to 9 months.'

This third type may be associated with marrow hypoplasia. The addition of testosterone to the therapeutic régime may accelerate erythropoiesis. Wardrop and Hutchison (1969) found that two-thirds of patients with untreated hypothyroidism had irregularly contracted red blood-cells which disappeared slowly with treatment.

Other changes are unusual, but there may be reduction of the plasma and total blood-volume. Red-cell survival is unimpaired. Abnormalities in serum proteins have been described. Buchanan, Koutras, Alexander, and Crooks (1962) found that the serum albumin was decreased in patients with auto-immune thyroiditis and those with primary hypothyroidism, possibly due to diminished synthesis by the liver. Similar results were obtained in thyrotoxicosis, perhaps accounted for by an increased breakdown in the peripheral tissues. Elevation of the gamma-globulin value was usually present in auto-immune thyroiditis, and to a lesser extent in primary hypothyroidism. They concluded that a 'raised gamma-globulin, abnormal findings in the thymol turbidity and flocculation tests, and an elevated E.S.R. are of value in the diagnosis of auto-immune thyroiditis'.

There is association with pernicious anaemia, and according to Tudhope and Wilson (1960) they occur together in 10 per cent of cases. Although chance relationship between them is greater at this age than in younger patients the explanation probably involves auto-immune mechanisms as gastric-cell antibodies may be present. Reduced vitamin-B_{12} absorption sometimes occurs when there is no deficiency of intrinsic factor and no evidence of a specific antibody.

Achlorhydria is present in over 50 per cent of cases of myxoedema, but according to Edward and Coghill (1966) this is the normal incidence in patients over 60.

GENERAL DISEASE

Adrenal Glands

It is well known that polycythaemia, though inconstant, is part of Cushing's syndrome, and that neutrophilia, lymphopenia, and eosinopenia can occur. When the adrenals are depressed the opposite is seen. Characteristically one finds leucopenia, relative lymphocytosis, eosinophilia, and a normocytic hypochromic anaemia. The difference is related to the adrenal response to pituitary adrenocorticotrophic hormone which stimulates leucocytosis. When injected into man there is increase of polymorphs and a reduction of lymphocytes and eosinophils. In hypoadrenalism there is only a neutrophilic response. It has been postulated that the neutrophilia is accounted for in part by mobilization from the marginal granulocyte pool and by a reduced egress into the tissues.

The blood-volume is markedly reduced in Addison's disease and this interferes with assessment of the anaemia.

There is no convincing association with pernicious anaemia, although gastric parietal-cell antibodies may occasionally be found in patients with Addison's disease and cortisone therapy can cause remission in patients with pernicious anaemia, presumably due to its effect on auto-immune mechanisms. When therapy is excessive or prolonged the adrenals are depressed, and this can result in blood-changes similar to those of Addison's disease.

Phaeochromocytomas may cause leucocytosis during phases of hypertension.

Pituitary Gland

The blood manifestations of Cushing's syndrome have been enumerated. Destruction of the anterior lobe, as in Simmonds's disease, leads to a normocytic anaemia of varying severity, together with leucopenia and eosinophilia. Hypoplasia of the marrow can occur, and sometimes a macrocytic anaemia is seen.

Diabetes Mellitus

In insulin-dependent diabetes there may occasionally be auto-immune mechanisms similar to those of pernicious anaemia. Not only may gastric parietal-cell antibodies be found, but pernicious anaemia occurs more often in them than it does in the general population and in those who are not insulin dependent. Ungar and others (1968) gave an incidence of 4 per cent.

The other blood-changes are related more to complications than to the disease itself. Diabetic acidosis usually produces leucocytosis, as does gangrene or infection.

REFERENCES

ALEXANDER, W. R. M., RICHMOND, J., ROY, L. M. H., and DUTHRIE, J. J. R. (1956), *Ann. rheum. Dis.*, **15**, 12.
AVERY JONES, F. (1947), *Br. med. J.*, **2**, 441.
— — (1969), *Ibid.*, **1**, 267.
BANNING, A., BARON, A., KOPELMAN, H., LAM, K. L., and WARREN, P. (1965), *Ibid.*, **2**, 781.
BERMAN, L., AXELROD, A. R., HORAN, T. N., JACOBSON, S. D., SHARP, E. A., and VONDER HEIDE, E. C. (1949), *Blood*, **4**, 511.
BETT, I. M. (1966), *Ann. rheum. Dis.*, **25**, 556.
BEUTLER, E., ROBSON, M. J., and BUTTENWIESER, E. (1958), *Ann. intern. Med.*, **48**, 60.
BLENDIS, L. M., ANSELL, I. D., LLOYD JONES, K., HAMILTON, E., and WILLIAMS, R. (1970), *Br. med. J.*, **1**, 131.

BOMFORD, R. R. (1938), *Q. Jl Med.*, N.S., **7**, 495.
BOTHWELL, T. H., and FINCH, C. A. (1962), *Iron Metabolism*. Boston: Little, Brown and Co.
BUCHANAN, W. W., KOUTRAS, D. A., ALEXANDER, W. D., and CROOKS, J. (1962), *Br. med. J.*, **1**, 979.
BYWATERS, E. G. L. (1957), *Ann. rheum. Dis.*, **16**, 84.
CALLEN, I. R., and LIMARZI, L. R. (1950), *Am. J. clin. Path.*, **20**, 3.
CANNON, P., and PENINGTON, D. G. (1967), *Lancet*, **2**, 1276.
CAROLI, J., and SALMON, C. (1969), *Liver Reactivity*, International Symposium (Ed. SHERLOCK, S., and DIOQUARDI, N.). Milan: Carlo Erba Foundation.
CARTER, M. E., ARDEMAN, S., WINOCOUR, V., PERRY, J., and CHANARIN, I. (1968), *Ann. rheum. Dis.*, **27**, 454.
CARTER, R. A., HAWKINS, J. B., and ROBINSON, B. H. B. (1969), *Br. med. J.*, **1**, 206.
CARTWRIGHT, G. E., and WINTROBE, M. M. (1949), *J. clin. Invest.*, **28**, 86.
CASTALDI, P. A., ROSENBERG, M. C., and STEWART, J. H. (1966), *Lancet*, **1**, 66.
CHAPLIN, H., and MOLLISON, P. L. (1953), *Clin. Sci.*, **12**, 351.
CHAKRABARTI, R., HOCKING, E. D., and FEARNLEY, G. R. (1969), *J. clin. Path.*, **22**, 659.
COWLING, D. C. (1956), *Ibid.*, **9**, 347.
COX, A. G., BOND, H. R., PODMORE, D. A., and ROSE, D. P. (1964), *Br. med. J.*, **1**, 465.
DAVIES, P. S., LUKE, C. G., and DELLER, D. J. (1966), *Lancet*, **2**, 1431.
DELLER, D. J., URBAN, E., IBBOTSON, R. N., HORWOOD, J., MILAZZO, S., and ROBSON, H. N. (1966), *Br. med. J.*, **1**, 765.
— — and WITTS, L. J. (1962), *Q. Jl Med.*, **31**, 71.
DIXON, A. St.J., RACHMARAN, S., and ROPES, M. W. (1955), *Ann. rheum. Dis.*, **14**, 51.
DOLLERY, C. T. (1969), *Br. med. J.*, **1**, 827.
DREYFUS, J. C., and SCHAPIRA, C. (1964), *Iron Metabolism*, International Symposium (Ed. GROSS, F., NAEGELI, S. R., and PHILPS, H. D.). Berlin: Springer-Verlag.
DRIVSHOLM, A. (1960), *Br. med. J.*, **2**, 1063.
DUBOIS, E. L., and ARTERBERRY, J. D. (1962), *J. Am. med. Ass.*, **181**, 366.
EDWARD, F. C., and COGHILL, N. F. (1966), *Br. med. J.*, **2**, 1408.
EKELÜND, C. (1962), *Rheumatism*, **18**, 4, 84.
ESCHBACH, J. W., FUNK, D., ADAMSON, J., KUHN, I., SCRIBNER, B. H., and FINCH, C. A. (1967), *New Engl. J. Med.*, **276**, 12, 653.
FEARNLEY, G. R. (1956), *Lancet*, **1**, 450.
FERGUSSON, D. A., and WYMAN, A. L. (1951), *Ibid.*, **1**, 814.
FORSELL, J. (1958), *Acta med. scand.*, **161**, 169.
GARDNER, D. L., and ROY, L. M. H. (1961), *Ann. rheum. Dis.*, **20**, 258.
GEILL, T. (1960), *Geront. clin.*, **2**, 195.
GIBBINS, F. J. (1966), *Br. J. clin. Pract.*, **20**, 1, 21.
GOUGH, K. R., MCCARTHY, C., READ, A. E., MOLLIN, D. L., and WATERS, A. H. (1964), *Br. med. J.*, **1**, 212.
GREEN, H. N., WAKEFIELD, J., and LITTLEWOOD, G. (1957), *Ibid.*, **2**, 779.
HALL, C. A. (1956), *J. Lab. clin. Med.*, **48**, 345.
HAMILTON, E., WILLIAMS, R., BARLOW, K. A., and SMITH, P. M. (1968), *Q. Jl Med.*, **37**, 171.
HAYHOE, F. G. T., and SMITH, D. R. (1951), *J. clin. Path.*, **4**, 47.
HINES, J. D., HOFFBRAND, A. V., and MOLLIN, D. L. (1967), *Am. J. Med.*, **43**, 555.
INNES, D., and SEVITT, S. (1964), *J. clin. Path.*, **17**, 1.
JANDL, J. H. (1955), *J. clin. Invest.*, **34**, 390.
JEFFREY, M. R. (1952), *Ann. rheum. Dis.*, **11**, 162.
LOEHRY, C. A., and CREAMER, B. (1966), *Br. med. J.*, **1**, 827.
LOGE, J. P., LANGE, R. D., and MOORE, C. V. (1958), *Am. J. Med.*, **24**, 4.
LOVGREN, O. (1959), *Acta rheum. scand.*, **5**, 66.
MACCARTHY, T. F., and THOMAS, J. H. (1963), VI International Congress of Gerontology, Copenhagen (unpublished).
MACDONALD, R. A. (1964), *Haemochromatosis and Haemosiderosis*. Springfield, Ill.: Thomas.
— — and MALLORY, C. K. (1960), *Archs intern. Med.*, **105**, 686.
MAILER, C., GODBERG, A., HARDEN, R. McG., GREY-THOMAS, I., and BURNETT, W. (1965), *Br. med. J.*, **2**, 784.
MILLER, A., CHODOS, R. B., EMERSON, C. P., and ROUS, J. F. (1956), *J. clin. Invest.*, **35**, 1248.

GENERAL DISEASE

NATHAN, D. G., SCHUPAK, E., and MERRILL, J. P. (1963), *Blood*, **22**, 811.
NEALE, G., ANTELIFF, A. C., WELBOURN, R. B., MOLLIN, D. L., and BOOTH, C. C. (1967), *Q. Jl Med.*, **36**, 464.
NIXON, R. K., and OLSEN, J. P. (1968), *Ann. intern. Med.*, **69**, 6, 1249.
OMER, A., and MOWAT, A. G. (1968), *Ann. rheum. Dis.*, **27**, 414.
DEN OTTOLANDER, G. J. H., SCHREUDER, J. TH. R., and HOORWEG, P. G. (1963), *Geront. clin.*, **5**, 103.
PARTRIDGE, R. E. H., and DUTHIE, J. J. R. (1963), *Br. med. J.*, **1**, 89.
PAULLEY, J. W., and HUGHES, J. P. (1960), *Ibid.*, **2**, 1562.
PENGELLY, C. D. R. (1966), *Ibid.*, **2**, 986.
PROUDFOOT, A. T., AKHTAR, A. J., DOUGLAS, A. C., and HORNE, N. W. (1969), *Ibid.*, **2**, 273.
QUICK, A. J. (1960), *Lancet*, **1**, 169.
RACHMILEWITZ, M., ARONOVITCH, J., and GROSSOWICZ, N. (1956), *J. Lab. clin. Med.*, **48**, 339.
RATH, C. E., and FINCH, C. A. (1948), *Ibid.*, **33**, 81.
RETIEF, F. P., and HUSKISSON, Y. T. (1969), *Br. med. J.*, **1**, 150.
RICHMOND, J., GARDNER, D. L., ROY, L. M. H., and DUTHIE, J. J. R. (1956), *Ann. rheum. Dis.*, **15**, 217.
ROBERTS, P. D., HOFFBRAND, A. V., and MOLLIN, D. L. (1966), *Br. med. J.*, **2**, 198.
ROY, L. M. H., ALEXANDER, W. R. M., and DUTHIE, J. J. R. (1955), *Ann. rheum. Dis.*, **14**, 63.
RUDERMAN, M., MILLER, L. M., and PINALS, R. S. (1968), *Arthritis and Rheumatism*, **11**, 3, 377.
SCHILLER, K., SPRAY, G., WANGEL, A., and WRIGHT, R. (1968), *Q. Jl Med.*, **37**, 451.
SEVITT, L. H., and HOFFBRAND, A. V. (1969), *Br. med. J.*, **1**, 18.
SEVITT, S. (1960), *Lancet*, **1**, 384.
SHERLOCK, S. (1968), *Diseases of the Liver and Biliary System*. Oxford: Blackwell.
SIMPSON, S. L. (1959), *Major Endocrine Disorders*. London: Oxford University Press.
SMITH, P. M., STUDLEY, F., and WILLIAMS, R. (1967), *Lancet*, **1**, 133.
STRANGE, S. L. (1963), *Geront. clin.*, **5**, 171.
SWEINSEID, M. E., HVOLBOLL, E., SCHICK, G., and HALSTED, J. A. (1957), *Blood*, **12**, 24.
THOMAS, J. H., and REES, W. E. (1954), *Gastroenterology*, **26**, 2, 260.
TUDHOPE, G. R., and WILSON, G. M. (1960), *Q. Jl Med.*, **29**, 513.
TURNBERG, L. A. (1967), *Glaxo Symposium* (Ed. KRIKLER, D. M.). London: Lloyd-Luke.
UNGAR, B., STOCKS, A. E., MARTIN, F. I. R., WHITTINGHAM, S., and MACKAY, I. R. (1968), *Lancet*, **2**, 415.
VAN DYKE, D., KEIGHLEY, G., and LAWRENCE, J. (1963), *Blood*, **22**, 838.
WALDENSTRÖM, J. (1964), *Acta med. scand.*, **176**, 3, 345.
WALTON, E. W. (1958), *Br. med. J.*, **2**, 265.
WARDROP, C., and HUTCHISON, H. E. (1969), *Lancet*, **1**, 1243.
WASTELL, C. (1969), *Ann. R. Coll. Surg.*, **45**, 193.
WEDGWOOD, J. (1955), *Lancet*, **2**, 1058.
— — (1961), *Geront. clin.*, **3**, 11.
WHELDON, E. J., VENABLES, C. W., and JOHNSTON, I. D. A. (1970), *Lancet*, **1**, 437.
WILKINSON, M., and SACKER, L. S. (1957), *Br. med. J.*, **2**, 661.
WILLIAMS, J. A., HALL, G. S., THOMPSON, A. G., and COOKE, W. T. (1969), *Ibid.*, **3**, 210.
WILLIAMS, R., MANENTI, F., WILLIAMS, H. S., and PITCHER, C. S. (1966), *Ibid.*, **2**, 78.
— — SMITH, P. M., SPICER, E. J. F., BARRY, M., and SHERLOCK, S. (1969), *Q. Jl Med.*, **30**, 149.
— — WILLIAMS, H. S., SCHEUER, P. J., PITCHER, C. S., LOISEAU, E., and SHERLOCK, S. (1967), *Ibid.*, **36**, 141, 151.
WILLIAMSON, J. M., GOLDBERG, A., and MOORE, F. M. L. (1967), *Br. med. J.*, **2**, 23.
WOODFORD-WILLIAMS, E., ALVAREZ, A. S., WEBSTER, D., LANDLESS, B., and DIXON, M. P. (1964), *Geront. clin.*, **10**, 86.

3

IRON DEFICIENCY

IRON ABSORPTION

THE iron content of various foodstuffs is known, but its availability for absorption and rate of incorporation into the red blood-cells have not been fully assessed. It is known that the iron in haemoglobin and liver is absorbed far more readily than that of eggs, but even with haemoglobin the rate at which the iron participates in erythropoiesis is slower than with inorganic iron salts.

The iron content of various common foodstuffs is given below in mg. per 100 g.

Brewers' yeast	18·2	Chicken	1·9	Milk	0·58
Fresh liver	12·1	Peas	1·9	Cheese	0·57
Beans	10·3	Fish	1·3–1·8	Oranges	0·4
Egg yolk	7·2	Cauliflower	1·1	Apples	0·3
Fresh eggs	2·7	Bacon	0·8	Butter	0·2
Steak	2·5	Potatoes	0·7	Cream	0·06

The low iron content of most foods is probably reduced by cooking. The average British daily diet contains about 10–12 mg. of iron and iron-deficiency anaemia does not arise as the amount of iron necessary is only 1 mg. a day under normal circumstances. When excretion of iron increases, as with blood-loss, considerably more than 1 mg. a day must be absorbed, if full erythropoiesis is to be maintained without depleting the stores. Absorption of dietary iron is less efficient than that of medicinal iron salts and great variation occurs, not only between individuals, but also in the same individual on different days.

Jacobs and Greenman (1969) measured the quantity of iron that could be extracted from common foods under laboratory conditions resembling those of the normal stomach. Factors determining ease of mastication and digestion played a part, as did the presence or absence of iron-binding substances. There was also variation caused by different methods of production, storage, and cooking. From their results it appeared that the amount available for absorption was often less than half the quantity present (*Table XVI*).

The site of absorption has been intensively studied. The whole intestine is capable of absorbing iron, although the duodenum and small intestine are the main sites. It is not clear why the iron does not precipitate as the hydroxide in an alkaline medium although the presence of iron-binding complexes, such as mucopolysaccharides, ensures that a proportion remains in the soluble state (Jacobs and Miles, 1969a). There are probably other factors in gastric juice that stabilize the iron and maintain it in a soluble form for absorption in the small intestine. Hydrochloric acid has a dubious role in the absorption of food iron, but increases that of ferrous and ferric iron salts, by preventing protein binding. The necessity of having an intact stomach for iron absorption is well recognized, but it appears that diminished absorption following partial gastrectomy is due to lessened secretion rather than altered anatomy. It has been suggested that possibly a factor is present in the gastric juice, known as 'gastroferrin', which becomes more active in the presence of iron deficiency and which is capable of enhancing iron absorption, but Jacobs and Miles (1969b) failed to find supporting evidence.

Table XVI.—SAMPLE FROM TABLE COMPILED BY JACOBS AND GREENMAN (1969) SHOWING IRON EXTRACTED FROM COMMON FOODS

Food	Total Iron Content (mg. per 100 g.)	Aqueous Extract		Peptic Digest	
		Iron (mg. per 100 g.)	Total Soluble (mg. per 100 g.)	Ionizable Iron (mg. per 100 g.)	Total Soluble (mg. per 100 g.)
Corned beef	4·51	0·16	0·45	0·71 (15·7 per cent)	1·84 (40·0 per cent)
Bacon	2·15	0·14	0·16	0·35 (16·3 per cent)	0·50 (23·2 per cent)
Peas	1·50	0·28	0·59	0·53 (35·4 per cent)	0·62 (41·3 per cent)
Potatoes (chips)	1·25	0·84	0·86	0·85 (68·0 per cent)	0·88 (70·5 per cent)
Egg (boiled)	2·35	0·06	0·14	0·35 (14·9 per cent)	0·78 (33·2 per cent)
Milk (dried)	0·90	—	—	0·14 (15·5 per cent)	0·16 (17·8 per cent)

Studies on pancreatic juice and bile have given conflicting results although there is some indication that the normal pancreas secretes an inhibitory substance, the absence of which, as in chronic pancreatitis, increases absorption (*Fig.* 10).

The form in which iron is presented to the mucosa is important, the ferrous ion being more easily absorbed than ferric ion and inorganic salts more easily than food iron, but the method by which the iron enters the mucosal cell is not understood, although it appears to be an active metabolic process. Presumably the iron enters the cell in a protein-bound form or in an ionized state. Ascorbic acid, in relatively large amounts, increases the absorption of inorganic iron, particularly in the presence of food, and so does alcohol, while phytates, phosphates, and food without vitamin C have the opposite effect. None of these influence the absorption of organic iron. Food contains both types, the inorganic being released by digestion as the ferric form and then reduced to ferrous prior to absorption.

It was thought until recently that the passage of iron within the mucosal cell stimulated the cell to form a special protein, known as 'apoferritin', which combined with iron to form ferritin. Accumulation of this ferritin within the cell blocked excess absorption. This view is not now accepted entirely. The rate of absorption seems proportional to the iron content of the body stores; when low, absorption is increased, and vice versa. The rate of erythropoiesis is also important, though how the stimulus is conveyed from the marrow to the intestinal wall is not known. Some form of erythropoietin may be implicated. In haemochromatosis, and to a lesser extent in cirrhosis of the liver, absorption appears to be independent of body requirements and presumably the mechanisms involved are different from those operating in iron-deficiency states.

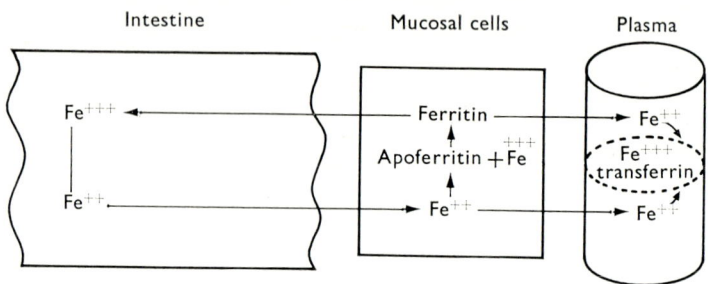

Fig. 10.—Schematic illustration of iron absorption.

The factors controlling iron absorption are tabulated below.

Factors increasing Absorption	*Factors decreasing Absorption*
1. Iron-deficiency anaemia	1. Transfusional polycythaemia
2. Acute blood-loss	2. Iron overloading
3. Iron deficiency without anaemia (low stores)	3. Hypoplastic anaemia
4. Haemochromatosis	4. Malabsorption syndrome
5. Cirrhosis of liver	5. High phytate and phosphate diet
6. Portacaval shunt	6. Gastro-intestinal surgery
7. Ascorbic acid, alcohol	

Organic iron is absorbed by a different mechanism. The haem ring of haemoglobin is separated from the globin in the intestine and then enters the mucosal cell where the iron is separated from the porphyrin and released into the plasma. Enzymes are probably implicated both in the separation of the haem and in its splitting.

When iron-deficiency anaemia is present the rate of absorption increases eight- to tenfold, but decreases as the haemoglobin level approaches normality. When iron salts are given orally the amount absorbed is directly proportional to the amount given.

Iron loss is mainly in the stools in the form of small amounts of blood (about 1 ml. daily) and within exfoliated intestinal cells. Very small amounts are also present in the urine, sweat, and bile. The total excretion amounts to around 1 mg. of iron a day. This has to be balanced by the intake. Departure from the normal, either by increased loss or diminished absorption, results eventually in iron deficiency.

IRON METABOLISM

TRANSFERRIN

Transferrin is a beta-globulin and has a molecular weight of nearly 90,000. One molecule can bind two atoms of ferric iron in a tight bond which confers increased stability on the transferrin-iron complex when exposed to heat or enzymatic digestion.

Plasma iron turnover is rapid (approximately 0·6 mg. per 100 ml. of whole blood per day) despite the firm bond that exists. At least fifteen distinct types of transferrin have been demonstrated electrophoretically, which are inherited as codominant alleles but behave identically in respect of iron transport and delivery. Transferrin constitutes 200–350 mg. per 100 ml. of normal plasma, and in health it is approximately one-third saturated with iron. Examples of hereditary absence of transferrin have been recorded. There may be a decrease shortly before death.

Transferrin conveys iron to developing erythroblasts of the marrow and cells of the reticulo-endothelial system. Iron is taken up without assimilation of the transferrin, part of which coats reticulocytes giving rise to the non-gamma-globulin Coombs's reaction that may be observed with reticulocyte-rich blood. It has been estimated that there are some 50,000 receptor sites to each reticulocyte (Katz and Jandl, 1964), and that the number occupied is proportional to the iron-transferrin concentration surrounding it. The extent of iron incorporation is regulated by the degree of transferrin saturation rather than the rate of haemoglobin synthesis. Direct transfer of iron can occur between clumps that have attached themselves to reticulo-endothelial cells.

HAEMOGLOBIN SYNTHESIS

The final stage of haemoglobin synthesis within the developing red cell involves the union of protoporphyrin III, globin, and iron. The first step in this reaction is probably the enzymatic incorporation of iron into the protoporphyrin molecule to form haem. Haemoglobin contains 0·34 per cent of iron.

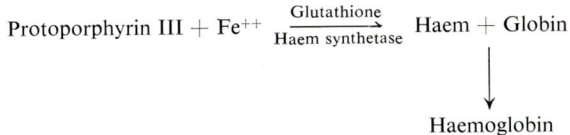

Most of the iron for haemoglobin synthesis is taken up by the pronormoblasts and basophilic normoblasts. Protoporphyrin synthesis is probably localized in the mitochondria.

Transferrin reverts to an unsaturated state following delivery of iron and is then available for its further uptake. The porphyrin component of the haemoglobin released from red-cell breakdown is largely converted to bilirubin; the globin forms part of the protein pool, and the iron is incorporated in the stores or is attached to transferrin.

STORAGE IRON—FERRITIN AND HAEMOSIDERIN

Storage iron may take one of two forms—ferritin or haemosiderin. Ferritin is water soluble and gives a diffuse positive Prussian blue reaction only when present in high concentration, while haemosiderin is insoluble in water and is readily visualized with the light microscope. Deposition of haemosiderin occurs when the ferritin concentration has reached a critical level. The iron content of haemosiderin is significantly greater than that of ferritin. Iron is stored in the parenchymal cells of the liver and the reticulo-endothelial cells of the marrow, liver, and spleen (*Fig.* 11).

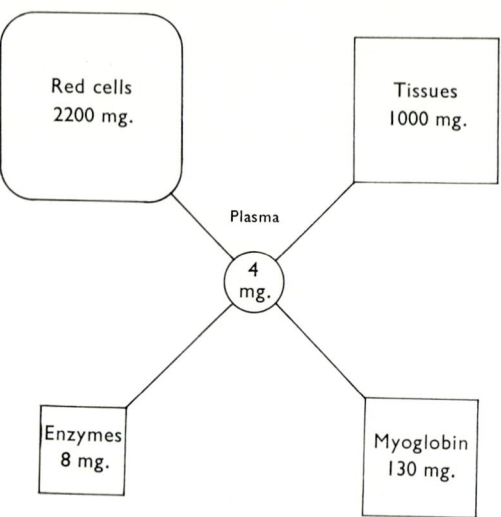

Fig. 11.—Distribution of body iron.

IRON-DEPENDENT ENZYME SYSTEMS

Iron functions as an oxygen transporter, being itself changed from the ferrous to the ferric form. It introduces oxygen indirectly into the organic substrate.

$$Fe^{++} \xrightarrow{+O_2} Fe^{+++}$$

Organic substrate

The major enzyme systems in which iron is involved are the cytochromes, catalases, and peroxidases. *Cytochromes* are conjugated proteins which carry iron-porphyrin prosthetic groups. The first of the cytochrome series functions by reduction of its iron from the ferrous to the ferric form, thereby carrying electrons from other enzyme systems, such as the flavoproteins. The terminal catalyst is cytochrome oxidase, which in the reduced state is readily oxidized by molecular oxygen.

Catalases and peroxidases are iron-porphyrin proteins in which the iron appears to remain in the ferric form. Both systems catalyse the reduction of substrate hydrogen peroxide and related peroxides by means of donated hydrogen atoms.

$$\underset{\text{Substrate}}{H_2O_2} + \underset{\text{Donor}}{H_2R} \xrightarrow{\text{Peroxidase or Catalase}} 2H_2O + R$$

The other iron-dependent enzyme systems include the flavin-linked dehydrogenases, oxidases, and hydroxylases. Thus, although the respiratory enzymes contain approximately only 0·2 per cent of the total body iron, their contribution is vital.

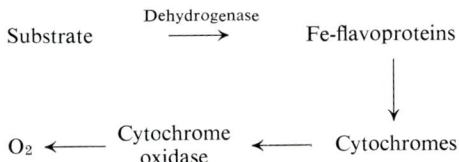

Myoglobin contains 3–5 per cent of the total body iron. It is an intracellular pigment, contains one haem group (as compared with four in haemoglobin), and has a molecular weight of approximately 18,000. Iron remains in the ferrous state when oxygen combines with the haem of myoglobin, which at a lower partial pressure has greater affinity for oxygen than haemoglobin.

CAUSES OF IRON DEFICIENCY IN THE ELDERLY

Iron deficiency may be absolute as when the body iron content is reduced, or relative when for some reason it cannot meet the demands of haemopoiesis or of tissue metabolism. The theoretical mechanisms are:—

1. Insufficient intake	Nutritional; disease of pharynx or oesophagus
2. Defective absorption	Chronic gastritis; achlorhydria; gastrectomy; malabsorption; steatorrhoea; diarrhoea
3. Defective utilization	Reduced binding capacity; inflammation; neoplasm
4. Increased demand	Chronic haemolysis; anoxic lung disease; polycythaemia; treated vitamin B_{12}, B_6, and folic-acid deficiency
5. Excessive loss	Acute and chronic blood-loss

LABORATORY FINDINGS AND DIAGNOSIS

Iron deficiency should always be regarded as a symptom rather than a final diagnosis—although this may sometimes be a counsel of perfection in the elderly. Whereas iron deficiency may be diagnosed and treated without further investigation in women during their reproductive years, this becomes a dangerous practice for both sexes in later life. The high incidence of iron deficiency in the elderly may well be a direct expression of the frequency of morbidity associated with ageing. Not only must a primary condition be excluded, but also associated deficiencies must be suspected.

HAEMOGLOBIN

Hypochromic anaemia is often taken to be synonymous with iron deficiency, and undoubtedly this is the commonest cause—although even this requires qualification with regard to pyridoxine-sensitive sideroblastic anaemia. Other forms of hereditary hypochromic anaemia are not likely to be found in the elderly. The significance and frequency of anaemia in the elderly are considered elsewhere. In a survey of elderly hospital patients we found that the haemoglobin level fell with age in men, but remained steady above 60 years in women until 90 years, after which the mean value rose. The M.C.H.C. showed no change (*Fig.* 12).

Although anaemia is common in the elderly there is no evidence that the 'normal' range for haemoglobin and red-cell indices are any lower than in younger patients. Furthermore, the frequent coexistence of cardiorespiratory disease may mean that normal or high haemoglobin values can occur with significant hypochromia.

The haemoglobin and packed-cell volume should be estimated and a blood-film examined in every patient. There is a considerable degree of observer variation in the assessment of hypochromia. The mean corpuscular haemoglobin concentration is valuable for this reason. We have found 32 per cent to be near the lower limit of normal.

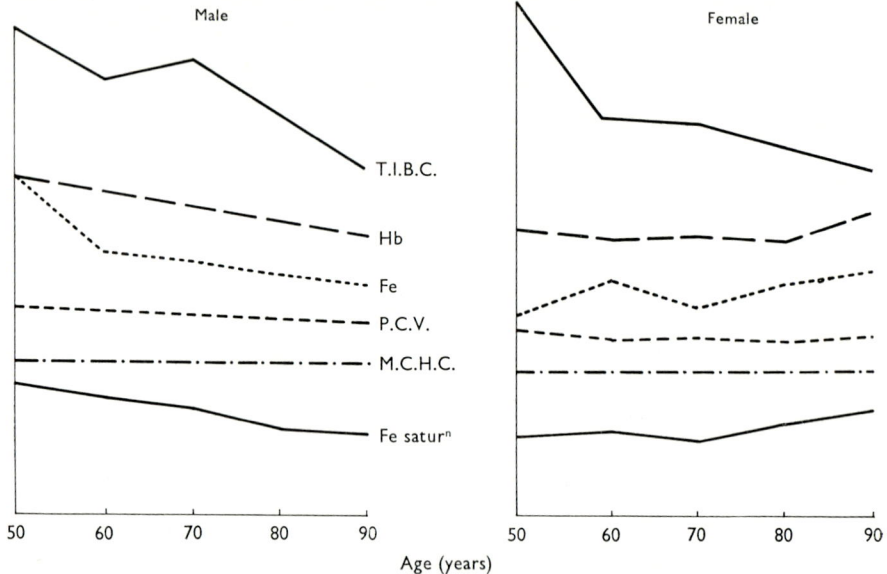

Fig. 12.—Comparison of Hb, M.C.H.C., serum iron, and T.I.B.C. with ageing.

Leucocytes

Usually these are not noteworthy, but hypersegmented neutrophils may be seen even when vitamin-B_{12} and folate deficiency have been excluded, and iron therapy causes the average lobe count to return to normal (Beard and Weintraub, 1969).

Serum Iron, Binding Capacity, and Saturation

Several technical factors influence the results. The appreciable diurnal and day-to-day variation in serum-iron levels makes it advisable that blood should be taken with the minimum of venous stasis in the morning fasting state. Fortunately, at levels below 50 μg. per 100 ml. the degree of variation becomes progressively smaller so that really low values can be accepted with greater confidence (*Figs.* 13, 14). The T.I.B.C. has the virtue of a much smaller degree of variability. The autoanalyser technique for serum-iron estimation described by Young and Hicks (1965) is one which we have found gives highly reproducible values, and is readily applicable to doing surveys of large numbers of patients. It may give elevated

T.I.B.C. levels, but Jordan and Podmore's modification (1963) of Ramsay's method for T.I.B.C. is reliable, and the final stage can be automated as described by Young and Hicks.

Serum-iron levels are lower in the elderly than in younger patients. Average levels for healthy adults are 125 µg. per 100 ml. for men and 110 µg. per 100 ml. for women. The reported mean values found in the elderly range from 60 to 80 µg. per 100 ml. We found (Powell, Thomas, and Mills, 1968) that the serum iron was below 50 µg. per 100 ml. in 40 per cent of men and women above 50 years

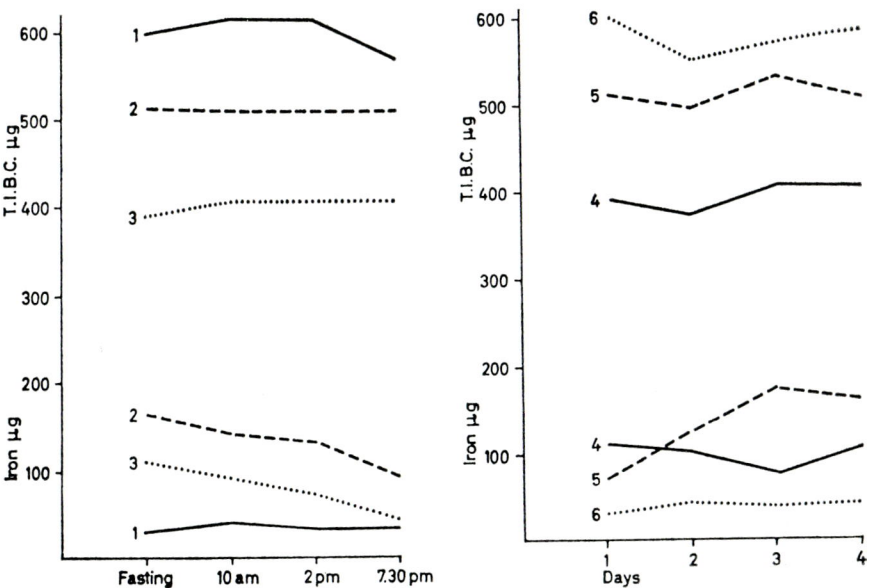

Fig. 13.—Diurnal variation in serum iron and T.I.B.C. (*From 'Gerontologia Clinica'.*)

Fig. 14.—Day-to-day variation in serum iron and T.I.B.C. (*From 'Gerontologia Clinica'.*)

old. After 60 years the level may rise in women, obliterating the previous sex difference (*Figs.* 12, 15).

An essentially similar picture is found with iron-binding capacity (T.I.B.C.) and saturation. The normal T.I.B.C. in healthy adults is approximately 300–340 µg. per 100 ml. Bothwell and Finch (1962) showed a progressive fall in T.I.B.C. with increasing years. There was no sex difference. In our study of hospital patients we found (Powell and Thomas, 1969) a T.I.B.C. greater than 400 µg. per 100 ml. in 46 per cent of both sexes. The highest levels were found at 50–60 years, following which there was a progressive fall with increasing age. The only other known causes of elevated values, apart from iron deficiency, are liver necrosis and hormone therapy. Elevated values are found in approximately half of an elderly population in hospital even when the primary diagnosis is an infective condition, which is reputed to lower T.I.B.C. levels. High T.I.B.C. values in the elderly appear to be uninfluenced by the primary diagnosis (*Fig.* 16).

Transferrin is normally one-third saturated with iron in the healthy adult. A saturation below 16 per cent is usually taken as a good index of iron deficiency (Bainton and Finch, 1964). If this is applicable to the elderly in hospital then approximately a half are iron deficient. A large proportion are below 10 per cent (35 per cent men and 25 per cent women).

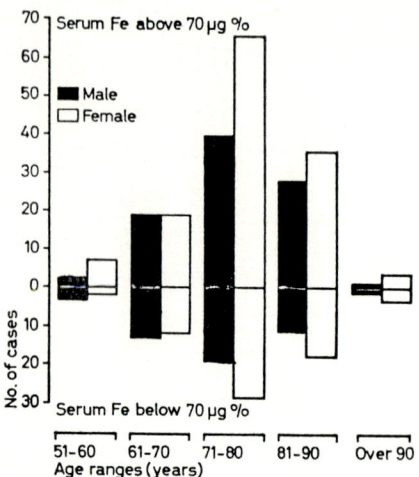

Fig. 15.—Proportion with serum iron above and below 70 µg. per 100 ml. in decades. (*From 'Gerontologia Clinica'.*)

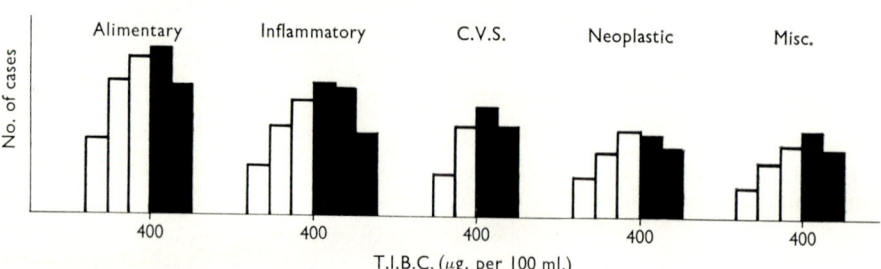

Fig. 16.—T.I.B.C. levels above 400 µg. per 100 ml. in different disease categories.

The interpretation of these values is peculiarly difficult because of doubt as to the normal range. The problem may be approached indirectly by attempting to correlate the measurements and relating them to the clinical state. High T.I.B.C. levels usually accompany low serum iron and saturation—but with many exceptions. The T.I.B.C. may be so elevated that even a 'normal' serum-iron level may give an abnormally low degree of saturation. Conversely, the T.I.B.C. may be sufficiently low to give a 'normal' saturation when the serum iron is below 50 µg. per 100 ml. Clearly it is imperative that serum-iron levels should only be interpreted in the light of the T.I.B.C. level. Serum iron and saturation show a significant correlation with the M.C.H.C. In 114 men the correlation between serum iron and M.C.H.C. was 0·220 ($P < 0.05$) and in 164 women it was 0·420

($P < 0.01$). The serum iron, however, showed a poorer correlation with haemoglobin ($r = 0.097$, not significant in men, and 0.256 with $P < 0.01$ in women only). This poor correlation is accounted for by the significant number that have sideropenia without anaemia—for example, we found that in a series of 333, 42 had a haemoglobin above 11·7 g. per 100 ml. with a serum iron below 35 µg. per 100 ml. Even with a haemoglobin above 14·6 g. per 100 ml., 15 per cent of the patients had a serum iron below 35 µg. per 100 ml. (*Fig.* 17). Therefore the peripheral blood-picture alone is not a reliable index of iron deficiency.

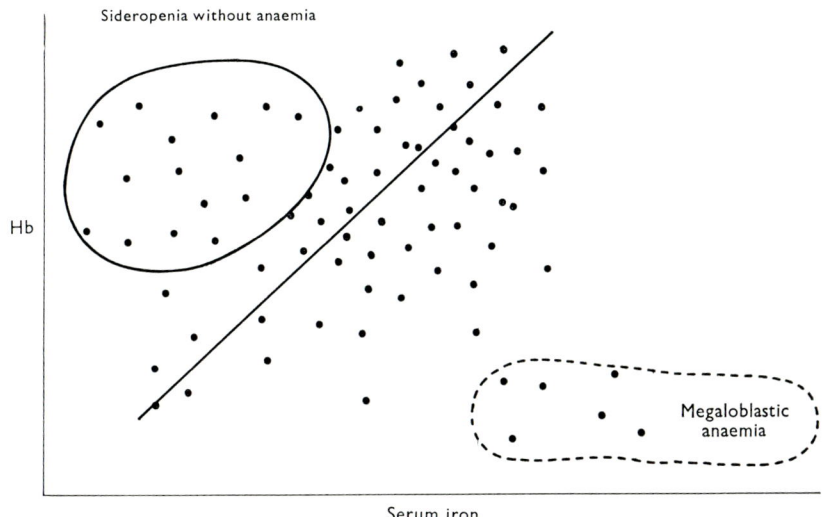

Fig. 17.—Serum iron in relation to haemoglobin. (*From 'Gerontologia Clinica'.*)

McFarlane, Pinkerton, Dagg, and Goldberg (1967) studied 500 women in general practice, 257 of whom were postmenopausal. They found an incidence of iron deficiency (a haemoglobin below 12·0 g. per 100 ml. and an iron saturation below 16 per cent) in 8·2 per cent of patients and 2 per cent in symptomless volunteers, and iron deficiency without anaemia (a haemoglobin over 12·0 g. per 100 ml. with an iron saturation below 16 per cent) in 22·2 per cent of patients and 16·3 per cent of the symptomless group. They found that iron deficiency with or without anaemia became slightly more common after the menopause.

BONE-MARROW

The frequency of osteoporosis in the elderly necessitates special care during marrow aspiration. Cytology should be assessed by a routine Romanowsky method; by Perls's technique for haemosiderin; and the aspirate sectioned at 6 µ and similarly stained. We have found Signy and Smith's procedure (1966) useful in routine work.

An assessment of marrow iron may be recorded in several ways. The amount present may be expressed on a roughly quantitative score, and the distribution between the cells and extracellular material noted. This procedure is not as easy as it is made to appear, because experience is required to differentiate artefact from true marrow iron. In some preparations this distinction cannot be made with confidence.

Haemosiderin can be readily identified in marrow by Perls's technique (*Figs*. 18, 19). Ferritin can only be seen when it is present in considerable excess. Haemosiderin granules are found in the erythroblasts and may also be seen in reticuloendothelial cells and extracorpuscular marrow material. Depletion or absence of stainable iron is frequently regarded as the hall-mark of iron deficiency against which all other indices are compared. This may well be a misleading oversimplification in the elderly. It is important to examine stained smears and sections of the marrow aspirate, because one may be more informative than the other. Stained sections are particularly useful because of the concentration of the material to be examined and the ease with which artefact staining can be recognized. However, apart from technical difficulties the marrow iron findings may fail to correlate with other indices. We found that smears may not show stainable iron when the saturation is above 20 per cent, but this does not occur so frequently with sections. When the saturation is below 10 per cent smears practically never show stainable iron, but

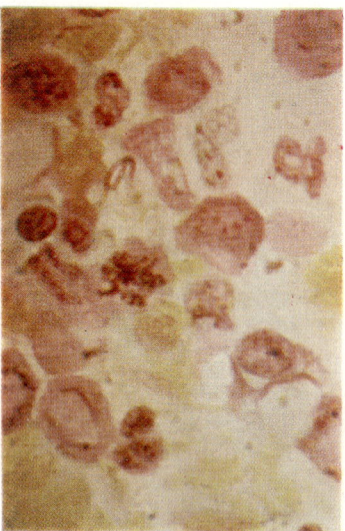 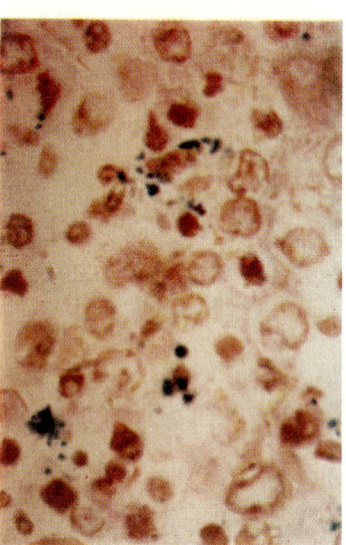

Fig. 18.—Perls's stain.   *Fig*. 19.—Perls's stain.

sections may do so in a few instances. Rath and Finch (1948) found an increased amount of stainable marrow iron in the presence of infection, but this is not a characteristic feature in the elderly. This may correlate with the finding that the T.I.B.C. in the elderly is elevated in infective conditions, as compared with the reduction observed in the younger patient.

Tissue Iron

It is no longer accepted that the iron-containing and iron-dependent enzyme systems are inviolate in iron depletion, although investigations give conflicting results. Several workers have reported a reduction of cytochrome-oxidase activity in iron deficiency (Beutler, 1959; Jacobs, 1961; Dagg, Goldberg, Gibbs, and Anderson, 1966). Balcerzak, Vester, and Doyle (1966) found a reduction in red-cell catalase which paralleled the lowering of haemoglobin and M.C.H.C. Tudhope (1967) failed to confirm this. None of these enzyme assays is as yet useful in the routine assessment of iron deficiency.

Structural changes in iron deficiency may be gross, as in koilonychia and cheilosis, or microscopic, as in atrophy of the epithelium and filiform papillae of the tongue. The changes in the gastric mucosa are of particular interest. Atrophic gastritis is a frequent finding although it is still debated whether these changes precede or follow the state of iron deficiency. Lees and Rosenthal (1958), in a clinical and histological study of 19 patients suffering from iron-deficiency anaemia, found that there was progression in the degree of gastritis and gastric atrophy 1 year after correcting the anaemia. Epithelial lesions elsewhere improved. The mucosa of the small intestine does not share in the histological abnormality. Achlorhydria may precede the onset of anaemia by many years, and once histamine-fast achlorhydria as assessed by the augmented histamine test is established, it is not reversed by iron therapy (Meulengracht, 1932; Witts, 1956). The evidence suggests strongly that the frequency of iron deficiency in the elderly is related to the progressive gastric atrophy that may occur with ageing.

Delamore and Shearman (1965) attempted to reconcile the differing views concerning the relationship of gastric abnormalities to iron deficiency by proposing that there are two groups of patients. In the first iron deficiency is primary, and acid secretion may improve after iron therapy, whereas in the second group the primary state is that of irreversible gastric atrophy with achlorhydria. These are the patients in whom circulating parietal cell antibodies are usually found. The prevalence of achlorhydria and gastric parietal cell antibodies increases with age (Wangel, Callender, Spray, and Wright, 1968).

Iron deficiency is often associated with other deficiency states in the elderly. Dagg, Jackson, Curry, and Goldberg (1966), in a study of 114 cases of iron-deficiency anaemia, found that 7 had latent pernicious anaemia as diagnosed by the Schilling test, and concluded that a patient with iron-deficiency anaemia had a 6 per cent chance of developing pernicious anaemia, and a 32 per cent chance if histamine-fast achlorhydria and circulating parietal cell antibodies were found.

The epithelial changes associated with iron deficiency are similar to those found in riboflavin and pyridoxine deficiency. This prompted Jacobs and Cavill (1968) to examine glutamic pyruvic transaminase levels as an index of pyridoxine nutritional status. They found reduced erythrocyte levels in iron-deficiency anaemia, which were related more to oral epithelial lesions than to the degree of anaemia. It would appear that the oral lesions often associated with iron depletion may be due to concomitant nutritional pyridoxine deficiency.

Radio-isotope Studies

Radio-isotope techniques have largely replaced chemical methods. Iron absorption can be assessed by measuring plasma radioactivity for 4 hours following an oral dose of ^{59}Fe, but the results have to be interpreted with considerable caution because of its unphysiological nature. The extent of plasma rise is a function of the degree of transferrin saturation and the marrow demand for iron—the maximal rise being obtained when the saturation is low and the patient not anaemic.

Iron turnover can be studied by following the rate of plasma clearance of radioactive isotope after administration of an intravenous dose of the radioactive isotope. In iron deficiency the iron disappears from the plasma at an increased rate. Unfortunately, this apparently simple approach is not a reliable test of iron deficiency.

Although radio-isotope studies have shed considerable light on many aspects of iron metabolism and haemopoiesis, they are not established as routine clinical tests on account of their specialized nature and the fallacies in their interpretation. If whole-body counting equipment should become more readily available this might well afford a useful routine procedure (Lunn, Richmond, Simpson, Leask, and Tothill, 1967).

DIFFERENTIAL FERRIOXAMINE TEST

Fielding (1965) described the use of a test whereby body iron is chelated by desferrioxamine. Desferrioxamine methanesulphonate is injected intravenously, together with a dose of ^{59}Fe-labelled ferrioxamine. A single 6-hour urine specimen is then collected and the amount of injected ferrioxamine excreted—Ft (as ^{59}Fe)—is compared with the total amount of ferrioxamine excreted—Fex (as estimated chemically).

The chelatable iron is calculated from the difference (Ft − Fex). In iron deficiency this approaches zero, or may give a negative quantity because of the variability of single observations. The test can be repeated.

Fielding, O'Shaughnessy, and Brumström (1965) used this test in an attempt to assess iron deficiency in the absence of anaemia, and suggested that 35 per cent of the non-anaemic women they tested were iron deficient.

ERYTHROCYTE-FREE PROTOPORPHYRIN

The claim of Dagg and others (1966) that erythrocyte-free protoporphyrin is increased in iron-deficiency anaemia is one which requires further evaluation as a routine investigation. The mean values in normal, sideropenic, and anaemic patients were 15·5, 93·3, and 159·2 µg. per 100 ml. respectively. This method has the further advantage that only a direct chemical estimation is required.

INVESTIGATION

The possible presence of bleeding must be investigated. The testing of faeces for occult blood yields such inconstant results that, although its simplicity ensures widespread use, undue importance must not be attached to the findings. Benzidine is no longer used, because of the high incidence of carcinoma in individuals concerned with its preparation, and the test has been replaced with the orthotolidine test, the Occultest tablet, and the Haematest tablet. This substance is also potentially carcinogenic, but the minute quantities present in these commercial preparations are acceptable although they should ideally be handled with gloves or forceps. Kay (1962) stated that the Haematest was not sensitive enough and that there was a risk of obtaining false-negative results, while the other two tests were oversensitive when patients were on an unrestricted diet. Ross, Gray, de Silva, and Newman

(1964) showed that none of the chemical tests was reliable when considered alone. Chemical tests can be replaced or supported by spectroscopic tests, such as examination for protoporphyrin or Snapper's test for pyridine-haemochromogen, but they are not suitable when many specimens are being examined. Where doubt exists intravenous administration of tagged patient's red cells with ^{51}Cr followed by faecal examination may resolve the problem.

If there is evidence of blood-loss a careful drug history is taken, particularly regarding the ingestion of aspirin, phenylbutazone, and cortisone, and a bleeding lesion of the mouth, throat, and anus is excluded.

When the source of bleeding is within the gastro-intestinal tract a conventional barium meal with follow-through radiograph is essential. This may have to be followed by a barium enema. When the cause is still not apparent oesophagoscopy, gastroscopy, proctoscopy, or sigmoidoscopy may be necessary. Where facilities exist, other procedures are also possible such as a small-bowel enema, the fluorescein string test, the serial testing of samples from the small intestine obtained by means of a Crosby capsule, or the use of optical instruments as in the fibrescope. Laparotomy is rarely justified.

The blood-urea and urine should always be checked. The possibility of malabsorption must be eliminated in refractory states. This may be present when there is no visible abnormality of the stools. A xylose-tolerance test may be of value, but direct measurement of faecal fat is usually required.

Serum vitamin-B_{12} activity (where no such therapy has been given), the Schilling test for vitamin-B_{12} malabsorption, serum folate, and possibly red-cell folate activity may also be required. Scorbutic features suggest the need for measuring leucocyte ascorbic acid content. The tryptophan-loading test may be useful in pyridoxine-deficiency states.

Most of the above investigations can be initiated while the patient is receiving iron therapy. The haemoglobin response should be followed rather than serial reticulocyte counts.

In practice we have found that estimation of the haemoglobin, M.C.H.C., serum iron, and T.I.B.C. enables a reliable assessment of a patient's iron status to be made. Further tests are either confirmatory or designed to eliminate other deficiencies.

Routine Investigations in Suspected Iron Deficiency

A. To establish the Presence of Iron Deficiency

1. Haemoglobin, M.C.H.C., blood-film.
2. Serum iron and T.I.B.C.
3. Examination of marrow, if indicated.
4. Other tests which may be available—radioactive isotopes, differential ferrioxamine, erythrocyte protoporphyrin.

B. To establish the Cause of Iron Deficiency

1. Search for systemic disease.
2. Test for blood-loss—faeces and urine.
3. Blood-urea.
4. Faecal fat.

C. TO ESTABLISH THE PRESENCE OF CONCOMITANT DEFICIENCIES
1. Parietal cell antibodies.
2. Diagnex blue. Augmented histamine test meal.
3. Serum vitamin B_{12}, folate (white-cell ascorbic acid).
4. Schilling test.

D. THE THERAPEUTIC TEST.—Assessment of response.

CLINICAL FEATURES

The presence of koilonychia, pale mucous membranes, smooth atrophic tongue, and dysphagia is usually stressed. Although these occur in the elderly the fully developed picture is rare in this country.

Pallor of the mucous membranes is always found, but the colour of the everted lower eyelid is sometimes a poor guide, because blepharitis may hide the pallor, while contraction of the capillaries and the presence of patchy xanthomata may accentuate pallor out of proportion to the anaemia. Severe anaemia can usually be diagnosed, but lesser degrees cannot. The tongue, lips, and creases of the hands are pale and sometimes these findings are present when the eyelid mucous membrane is of normal colour, but here again the physical signs are too variable to be reliable.

Koilonychia is uncommon in our experience and is not related to the degree of anaemia. Perhaps additional factors, such as amino-acid deficiency, must be present before the sign appears. Sometimes the nails are flattened or brittle, but these changes are seldom noteworthy. A smooth tongue is common in the elderly and is not limited to those with iron deficiency. Indeed, the tongue surface may be normal when anaemia is marked.

Sideropenic dysphagia is infrequent, but Jacobs and Kilpatrick (1964) found 11 patients over the age of 60 years among 55 with difficulty in swallowing localized to the postcricoid region. There was a high incidence of iron deficiency, achlorhydria, and subnormal vitamin-B_{12} absorption, and they suggested that iron deficiency was a secondary feature of a genetically determined gastric atrophy. In these patients the Paterson-Kelly syndrome may precede or follow the anaemia, and the gastric atrophy can also lead to latent or frank pernicious anaemia. The most common causes of dysphagia in an anaemic elderly patient are either neurological in origin or related to an oesophageal lesion—usually a stricture or neoplasm.

The presence of a palpable spleen almost invariably indicates some other disease.

Excessive reliance is being placed on physical signs in the diagnosis of anaemia so that the condition is often missed. Iron deficiency should be looked for, not only when it is suspected, but also in those with unconnected diseases. Even minimal anaemia is of considerable importance in the elderly owing to the diminished reserve power of organs. Blood examination is always necessary whatever the symptom.

It is sometimes difficult to separate the symptoms of the anaemia from those of the underlying cause, especially when the anaemia is due to blood-loss from the alimentary tract. Iron therapy may render the patient symptomless even when a peptic ulcer is still present. This may be related to the natural history of pain in that condition, but similar improvement may occur with carcinoma of the stomach.

Anorexia, flatulence, and vague indigestion can result from iron deficiency and will disappear when this is corrected, but nevertheless, if these symptoms are present, a radiological examination should be carried out. Carcinoma of the stomach or colon may be symptom free and often iron-deficiency anaemia is the first abnormality noted. Diarrhoea due to oral iron therapy can complicate the issue. These patients may be admitted with mental confusion and incontinence.

An understanding of the complex picture frequently demands persistence. Despite the tendency to multiple pathology in the elderly, there is evidence that iron deficiency gives rise to distinct clinical syndromes. Anaemia is not invariable and therefore it is justifiable to consider two groups, namely, those with anaemia and those without.

Iron Deficiency with Anaemia

Before describing the symptoms found in anaemic patients, the difficulty of assessing their attributability to anaemia should be stressed. Thus Dawson, Ogston, and Fullerton (1969) studied 133 anaemic and 111 non-anaemic patients. These groups included 39 and 30 patients over 70 years respectively. Each patient was questioned as to the presence of symptoms such as fatigue, pallor, recent headache, recent insomnia, paraesthesia, dizziness, etc. The only feature which was significantly associated with the severity of the anaemia was pallor of recent onset. Acute blood-loss was associated with dizziness, and anorexia and painful tongue with vitamin-B_{12} deficiency. Therefore, although symptoms such as those listed below are commonly found in anaemic patients, these should not necessarily be attributed directly to the anaemia.

Although the extent and duration of anaemia influence the clinical picture the symptoms associated with severe anaemia should not be separated from those of mild anaemia, because the underlying integrity of organ or organs varies considerably. In a series of individuals no definite association between symptoms and the degree of anaemia can be demonstrated. All those with severe anaemia are ill, but so are many with mild anaemia, despite the fact that others may be reasonably healthy.

For the sake of convenience and clarity the relevant symptoms will be considered under specific organ defects. Although overlapping occurs it is surprising how often individual systems are involved and also how variable the presentation may be among those with a similar degree of deficiency.

1. Central Nervous System

Apathy and loss of interest in the environment are probably the most common symptom complex encountered. They may manifest themselves by a lowering of social standards. Body cleanliness is ignored and the condition of the home deteriorates. Gradually the patient stays more and more in bed with consequent reduction of mobility and of ability to perform daily activities. Cooking and eating become a drudgery so that malnutrition is superimposed. Judgement becomes faulty and the apathy may gradually merge into negativism, which results in the patient resisting all efforts at improving his or her lot.

Case 1.—A female, aged 72 years, who had been caring for her bachelor son began to neglect both house and meals. She went to bed early and got up late. Despite her objections a doctor was informed, but she then refused treatment and admission to hospital. Illness was denied. A 'special order' had to be invoked before she came into hospital. It was then found that she had a Hb of 35 per cent and M.C.H.C. of 29—due to bleeding haemorrhoids. She was given blood transfusion followed by intramuscular iron therapy and 3 weeks later her Hb was 80 per cent. At no time was she confused but there was no recollection of what had taken place, and when informed of her behaviour she was most apologetic.

This degree of resistance is unusual, but lesser degrees are common and can be a problem, not only regarding admission and medical treatment, but also when surgery is indicated.

Depression may follow prolonged apathy, but often there is no obvious prodromal feature. A morose premorbid personality seems characteristic and usually the person is either living alone, or is the centre of controversy in the household. Sometimes mild physical or mental trauma may be a precipitating agent. The patient becomes withdrawn and dementia may be simulated.

Case 2.—A woman, aged 68 years, with Paget's disease was living alone, surprisingly well and active, when she fell, injuring her leg. Severe pain developed but there was no fracture. She then became depressed and this progressed rapidly with persistent weeping and suicidal tendencies. Imipramine and analgesics were prescribed and local authority home services arranged. As there was no improvement after 14 days she was admitted to hospital where the presence of iron-deficiency anaemia was detected. Her Hb was 60 per cent. Rapid improvement occurred with iron therapy alone and she was discharged 3 weeks later. There was no recurrence of depression during the next 5 years.

Although it is difficult to evaluate the role of iron deficiency in the depression, this and comparable cases suggest a possible association.

Dementia may be wrongly diagnosed in a patient with severe depression. True dementia does not appear to be caused by pure iron deficiency, though clinically there is probably an association between them because correction of such a deficiency in the early stages of dementia has a beneficial effect and seems to delay progression. The relationship is not as definite as it is with vitamin B_{12} or folate deficiency.

Agitation is a common feature and may be accompanied by insomnia or early depression. Constant wandering may be troublesome and for brief periods there may be loss of awareness of surroundings. Loneliness is often present. Like apathy and depression this symptom complex has many medical and psychiatric causes, but it is surprising how often iron-deficiency anaemia has a significant role.

Mental confusion occurs commonly but a reliable history is often unobtainable and physical examination unrewarding in many instances.

Sometimes iron deficiency is the main cause of the disturbance, but anaemia need not be a prominent feature, although some degree is usually present. A haemoglobin level below 80 per cent was obtained in 17 of 50 consecutive admissions with unexplained confusion, but this incidence is the same as that among other elderly patients.

The effect on the confusion of correcting the anaemia cannot be predicted. Sometimes return to normality can be achieved with fair rapidity; in others improvement is slow while there are some whose confusion persists. Occasionally, difficulties arise because of physical improvement without mental change. A confused anaemic patient, easily managed in a general ward, may thus be rendered unmanageable and require transfer to a mental hospital.

Behavioural problems, usually of an antisocial kind, may be caused or accentuated by iron deficiency. There are sometimes abnormal dietary proclivities. Usually mild dementia is present, although the personality may be well maintained.

Other mental disturbance such as feelings of persecution, delusions, and hallucinations may be precipitated or aggravated, but these manifestations are rarer than those previously described.

Paraesthesiae of the hands and, to a lesser extent, of the feet may be admitted, although seldom volunteered. The symptom is common in the elderly and is accepted as being due to ageing, or is mild in nature and considered unimportant.

Patchy anaesthesia may be present over the hands. Clumsiness of finger control, morning stiffness, and a burning sensation of the finger-tips are unlikely to be commented upon. Peripheral nerve involvement is unusual and we have not seen a case where peripheral neuritis could be diagnosed, though muscle tenderness is common.

Cranial nerve involvement is exceedingly rare and we have not seen papilloedema. Linear retinal haemorrhages, soft exudates, and deeper round haemorrhages may occur when the anaemia is severe.

Headache may be described as a 'heavy' or a 'muzzy' feeling, or as a throbbing sensation behind the eyes, around the forehead, or on top of the head. It may persist as a dull ache or be interrupted by short stabs of pain, particularly when the head is turned quickly, or the person bends forward. A migrainous quality may be evident. This may develop in a person who has hitherto been free from migraine, or it may increase the frequency and severity of attacks.

Vertigo and light-headedness often form part of the clinical picture, sometimes alone, but usually in association with other subjective phenomena.

2. CARDIOVASCULAR SYSTEM

Coronary atheroma of variable degree is common in the elderly. Usually anaemia merely acts as a superimposed factor, though sometimes the heart appears basically healthy.

Dyspnoea occurs, but is not complained of as often as one would expect in this age-group. It is only when mobility is severely restricted because of the dyspnoea that the symptom is usually mentioned. Even then it may be ascribed to ageing. Those with normal mobility soon notice the difference if the anaemia is of rapid onset, but when the development is slow, as it often is, dyspnoea on exertion is less evident.

General weakness is a symptom which is clinically ill defined and difficult to separate from apathy. A complaint of general weakness often means inability or lack of desire to carry out customary activities. The patient may state that he is too weak to get out of bed in the morning, or to go for a walk, but on closer questioning may admit that he has no desire to get out of bed or that he gets too short of breath if he does.

Angina is relatively rare in the elderly and there are many pitfalls in its diagnosis. Typical histories of angina may be obtained in patients with oesophageal diverticula or gastric hernia, and anaemia is common in these conditions. Despite these difficulties, however, undeniable evidence of angina pectoris may be obtained, even at an advanced age. Iron-deficiency anaemia is sometimes present in these patients, and if so should be treated, irrespective of its degree. Improvement, as judged by diminution in the severity of the angina, is common and sometimes there is complete relief.

Palpitations may be present. Although usually of no particular significance they may be a presenting symptom of anaemia. Frequent multifocal extrasystoles, bouts of atrial fibrillation, and brief periods of paroxysmal tachycardia have been observed.

Tachycardia is often present and a ventricular rate of around 110–120 per minute is common. Response to therapy is relatively slow and it may take several weeks before the heart-rate returns to normal.

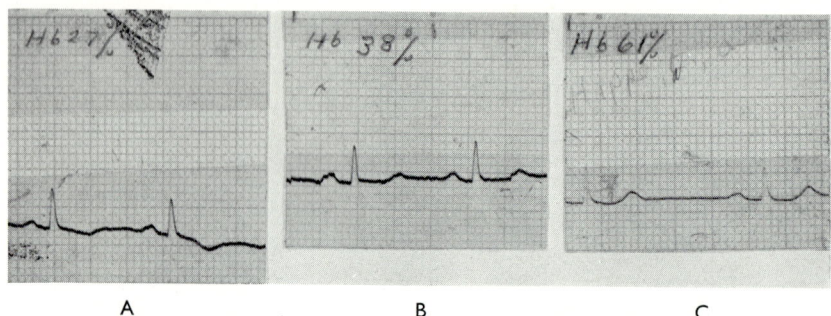

Fig. 20.—Female, 72 years old, admitted from out-patient department, complaining of headache and paraesthesiae of hands and feet. Hb, 32 per cent; serum vitamin B_{12}, 40 pg. per ml.; serum folate, 2·5 ng. per ml.; serum iron, 40 μg. per 100 ml. Next day she had melaena and Hb was 27 per cent (A). E.C.G. showed inverted T waves. Transfused with 1 pint of blood. E.C.G. next day showed upright T waves. Hb, 38 per cent (B). Treatment continued with vitamin B_{12} and iron (C).

Atrial fibrillation is another common manifestation. It is unusual for the fibrillation to disappear with iron therapy, although an associated rapid ventricular rate may respond.

A systolic murmur over the precordium may be heard when anaemia is severe. It usually disappears when the haemoglobin level reaches 50–60 per cent. Systolic murmurs are, however, common in the elderly and one should not regard a murmur as 'haemic' in origin unless it disappears when the anaemia is corrected. Atherosclerosis of the aorta, aortic stenosis, and rheumatic valvular diseases are common causes of murmurs and when anaemia is present the loudness is accentuated.

Generalized cardiac enlargement may be detected, but if considerable another cause should be suspected, including bacterial endocarditis.

Congestive cardiac failure is a frequent manifestation. A low haemoglobin may be attributed to haemodilution, when in fact anaemia is present. Severe anaemia is accepted as a primary cause or as a precipitating cause of congestive failure, but a mild degree may be neglected.

In a series of 50 consecutive admissions with congestive cardiac failure a haemoglobin level of 80 per cent or below was obtained in 21 (42 per cent), 70 per cent or below in 12 (25 per cent), and 60 per cent or below in 6 (12 per cent). The lowest level was in a female of 82 in whom the haemoglobin was 37 per cent due to iron and folate deficiency. It reached 86 per cent with appropriate therapy. Twenty-nine patients had a haemoglobin level of 81 per cent or above, and of these 12 were above 100 per cent, the highest being 120 per cent. Only 2 patients gave a history of previous blood-loss and in both the haemoglobin was within the accepted normal limits.

Left ventricular failure and pulmonary oedema may also be caused or aggravated by anaemia. The patient may be in an acute attack of failure when first seen. Recovery is often incomplete, but there are many exceptions.

Electrocardiographic changes due to anaemia are often present, but sometimes a haemoglobin as low as 40 per cent is unaccompanied by any alteration, while in others changes may be present when anaemia is minimal (*Fig.* 20).

The most common abnormality is flattening of the T wave, but others also occur, such as inversion of the T wave and elevation or depression of the ST segment. Convincing evidence of conduction defects has not been obtained.

These changes may suggest ischaemia and be wrongly interpreted as contraindicating surgery.

3. Respiratory System

Dyspnoea may be due to cardiac or respiratory embarrassment. Hypoxia often results in an elevated haemoglobin and an increase in red-cell count, so that a patient with chronic pulmonary disease and a haemoglobin of 90 per cent may be 'anaemic'. Elevation of the haemoglobin to well above 100 per cent may follow iron therapy. Frequently the patient improves and dyspnoea diminishes.

4. Renal System

Azotaemia may diminish when anaemia is treated. Lowered renal reserve, possibly due to atherosclerosis of the renal arteries or chronic pyelonephritis, is often present, and when anaemia is superimposed renal failure may result. A blood-urea as high as 250 mg. per 100 ml. may be consistent with recovery when anaemia is corrected. In others there is no response.

Sideropenia is common when the blood-urea is elevated. Measurement in a series of 298 patients (125 males and 173 females) gave the following results:—

Fifty-two patients (19 male and 33 female) had a blood-urea of 60 mg. per 100 ml. or above. In these 46 had a serum iron of 70 μg. per 100 ml. or below and only 6 above; whereas of 246 patients with blood-urea below 60 mg. per 100 ml. the relative numbers were 150 and 96.

5. Skin

Pallor of the skin may be noted, and in severe iron-deficiency anaemia there may be slight subcutaneous oedema, suggestive of water retention.

Coldness of the trunk and the extremities combined with slight puffiness of the face may superficially resemble myxoedema.

Bruising, arising spontaneously or from minimal trauma, is sometimes seen.

When a dermatological disease is present there may be superadded iron deficiency from malabsorption or desquamation. In these the serum iron is low and the binding capacity raised, but sideropenia can occur with a decreased binding capacity—as in classic chronic infection (Marks and Shuster, 1968).

6. Intestine

Mild steatorrhoea may be present as a result of the anaemia.

Iron Deficiency without Anaemia

Sideropenia without anaemia occurs frequently in the elderly, but there is difficulty in defining anaemia because a level within normal limits may be low for the individual concerned. If iron therapy elevates the haemoglobin a degree of anaemia was presumably present. Nevertheless, the effect of haematinic drugs is not usually ascertained when the haemoglobin level is above 80 per cent. If sideropenia persists definite anaemia may develop and progress within a few months.

Patients with sideropenia in the absence of anaemia should be investigated and treated. An underlying neoplasm may be present as was observed in a third of 21 non-anaemic patients whose serum-iron level was below 35 μg. per 100 ml.

Following iron therapy there is often a reduction of fatigue, lassitude, general weakness, and irritability. Occasionally the mental faculties improve. The patient feels better, although another disease may still be present.

TREATMENT

The treatment of uncomplicated iron-deficiency anaemia is as satisfactory in the elderly as it is in younger patients, unless there is continuing blood-loss, additional haematinic deficiencies, hypoplastic marrow, renal failure, or an underlying disease, such as a neoplasm or infection. Care is necessary to ensure that the prescribed treatment is being followed.

Iron therapy often leads to subjective improvement before a haemoglobin response is noted. The reticulocyte count may increase from the fifth to the seventh day, reaching a figure as high as 20 per cent (of R.B.C.) by the tenth day or so. Thereafter, the haemoglobin level rises progressively until normality is reached. The rapidity of the increase is related to the degree of the anaemia, being highest when the anaemia is severe, although occasionally the haemoglobin level does not change appreciably until about the third week. Presumably in these patients the marrow is less active initially, or the stores require more iron. When judging the efficacy of treatment reliance should be placed on improvement in the haemoglobin level rather than on the extent of the reticulocyte response.

When a patient with iron-deficiency anaemia in this age-group is treated, the levels of vitamin B_{12} and folate should ideally be assessed, even though the blood-film shows hypochromia. A poor response indicates the presence of a complicating factor, but serious disease may still be present when the response is satisfactory. No patient is too ill for treatment and in severe cases urgent therapy is required, as rapid deterioration leading to death may occur unexpectedly.

1. Oral Therapy

The administration of iron salts by mouth in sufficient dosage is the standby of therapy. Other routes become necessary only when the patient cannot tolerate the dosage prescribed, or is too ill to allow an interval of 2 weeks or so to elapse before improvement occurs.

The ferrous salt is absorbed three to seven times as readily as its ferric counterpart (Brise and Hallberg, 1962). Approximately 200 mg. a day of elemental iron are necessary, but it is sometimes preferable to commence with 100 mg. a day and then gradually increase the dose. The same quantity is necessary for mild anaemia as for severe anaemia. The salt should be taken between or before meals, because

Brise (1962) showed that absorption was reduced by half when it was given half an hour after a light meal, and by 30–60 per cent when given with meals. However, when troublesome gastro-intestinal side-effects are produced it is justifiable to do otherwise provided the dose is increased in order to compensate for the diminished absorption.

Many products contain insufficient iron and should be avoided. Their reduced side-effects are almost certainly due to this. Some patients can tolerate more than 250 mg. a day and there is no reason why it should not be given, provided the quantity is not continued indefinitely.

IRON PREPARATIONS

Ferrous Sulphate has stood the test of time and is the standard by which other preparations are measured. It is also the least expensive and contains 30 per cent of elemental iron. The usual dose is 200 mg. three times a day.

Ferrous Gluconate is reputed to be less irritant to the gastro-intestinal tract than ferrous sulphate. There is no definite evidence to substantiate this when the same amount of elemental iron is given. Its efficacy is similar. An average dose is 5 tablets daily, each tablet containing 36 mg. of iron.

Ferrous Fumarate.—The average dose is 3–4 daily of the 0·2-g. tablets, each containing 65 mg. of iron. It is claimed that tests for occult blood in the stools may be strongly positive when benzidine or orthotoluidine is used. Its superiority over ferrous sulphate has not been proven.

Ferrous Carbonate contains 25 mg. of elemental iron per tablet of 300 mg. Eight tablets a day are therefore necessary. Its solubility is low.

Ferrous Succinate.—This preparation has no practical advantage over ferrous sulphate, although its absorbability is a little more (Brise and Hallberg, 1962).

Ferrous Calcium Citrate.—Each tablet contains 25 mg. of elemental iron and absorption appears to be less than with ferrous sulphate.

Ferrous Hydroxide.—Sixty milligrams of elemental iron are contained in each capsule, but absorption is poor.

Ferroglycine Sulphate.—This is available in 250-mg. tablets (40 mg. elemental iron). Early claims of a marked diminution in side-effects have not been confirmed.

Iron with Other Haematinics.—These cannot be recommended. A better approach is to estimate the serum iron, vitamin B_{12}, and folate and in severely anaemic patients to prescribe all three separately, in adequate amounts. The inappropriate haematinic or haematinics can be discontinued when the serum level is known.

Prolonged-release Iron Preparations.—These were developed to combat gastric symptoms by not releasing iron until the lower intestine had been reached, but, as the main site of absorption is therefore by-passed, rapid, reliable, and adequate iron absorption cannot be guaranteed. However, Israëls and Cook (1965) suggested that a daily tablet of Ferro-Gradumet (a slow-release ferrous sulphate preparation containing 105 mg. of iron) was as effective as 1 tablet three times a day of ferrous sulphate (180 mg. of iron) taken after meals, but Callender (1969) found that 100 mg. of iron in the form of ferrous fumarate as a single morning dose gave comparable results and was not associated with a higher incidence of side-effects. She stated that 'the idea of being able to treat patients with a single daily dose is attractive, but it would appear from the present data that no specific benefit is to be derived by using a slow release preparation'.

Adjuvant Substances

Ascorbic acid increases the absorption of iron. Brise and Hallberg (1962) produced evidence that iron absorption was enhanced when 200 mg. of vitamin C a day were given, and that the benefit was more marked when the dose was increased. They felt that this was due to its reducing action. Despite this effect vitamin C supplementation is seldom valuable in the treatment of resistant iron-deficiency anaemia. Deficiency of the vitamin, however, is common, and the giving of ascorbic acid for this, in a dosage of 100–200 mg. a day, is logical.

Cobalt salts have been reported as giving encouraging results in the treatment of refractory anaemias, but their toxicity is a major obstacle. Hyperglycaemia, weight-loss, anorexia, nausea, vomiting, and enlargement of the thyroid can occur, particularly when the daily dose exceeds 100 mg. of cobalt chloride. Cobalt alone does not appear to possess a definite anti-anaemic effect, and it was suggested by Geill (1969) that it probably stimulated the liberation of erythropoietin from the kidneys, which could then act if the marrow contained sufficient iron. He treated 107 persons (ranging in age from 70 to 97 years, all of whom had an anaemia refractory to simple iron medication) with tablets of cobalt chloride (20 mg.) combined with ferrous tartrate (250 mg.). Three tablets were taken daily, together with ascorbic acid (300–450 mg. per day). A good response was obtained in 99 patients despite the fact that the majority were suffering from various degrees of chronic pyelonephritis. Increase in serum-iron levels was greater than when iron alone was administered, although in most instances the effect was sluggish, probably due to underlying infection.

Succinic acid has an enhancing effect on iron absorption when the iron is in a liquid preparation, but is less definite when the iron is in tablet form, although Hallberg and Sölvell (1966) considered that the enhancing effect was still present when ferrous sulphate was given.

Copper has no place in therapy other than as a trace substance and *arsenic* has outlived its popularity and usefulness.

Side-effects

Side-effects occur in about 30 per cent but usually they are mild and transient. In the General Practitioner Clinical Trials (1966) constipation was noted in 5 per cent with Sidros—ferrous gluconate 300 mg. + ascorbic acid 30 mg.—and in 18 per cent with ferrous gluconate alone. Vague headache, 'muzziness', nausea, vomiting, a bloated feeling in the abdomen, anorexia, diarrhoea, and cramps may develop. Severe headaches, persistent vomiting, and troublesome diarrhoea are distinctly rare, unless the patient is subject to frequent headaches or has a gastro-intestinal disturbance before therapy commenced. Changing to another oral preparation containing the same amount of elemental iron has no advantage. Assessment is difficult when the quantity is reduced. Elevation of a low haemoglobin can still be satisfactory in the early stages, although absorption may be insufficient for normality to be reached and for the iron stores to be replenished. The fact that iron absorption decreases as the haemoglobin rises is not sufficiently recognized.

Intramuscular Therapy

Parenteral therapy should be given when patients are unable to tolerate or unwilling to take adequate doses orally, or when malabsorption is present.

Occasionally anaemia, shown to be resistant to oral iron, in patients with chronic infection or rheumatoid arthritis responds, temporarily at least, to intramuscular (or intravenous) iron therapy—even when there is no evidence of impaired absorption.

The preparations most commonly used in this country are Jectofer and Imferon.

Jectofer.—The iron is present as a sterile solution of an iron–sorbitol–citric acid complex with dextrin as a stabilizer, each millilitre containing 50 mg. of elemental iron. About 70 per cent of an injected dose is absorbed within 3 hours and approximately 30 per cent is excreted in the urine. An intramuscular injection, in a dose corresponding to 100 mg. iron, elevates the haemoglobin approximately 0·39 g. per 100 ml., which is about 40 per cent less than that produced when a similar quantity is given intravenously. According to Anderson (1961) 60 per cent of the iron is utilized in haemoglobin synthesis.

Imferon.—This contains 50 mg. of elemental iron per millilitre, in the form of ferric hydroxide combined with a low molecular weight dextran. The complex is transported by the lymphatics and enters the reticulo-endothelial system where it is broken down and the iron released. The same product, when diluted, can be given intravenously, either in divided doses or as a total dose infusion.

Calculation of the quantity necessary is based on the haemoglobin percentage deficit and the weight of the patient in pounds. Various amounts can be given intramuscularly, but our usual method is to inject 2–4 ml. daily or on alternate days until the calculated iron dose is given.

Staining of the skin is not troublesome when the injection is given deeply and rubbing omitted. Sarcomatous lesions, such as occurred with relatively large quantities in mice, have not been recorded in man.

Rees and Coles (1969) suggested that caution was necessary when uraemic patients were treated, for fear the iron dextran acted as a 'challenger' and precipitated soft-tissue calcification in those who might be sensitized by high serum parathyroid hormone levels.

Intravenous Therapy

Intravenous therapy with *saccharated iron oxide* (Ferrivenin) has been used occasionally in our patients, but not during the past 2 years. After a test dose of 50 mg. the required amount of elemental iron is given in divided doses over the ensuing 7–10 days, no more than 200 mg. of elemental iron in a 1 per cent solution being given on any one occasion. The calculated amount required takes into consideration the quantity necessary for replenishing the body stores as well as that for the haemoglobin mass. The total iron in the haemoglobin is taken to be 2·5 g. This figure is multiplied by the per cent haemoglobin deficit and 1·2 g. of iron is added as replacement for the body stores.

Severe pain results if the preparation leaks into the surrounding tissue; thrombophlebitis has occurred and also painful venous spasm. Headache, vomiting, tachycardia, fever, and abdominal cramp have occasionally developed, usually soon after the injection, but sometimes a few hours later. Pain in the extremities, lumbar region, and chest are recorded, and deaths have been described.

The response is comparable to that obtained by the intramuscular route, but the complications are more numerous and troublesome.

Iron-dextrin in a preparation known as Astrafer may also be given. This is a high molecular weight iron-carbohydrate complex, containing 20 mg. per ml., in isotonic solution with a pH of 7·3. It is purported to be stable in saline and plasma. The iron is trivalent. It differs from iron-dextran (Imferon) in having a lower molecular weight carbohydrate-dextrin as protective carrier for the colloidal ferric hydroxide. Fielding (1961) obtained a satisfactory haemoglobin response in 49 of 51 anaemic patients, between 19 and 40 years of age, with doses of 100 mg. given daily or on alternate days. Clinical toxicity was infrequent and mild, and no instance of thrombophlebitis was seen.

Total Dose Infusion with Iron-dextran (Imferon)

The preparation has a pH of 5·2–6·5, is isotonic with tissue fluids, and is less toxic than ferrous sulphate. The quantity of free ionic iron is very small. Fifty milligrams of elemental iron are present per ml.

The amount necessary is based on the following formula:—

$$\text{Total iron required} = 0\cdot 3WD,$$

where W = body-weight in pounds and D = haemoglobin percentage deficit.

The required dose is then given in normal saline at 45–60 drops per minute. The concentration should not exceed 5 per cent, and the flow is regulated to 10 drops per minute for the first 10 minutes, this being regarded as a test dose. If nothing untoward happens the drip is quickened. The method is valuable because treatment can be given in out-patients without the need for repeated attendances, and in selected cases it can replace blood transfusion. Another advantage is that the body stores are replenished. The procedure is reasonably safe in the elderly, but is not widely used at present.

Andrews, Fairley, and Barker (1967) treated 22 elderly in-patients and 21 elderly day-hospital patients. They noted that there was a linear haemoglobin response directly related to the severity of the anaemia. There were no serious side-effects and they concluded that 'total dose infusion is an effective method of administering iron to elderly patients in those cases where oral or intramuscular iron is considered to be less suitable and/or a rapid response is required'.

Reactions are uncommon and consist mainly of vomiting, arthralgia, headache, fever, and rashes. Severe reactions of the anaphylactoid type have occurred and circulatory collapse has been described, but the incidence is estimated to be less than 0·5 per cent. Wright (1967) noted the following side-effects in 68 patients ranging in age from 65 to 90 years: slight breathlessness in 1; restlessness in 2, which responded to reassurance; and local phlebitis in 5. None of the other patients had any local or general symptoms that could be related to the treatment.

Duration of Therapy

The haemoglobin usually returns to normal in 6–8 weeks depending on its original level but may take considerably longer. Among 58 patients over the age of 60 in the General Practitioner Clinical Trials (1966) the rise in haemoglobin varied from 7 to 13 per cent in a mean time of 4 weeks. Oral therapy should be continued in the same dosage for another year to replenish the body stores.

When iron is given intramuscularly or intravenously the theoretical quantity necessary for the body stores is included in the calculation.

Whenever possible, the patients should be followed up at 4–6-monthly intervals and the haemoglobin checked. Relapse requires suitable therapy, but the development of disease may be insidious and it is unwise to give repeated courses of intramuscular iron without further investigation. Moreover, the development of anaemia in a treated iron-deficient patient is often due to folate or vitamin-B_{12} deficiency.

Blood Transfusion

Recourse to blood transfusion is seldom necessary unless the patient has had a severe haemorrhage. Increasing the blood-volume is a more serious hazard in the elderly than in younger patients, because the elderly are normally relatively dehydrated. Their cardiac reserve may be overwhelmed, resulting in pulmonary oedema. Cerebral oedema may also develop. Nevertheless, in practice, slow transfusion of packed red cells may be life-saving and in others accelerate recovery. Each case has to be considered on its merits and due consideration given to the expected benefit and the possible danger. The giving of blood merely to diminish the patient's stay in hospital is not clinically justifiable.

We have occasionally transfused patients when the following features have predominated:—

1. Acute left ventricular failure associated with a haemoglobin level below 50 per cent, when the anaemia is considered to be the primary cause. Severe congestive failure is similarly assessed. Bedford and Caird (1960) discussing blood transfusion in patients with heart failure and anaemia wrote, 'packed red cells given slowly (e.g., cells from 1 litre in 6–8 hours) are extremely well tolerated ... and may need to be repeated every 1–3 days until a haemoglobin concentration of 10 g. per 100 ml. is reached'.

2. Mental confusion of recent origin when no cause can be implicated other than the anaemia. We have felt that a haemoglobin below 50 per cent sometimes merits this approach.

3. When the anaemia is not responding satisfactorily to adequate therapy. Investigation of blood-loss, marrow content, and renal function is imperative, but detailed study of the alimentary tract may be necessary and this is often tedious and difficult in the ill elderly. Indeed, it is essential sometimes to transfuse patients before adequate gastro-intestinal radiology becomes possible. The reason for the poor haemoglobin response may be blood-loss from a carcinoma of the colon.

4. The preparation of an anaemic patient for surgery requires blood transfusion, if delay is undesirable.

Packed red cells are given, except after haemorrhage when whole blood is transfused. One litre of blood contains 500 mg. of elemental iron. The rate of transfusion must be slow and sometimes it is necessary, if the patient is very ill, to give small quantities, such as 4 oz. (112 ml.) on three or four separate occasions.

Iron therapy should also be administered. We usually continue with intramuscular iron as the patients requiring blood transfusion are too ill for risks to be taken regarding possible malabsorption.

Proprietary Preparations

A large number of proprietary preparations have become available and the compiling of a complete list would be a formidable task. Those fairly commonly prescribed are given in *Table XVII*:—

Table XVII.—Proprietary Iron Preparations

Official Preparation	Proprietary Preparation	Elemental Iron	Folic Acid	Vitamin B₁	Vitamin C	Vitamin A
Ferri et ammon. cit.		600 mg. per 3 g.				
Ferrous gluconate	Fergon	35 mg. per 300 mg.				
	Ferlucon	29 mg. per 250 mg.		+		
	Folex	35 mg. per 300 mg.	+			
	Gluferate	35 mg. per 300 mg.			+	
	Sidros	35 mg. per 300 mg.			+	
Ferrous sulphate		60 mg. per 200 mg.				
	Fefol } slow	45 mg. per 150 mg.	+			
	Feospan } release	45 mg. per 150 mg.		+		
	Ferraplex	46 mg. per 167 mg.		+	+	
	Ferrograd	105 mg. per 350 mg.				
	Ferro-Redoxon	30 mg. per 120 mg.			+	
	Pregfol	60 mg. per 200 mg.	+			
	Pregnavite	60 mg. per 200 mg.		+	+	+
Ferrous fumarate		65 mg. per 200 mg.				
	Ferro-Mandets	20 mg. per 61 mg.			+	
	Fersamal	65 mg. per 200 mg.				
	Pregamal	65 mg. per 200 mg.	+			
Ferrous aminoates	Ferroids	35 mg. per 350 mg.		+		
	Folaemin	35 mg. per 350 mg.	+			
Ferrous carbonate		450 mg. per 29 g.				
Ferrous succinate	Ferromyn	37 mg. per 150 mg.				
Ferrous tartrate		70 mg. per 250 mg.				
Iron dextran	Imferon	50 mg. per ml.				
Iron dextrin injection	Astrafer	20 mg. per ml.				
Saccharated iron oxide injection	Colliron	20 mg. per ml.				
	Ferrivenin	20 mg. per ml.				
Iron sorbitol injection	Jectofer	50 mg. per ml.				
Sodium ironedetate	Sytron (children)	27·5 mg. per ml.				
Ferrous calcium citrate	Rarical	25 mg. per tablet	+			

REFERENCES

Anderson, N. S. E. (1961), *Br. med. J.*, **1**, 275.
Andrews, J., Fairley, A., and Barker, R. (1967), *Scott. med. J.*, **12**, 208.
Bainton, D. F., and Finch, C. A. (1964), *Am. J. Med.*, **37**, 62.
Balcerzak, S. P., Vester, J. W., and Doyle, A. P. (1966), *J. Lab. clin. Med.*, **67**, 742.
Beard, M. E. J., and Weintraub, L. R. (1969), *Br. J. Haemat.*, **16**, 161.
Bedford, P. D., and Caird, F. I. (1960), *Valvular Disease of the Heart in Old Age*. London: Churchill.
Beutler, E. (1959), *Acta haemat.*, **21**, 371.
Bothwell, T. H., and Finch, C. A. (1962), *Iron Metabolism*. Boston: Little, Brown.
Brise, H. (1962), *Acta med scand.*, **171**, Suppl. 376.
— and Hallberg, L. (1962), *Ibid.*, **171**, Suppl. 376.
Callender, S. T. (1969), *Br. med. J.*, **4**, 531.
Dagg, J. H., Goldberg, A., Gibbs, W. N., and Anderson, J. R. (1966), *Ibid.*, **2**, 619.
— — Jackson, J. M., Curry, B., and Goldberg, A. (1966), *Br. J. Haemat.*, **12**, 331.
Dawson, A. A., Ogston, D., and Fullerton, H. W. (1969), *Br. med. J.*, **3**, 436.
Delamore, I. W., and Shearman, D. J. C. (1965), *Lancet*, **1**, 889.
Fielding, J. (1961), *Br. med. J.*, **2**, 279.
— — (1965), *J. clin. Path.*, **18**, 88.
— — O'Shaughnessy, M. C., and Brumström, G. M. (1965), *Lancet*, **2**, 9.
Geill, T. (1969), *Geront. clin.*, **11**, 48.
General Practitioner Clinical Trials (1966), *The Practitioner*, **197**, 233.
Hallberg, L., and Sölvell, L. (1966), *Acta med. scand.*, Suppl. 459, 23.
Israëls, M. C. G., and Cook, T. A. (1965), *Lancet*, **2**, 654.
Jacobs, A. (1961), *Ibid.*, **2**, 1331.
— and Cavill, I. (1968), *Br. J. Haemat.*, **14**, 291.
— and Greenman, D. A. (1969), *Br. med. J.*, **1**, 673.
— and Kilpatrick, G. S. (1964), *Ibid.*, **2**, 79.
— and Miles, P. M. (1969a), *Gut*, **10**, 3.
— — — — (1969b), *Br. med. J.*, **4**, 778.
Jordan, A., and Podmore, D. A. (1963), Broadsheet No. 46. Assoc. of Clin. Pathologists.
Katz, J. H., and Jandl, J. H. (1964), *Iron Metabolism* (Ed. Gross, F., Naegeli, S. R., and Philps, H. D.). Berlin: Springer-Verlag.
Kay, A. W. (1962), *Br. med. J.*, **2**, 1709.
Lees, F., and Rosenthal, F. D. (1958), *Q. Jl Med.*, **28**, 19.
Lunn, J. A., Richmond, J., Simpson, J. D., Leask, J. D., and Tothill, P. (1967), *Br. med. J.*, **3**, 331.
McFarlane, D. B., Pinkerton, P. H., Dagg, J. H., and Goldberg, A. (1967), *Br. J. Haemat.*, **13**, 790.
Marks, J., and Shuster, S. (1968), *Arch. Derm.*, **98**, 469.
Meulengracht, F. (1932), *Acta med. scand.*, **78**, 387.
Powell, D. E. B., and Thomas, J. H. (1969), *Geront. clin.*, **11**, 36.
— — — — and Mills, P. (1968), *Ibid.*, **10**, 21.
Rath, C. E., and Finch, C. A. (1948), *J. Lab. clin. Med.*, **33**, 81.
Rees, J. K. H., and Coles, G. A. (1969), *Br. med. J.*, **2**, 670.
Ross, G., Gray, C. H., de Silva, S., and Newman, J. (1964), *Ibid.*, **1**, 1351.
Signy, A. G., and Smith, D. R. (1966), Broadsheet No. 53. Assoc. of Clin. Pathologists.
Tudhope, G. R. (1967), *Clin. Sci.*, **33**, 165.
Wangel, A. G., Callender, S. T., Spray, G. H., and Wright, R. (1968), *Br. J. Haemat.*, **14**, 161.
Witts, L. J. (1956), *Anaemia and the Alimentary Tract*. R. Coll. of Phys. Ed. Publication, No. 7.
Wright, W. B. (1967), *Geront. clin.*, **9**, 107.
Young, D. S., and Hicks, J. C. (1965), *J. clin. Path.*, **18**, 98.

4

MEGALOBLASTIC ANAEMIAS

Vitamin-B_{12} Deficiency
  Pernicious anaemia.
  Nutritional. Veganism.
  'Refractory'.

Folate Deficiency
  Nutritional.
  Drugs.
  Chronic liver disease.
  'Refractory'.

Mixed Vitamin-B_{12} and Folate Deficiency
  Nutritional.
  Gastro-intestinal disease.—
    Carcinoma.
    Blind loop.
    Intestinal fistula and stricture.
  Malabsorption. Steatorrhoea.

Other Deficiencies
  Vitamin C. Pyridoxine.

Sideroblastic

VITAMIN-B_{12} METABOLISM

Vitamin B_{12} has a molecular weight of approximately 1357. It consists of a modified porphyrin ring which is linked to the ribonucleoside of 5,6-dimethylbenzimidazole by a phosphate-ester bond. A cobalt atom occupies the central position in the porphyrin ring, corresponding to that occupied by iron in haem. One of the remaining two cobalt valencies is linked to the imidazole ring, and the other link determines the various forms, such as —CN in cyanocobalamin; —OH in hydroxocobalamin, and —NO_2 in nitrocobalamin. All these forms have anti-pernicious anaemia activity. The active form of vitamin B_{12} in the body may be the coenzyme, deoxyadenozyl B_{12} in which 5′-deoxyribose is attached to the cobalt valency (*Fig. 21*).

Intake and Absorption of Vitamin B_{12}

It is present in liver, kidney, milk, eggs, and muscle tissue. The minimal adult daily requirement is 0·6–1·2 μg. It is not found in higher plants, but is synthesized by bacteria and fungi. Although produced in this way in the human colon it is doubtful whether a significant quantity is absorbed. Animals, such as rabbits, on a vitamin-B_{12}-deficient diet do not develop deficiency states if they are allowed to eat their faeces.

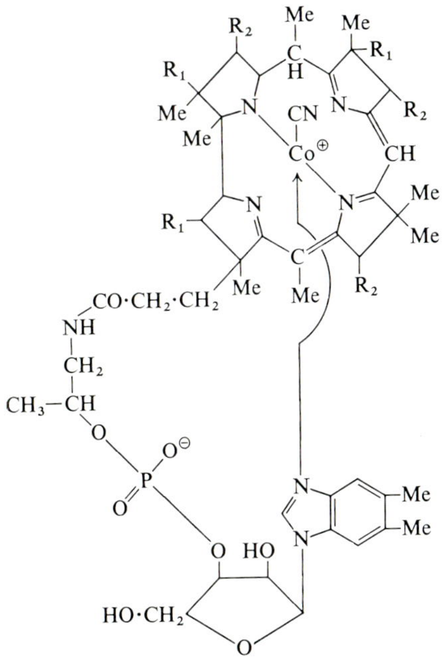

Fig. 21.—Vitamin-B_{12} (cyanocobalamin) molecule. Me = CH_3; R_1 = $NH_2.CO.CH_2$; R_2 = $NH_2.CO.CH_2.CH_2$.

Although the daily adult requirement is approximately only 1 μg. of vitamin B_{12}, gastric intrinsic factor is essential for its absorption, but if present in excessive amounts absorption is not significantly increased. A large unphysiological dose of vitamin B_{12} administered orally is absorbed by mass action independently of the presence of intrinsic factor.

Intrinsic Factor

Intrinsic factor may be a mucoprotein with a molecular weight of approximately 600,000. It is non-dialysable, thermolabile, and inactivated by pepsin. In man, secretion is by the parietal or chief cells of the fundus and body of the stomach, which can be stimulated by histamine or gastrin. Normally far more is present than is essential. One milligram of intrinsic factor binds 25 μg. of vitamin B_{12} (Chanarin, 1968). Impaired absorption of vitamin B_{12} does not occur until the intrinsic factor is nearly 99 per cent depleted. There is a close correlation between acid and intrinsic factor secretion (Irvine, Davies, Haynes, and Scarth, 1965)—possibly because both are produced by the gastric parietal cells. This becomes of great significance in the elderly where the secretory ability for both declines.

The existence of intrinsic factor has been deduced from its ability to promote the absorption of extrinsic factor (vitamin B_{12}). They are bound by a specific and a non-specific mechanism, and the latter can be completely inhibited by anti-intrinsic factor antibody. Hydrochloric acid facilitates the binding of vitamin B_{12} and intrinsic factor. Together they form a complex which reaches the mucosal cells of the ileum where absorption takes place (Booth and Mollin, 1959). It appears that vitamin B_{12} is released from the complex at the mucosal cell surface, where a 'releasing factor' may be operative (Hippe, 1966). This is suggested by the occurrence of vitamin-B_{12} deficiency states in the presence of adequate intake and intrinsic factor. Food may affect vitamin-B_{12} absorption. Deller, Germar, and Witts (1961) found that absorption of oral vitamin B_{12} after partial gastrectomy was much enhanced when food was given, although they did not find this in normal subjects, or in those with pernicious anaemia. The released intrinsic factor probably enters the villus cells, but its fate thereafter is not known.

After absorption, vitamin B_{12} is bound to plasma proteins. Endogenous vitamin B_{12} is bound to an alpha-1-globulin (transcobalamin I), but vitamin B_{12} added to serum *in vitro* binds with beta-globulin (transcobalamin II). Herbert (1968) suggested that the vitamin B_{12}-binding betaglobulin functioned as a transport protein, whereas the alpha-1-globulin conserved the vitamin B_{12} and was normally almost saturated with it. In vitamin-B_{12} deficiency, where the alpha-1-globulin is relatively unsaturated, administered vitamin B_{12} is taken up by the alpha-1-globulin which delivers it slowly to the tissues. Vitamin B_{12} is therefore cleared more slowly from the blood-stream when there is depletion of the body stores. The total vitamin-B_{12} binding capacity is normally one-third saturated. The percentage saturation falls and the total binding capacity tends to rise in vitamin-B_{12} deficiency. Previous reports of an extragastric intrinsic factor promoting tissue uptake of vitamin B_{12} are probably explained by variations in the vitamin-B_{12} binding of globulin fractions.

The liver contains 0·5–1·2 μg. per g., and holds most of the reserve vitamin B_{12} which is normally 1000–2000 μg. (Girdwood, 1952).

Vitamin B_{12} is excreted in the bile, but most of this is reabsorbed, there being a closed enterohepatic circulation. Adams and Boddy (1968) have used whole-body monitoring techniques to estimate the daily loss of cobalamins. The daily loss in healthy individuals and in vitamin-B_{12} deficient patients was found to be 0·1–0·2 per cent of the administered dose of ^{58}Co-cyanocobalamin. Three out of 5 patients with renal or hepatic disease showed increased loss. In general, urinary excretion is not increased unless the serum level is greatly elevated. This suggests that the circulating protein–vitamin-B_{12} complex is fairly stable (Retief and Huskisson, 1969).

Liver disease, renal failure, and chronic myeloid leukaemia are associated with raised serum vitamin-B_{12} levels. Acute viral hepatitis gives rise to a raised level with a diminished unsaturated vitamin-B_{12} binding capacity, in contrast with cirrhosis where the latter is also raised. In chronic myeloid leukaemia the vitamin-B_{12} level and binding capacity may both be markedly increased.

PERNICIOUS ANAEMIA

Laboratory and Diagnostic Features

The clinical and laboratory findings in pernicious anaemia do not bear a strict relationship to the severity of the depletion as measured by serum vitamin-B_{12} levels or its malabsorption. The diagnosis differs from that of iron deficiency in that it is not quantitative. Serum vitamin-B_{12} levels and impaired vitamin-B_{12} absorption show an inconstant relationship to the severity of the clinical features and the degree of anaemia.

Blood-picture

Red Blood-cells and Haemoglobin.—When anaemia is present the fall in the number of red cells is disproportionately greater than the fall in haemoglobin. The haemoglobin concentration of each red cell remains normal (unless there is associated iron deficiency), although the haemoglobin content is raised because of the increase in erythrocyte volume. The increased mean corpuscular volume is probably the most valuable of the various red-cell indices.

Typical red-cell indices in established pernicious anaemia are:—

	Normal	Pernicious Anaemia
Mean corpuscular volume (M.C.V.)	75–95 c.μ	110 c.μ <
Mean cell haemoglobin (M.C.H.)	27–32 μg.	35–50 μg.
Mean cell haemoglobin concentration (M.C.H.C.)	32–36 per cent	32–36 per cent unless iron deficient

Visual counting of red cells is a tedious and relatively inaccurate procedure and as a result had fallen largely into disuse in many routine laboratories, but with the introduction of electronic cell counters the position has changed. The red-cell count and M.C.V. can be useful measurements particularly when the anaemia is slight and the blood-film difficult to interpret. Nevertheless, examination of the stained blood-film remains essential. The degree of macrocytosis, anisocytosis, and poikilocytosis can be assessed visually. Hypochromia will also be detected. Fragmented and spherocytic cells will suggest significant haemolysis. Nucleated red blood-cells and Howell-Jolly bodies may be seen. Examination of a blood-film will help in differentiating from other causes of macrocytosis—as, for example, the numerous polychromatic macrocytes seen in the regenerative phase after haemorrhage or haemolysis.

White Blood-cells.—The total white-cell count is usually reduced and values are often in the range 2000–3000 per c.mm. This is associated with a true neutropenia and relative lymphocytosis. Examination of the stained blood-film may show large hypersegmented neutrophils even when anaemia is minimal, although this may also be found in uncomplicated iron deficiency (Beard and Weintraub, 1969). Eosinophilia has been reported.

Platelets.—Significant thrombocytopenia may be a pronounced feature, with values well below 100,000 per c.mm. Giant abnormal platelet forms may be seen in the film. Values below 50,000 per c.mm. can be associated with purpura and a prolonged bleeding time.

Buffy Coat.—The leucocyte-rich layer of a centrifuged sample of blood helps in the examination of cases where bone-marrow aspiration is not possible. The neutrophil changes are more readily seen and nucleated red blood-cells may be identified as late megaloblasts.

BONE-MARROW

The bone cortex is thin and soft and the marrow highly cellular. The red-cell series forms up to 50 per cent of the cells present. In the absence of anaemia bone-marrow examination does not help in the diagnosis of latent pernicious anaemia. When mild anaemia is present macropolycytes and giant metamyelocytes may be noted. The degree of megaloblastosis observed is usually approximately proportional to the severity of the anaemia—all stages of megaloblastic erythropoiesis can be seen in untreated severely anaemic patients (*Fig.* 22). Abnormal megakaryocytes and an increased number of reticulum cells may be seen.

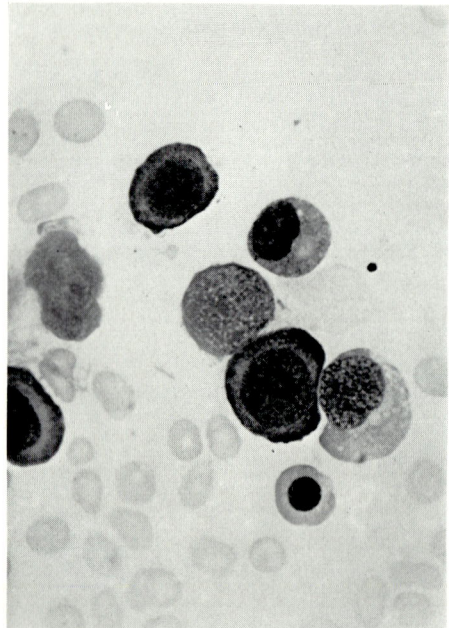

Fig. 22.—Megaloblasts in the marrow of a woman aged 86 years, Hb 39 per cent and typical macrocytic peripheral blood picture. ($\times$1100.)

Marrow smears should always be stained for iron and sections of the aspirate cut and similarly treated. Concomitant iron deficiency is common in the elderly, otherwise an excess of stainable iron can be seen.

GASTRIC ACID SECRETION

Diagnex Blue.—A carboxylic cation-exchange resin is reacted with azure A to form Diagnex Blue (Squibb) which is given orally. In the presence of free gastric hydrochloric acid the azure A is released, absorbed, and excreted in the urine. The colour is compared with that of a control. Caffeine sodium benzoate (500 mg.) is given 1 hour before the Diagnex Blue as a stimulant to gastric acid secretion.

The test is not designed for quantitative evaluation of acid secretion and can provide only *presumptive* evidence of achlorhydria. However, it is still a valuable screening procedure, particularly in the elderly.

Gastrotest (Ortho) is a similar test where instead of azure A, 2,6-diamino-3-phenyl azopyridine is used.

Augmented Histamine Test.—Maximal histamine stimulation is required to demonstrate complete achlorhydria. The test as described by Kay (1953) uses 0·04 mg. histamine acid phosphate per kg. body-weight. The extra-gastric side effects are obviated by the use of an antihistamine. It is doubtful whether it is justified or necessary to use this test routinely in the investigation of megaloblastic anaemias in the frail elderly. The Diagnex Blue test fails to detect acid deficiency in only about 3 per cent of cases, and can also be improved if used in conjunction with stronger gastric stimulants such as histamine.

Synthetic gastrin (Peptavlon, I.C.I.) is claimed to be a much more potent stimulant of gastric secretion than histamine, but without its side-effects. The recommended subcutaneous dose is 6 μg. per kg.

A multicentre study (1969) compared the gastric-acid output in response to subcutaneous histamine (40 μg. per kg.), intravenous histamine (40 μg. per kg. per hour), subcutaneous Histalog (2 mg. per kg.), and intramuscular pentagastrin (6 μg. per kg. per hour). It was found that the 30-minute response from intramuscular pentagastrin underestimated the peak acid output by only 2·7 per cent from the mean, and therefore it was recommended that this method was reliable and acceptable to the patient.

Pepsin and rennin secretion are also impaired but testing for these is unnecessary because achlorhydria precedes the loss of these enzymes. Serum pepsinogen levels are lower in the elderly.

BIOCHEMICAL CHANGES

A large number of abnormal biochemical results have been reported in pernicious anaemia, such as increased uric acid excretion, low plasma cholesterol and alkaline phosphatase, increased methylmalonic acid excretion, and raised serum lactic dehydrogenase activity. The indirect reacting serum bilirubin and urinary urobilinogen are raised in proportion to the degree of red-cell destruction. Most of these are of no diagnostic value, but Green and Pegrum (1968) suggested that the 24-hour urinary excretion of methylmalonic acid after loading with 10 g. of valine distinguished between true vitamin deficiency and a low serum level. However, Brozović, Hoffbrand, Dimitriadou, and Mollin (1967) showed an increased excretion with borderline serum vitamin-B_{12} levels and without critical liver vitamin-B_{12} depletion.

Serum Iron.—Unless there is associated iron deficiency the serum iron is raised, giving average levels of 150–300 μg. per 100 ml. The total iron-binding capacity is normal or reduced so that very high saturation levels result. This is a useful diagnostic feature, and the finding of high saturation levels (above 50 per cent) in the presence of severe anaemia is itself highly suggestive of a megaloblastic reaction. This is particularly noteworthy in the elderly who otherwise have a much higher incidence of low serum iron and saturation levels.

Serum Folate.—Normal or raised values may be found in pernicious anaemia. However, many of these elderly patients have associated folate deficiency which is reflected in reduced serum and red-cell folate levels and a positive FIGLU test (*see* Chapter 5).

Serum Vitamin B_{12}.—The level of serum vitamin B_{12} is one of the most useful tests that can be carried out in untreated pernicious anaemia both in the latent and anaemic phases.

The normal range should be interpreted in the light of the method and laboratory carrying out the test. The three methods in common use are microbiological assays using either *Lactobacillus leichmanii* or *Euglena gracilis*, and the radioassay procedure using radioisotopically labelled vitamin B_{12}.

If levels are assayed using the *L. leichmanii* method, care should be taken to account for the possible inhibitory effect of some antibiotics. Powell, Thomas, Mandal, and Dignam (1969) showed that ampicillin was particularly important in this respect, and deceptively low levels are sometimes due to the effect of this drug. *E. gracilis* was unaffected, but the organism has the disadvantage that it cannot be used to measure the hydroxocobalamin levels. Furthermore, Lie, Ungar, and Cowling (1969) have shown that antimicrobials such as sulphonamides may suppress *Euglena* in concentrations attainable in the serum during treatment.

VITAMIN-B_{12} ABSORPTION STUDIES

A variety of tests have been described for the measurement of vitamin-B_{12} absorption. The one most commonly used is the urinary excretion test (Schilling). A $1 \cdot 0$-μg. dose of radioactive vitamin B_{12} (^{57}Co) is given in a morning drink of water after an overnight fast. At the same time 1000 μg. of non-radioactive vitamin B_{12} is given intramuscularly ('flushing dose'). Urine is collected over the ensuing 24 hours. The percentage excretion is expressed as:—

$$\frac{\text{Counts per minute in 24-hour urine}}{\text{Counts per minute of standard dose}} \times 100.$$

The normal range is over 12–15 per cent. In pernicious anaemia it is below 5 per cent. Confirmation can be obtained by repeating after giving intrinsic factor (for example 100 mg. concentrate of hog stomach or normal human gastric juice). This should result in a normal excretion level. Renal disease may give low values. The test may be difficult to control in some elderly patients when there is confusion or incontinence. If there is doubt as to the completeness of the urinary collection the urinary creatinine content (15–25 mg. per kg. per 24 hours) provides a useful check.

'Dicopac' (The Radiochemical Centre, Amersham) is based on the principle of giving one capsule containing ^{57}Co-cyanocobalamin bound to gastric juice, and another containing ^{58}Co-cyanobalamin. A flushing parenteral dose is given and the excretion of the two isotopes counted differentially (Bell, Bridges, and Nelson, 1965; Katz, Dimase, and Donaldson, 1963). This combined test saves time; complete urine collection is not so critical; it is not affected by moderate renal dysfunction; and can be used if the patient is refractory to hog intrinsic factor.

ANTIBODIES

Parietal-cell Antibody.—This can be tested for by treating cryostat sections of gastric mucosa with the patient's serum and demonstrating the fixation of gamma-globulin to the cytoplasm of the parietal cells by fluorescence. Alternatively a complement-fixation test against saline extracts of the mucosa of the body of the human stomach can be used. Both techniques give positive results in approximately 80 per cent of patients with pernicious anaemia.

This test, however, is of little diagnostic value in the elderly as other conditions which may give a positive result such as iron deficiency, thyroid disease, and diabetes mellitus are common. There is also an increased prevalence of parietal-cell antibodies in the elderly probably related to the increased incidence of gastric atrophy. It can be used as a non-specific screening test.

Intrinsic Factor Antibody.—Lack of response of pernicious anaemia to treatment with oral vitamin B_{12} and hog intrinsic factor is associated with the presence of a serum factor. Two types of intrinsic factor antibody are recognized—one blocks the attachment of vitamin B_{12} to intrinsic factor; the other binds the vitamin-B_{12}-intrinsic factor complex, preventing its absorption by the intestinal mucosa. Intrinsic factor antibody is present in over 50 per cent of patients with pernicious anaemia and is rarely found in healthy persons. The method can also be varied for the quantitative estimation of intrinsic factor in the gastric juice.

$$B_{12} + serum + gastric\ juice \longrightarrow [B_{12} - serum],$$
$$B_{12} + serum + gastric\ juice + I.F.\ antibody \longrightarrow B_{12} + serum + [gastric\ juice - I.F.].$$

Pernicious anaemia patients show an increased incidence of complement-fixing and haemagglutinating auto-antibodies to thyroid antigens.

PATHOLOGY

The chief pathological findings are seen in the gastro-intestinal tract, central nervous system, and bone-marrow.

Gastro-intestinal Tract.—The epithelium of the tongue, mouth, stomach, and intestine is atrophic. Gastric biopsy studies have shown that the secretory tubules are also atrophied, although this histological change does not always accompany deficiency of intrinsic factor. Atrophy is most severe in the upper two-thirds of the body of the stomach, leaving the pyloric antrum and duodenum histologically normal. Inflammatory changes denote atrophic gastritis, but are not invariably present in uncomplicated pernicious anaemia.

Central Nervous System.—In subacute combined degeneration the most severe lesions are found in the mid-thoracic segments of the spinal cord. Primary demyelination takes place in the centre of the white columns. The damage is less in the cervical segments and usually confined to the dorsal columns, especially the funiculus gracilis. Similarly on passing down the cord the disease becomes more limited until in the lower lumbar region only the pyramidal tracts are affected.

Axon lesions develop soon after the primary degeneration of myelin. Neurological scarring and astrocytic reaction occur later.

The brain may be extensively affected in rare instances. Small, ill-defined areas of demyelination are seen in the cerebral white matter. The large ascending and descending tracts are mostly spared. Ischaemic cortical necrosis and Wernicke's syndrome have also been reported.

Bone-marrow.—There is a marked increase in red bone-marrow. The marrow of the long bones becomes dark red and gelatinous with interspersed pale fatty areas. When hyperplasia is severe cortical bone absorption may take place. Histological sections confirm the hypercellularity in which there is a preponderance of immature red-cell precursors and numerous reticulo-endothelial cells. However, cytological details are far more readily characterized in smear preparations.

The other pathological findings are the result of severe anaemia (fatty degeneration of parenchymal organs), increased erythropoiesis, and excessive blood destruction.

Clinical Features

Pernicious anaemia is a disease of gradual onset and anaemia may be profound before diagnosis is made. In others, symptoms may be present when anaemia is minimal or absent. Approximately half the patients have passed their sixtieth year at the time of onset (Cantor, 1963).

The clinical features can be considered under the following headings:—

1. Those due to the causative factors.
2. Those due to the anaemia.
3. Those due to cellular changes consequent upon hypoxia.
4. Those due to changes in the body from vitamin deficiency.

Symptoms due to gastric atrophy are not prominent, but there may be anorexia, flatulence, vague indigestion, and loss of weight which may simulate a carcinoma. Indeed, carcinoma of the stomach may be present, as the incidence is higher than in the general population. In rare instances such a carcinoma causes a megaloblastic anaemia, but usually it is a complication of the gastric atrophy. A barium meal X-ray is necessary, particularly if response to treatment is unsatisfactory or the anaemia recurs despite adequate therapy.

The effects of reduced oxygen-carrying power of the blood cannot be clearly separated from those caused by diminution of the vitamin. Both are probably implicated in the mental changes that may be present, but when cardiac failure is the presenting feature it is unlikely that absence of vitamin B_{12} is in itself important.

Apathy, loss of memory, and *failure of concentration* are often present and may lead to psychiatric referral. Social habits may deteriorate and *dementia* develop. Frequently *mental confusion* appears, and occasionally the person becomes hypomaniacal.

Case 1.—A man, aged 68 years, with a year's history of angina pectoris, became confused over a month and then suddenly maniacal. The family doctor requested a home visit before referral to a psychiatrist. Owing to the short history and the fact that he was pale, admission to a general hospital was arranged. His Hb level was 24 per cent and the blood-picture consistent with pernicious anaemia. Response to vitamin-B_{12} therapy was satisfactory. Chlorpromazine was given during the first fortnight of in-patient stay. It was subsequently discovered that he had complete amnesia covering a period of 6 weeks. When discharged he was mentally sound, with a normal blood-picture and electrocardiograph. He was well, both mentally and physically, 5 years later, and there was no angina.

Depression, which may be acute in onset, is another recognized presentation. In one series 82 per cent of the patients had psychiatric symptoms (Shulman, 1967). Anaemia may be obvious in these cases, but it is not an invariable finding.

Despite the frequent occurrence of mental symptoms in patients with pernicious anaemia the relationship is not as definite as one might suppose. Several possibilities complicate the issue. Apathy and depression are common in the elderly and are often of long duration, so that chance association with anaemia can presumably occur. Reduced food intake, particularly of protein, is a frequent sequel of apathy, and this leads to a lowered consumption of vitamin B_{12} and iron. Although nutritional vitamin-B_{12} deficiency is unlikely to develop iron deficiency may result, particularly if iron loss is increased, and a number of such patients—about 6 per cent—develop associated vitamin-B_{12} deficiency from gastric mucosal changes. There is a familial tendency not only in depression and dementia but also in pernicious anaemia. The two may coincide.

Serum vitamin-B_{12} levels tend to be lower in the elderly than in the young, although the evidence for this is somewhat contradictory. We found that the mean serum level diminished at around 70 years of age in patients admitted to the neighbouring mental hospital, and around 80 years of age in the general hospital (Nam, Powell, and Thomas, unpublished). We compared 750 routine admissions to a psychiatric hospital with 241 consecutive admissions to the acute geriatric unit of a general hospital (*Table XVIII*). There was no clear-cut difference in serum level between the two groups, but this could be due to overlap in the type of cases admitted.

Table XVIII.—Comparisons of Serum Vitamin-B_{12} Levels in Groups of Psychiatric and Medical Patients

Age (years)	750 Psychiatric Patients		241 Medical Patients	
	Mean Serum Vitamin B_{12} (pg. per ml.)	S.D.	Mean Serum Vitamin B_{12} (pg. per ml.)	S.D.
11–30	217	80		
31–50	219	75		
51–60	205	83		
61–70	200	85	196	82
71–80	166	79	195	83
81–90	163	75	156	82

A comparison between those who are mentally and physically normal and those who are confused or demented tends to show a higher incidence of low and intermediate levels in the latter. Droller and Dossett (1959) found that of 22 'normal' patients all had a serum level above 180 pg. per ml., whereas of 18 with dementia 10 were below 180 pg. per ml. (2 below 110 pg. per ml.) and of 18 confused patients 5 were below this level (0 below 110 pg. per ml.). The numbers are small, but the authors were painstaking in their assessment of cases and excluded those with physical disease.

It could be argued that when mental disturbance is due to vitamin-B_{12} deficiency correction of the deficiency should result in a return to mental normality. Unfortunately, this does not necessarily follow, because similar irreversible changes can take place in the brain as in the spinal cord. Most patients do in fact recover mentally when severe anaemia is treated, unless the anaemia is of long duration, or the patient was mentally disturbed before the illness developed. Recovery is less likely when the anaemia is mild, but may still occur. On the other hand, the results of vitamin B_{12} therapy in non-anaemic, confused, or demented patients with low serum levels are disappointing. Mental disturbance is not proportional to the anaemia, presumably because other factors are present, such as cerebral atherosclerosis.

The development of *congestive failure* or of *left ventricular failure* may be rapid and results in a critical state demanding urgent treatment.

There is sometimes a preceding history of *angina pectoris*. Usually the presence of anaemia has been noted and iron medication prescribed. While waiting 2 or 3 weeks for improvement the patient's condition deteriorates over a few days and anaemia becomes profound. Often left ventricular failure is the first indication that treatment is unsuccessful. The onset of congestive failure is less dramatic and usually these patients have had mild failure before becoming anaemic. Cardiac output is increased in anaemia and circulation time shortened, but the rapid development of failure is probably due to hypoxia of the myocardium. Dilatation may be considerable. The critical haemoglobin level at which these changes occur is not constant, presumably because the severity of coronary atheroma varies. The same variability of quality applies to the myocardium. Although severe cardiac embarrassment may develop when the haemoglobin level is in the region of 50 per cent, usually a much lower level is present, often 30 per cent or less.

Electrocardiographic changes of flattened or inverted T waves are almost invariably present, but these changes can occur when there is no clinical evidence of cardiac failure. As the haemoglobin level rises these changes disappear, unless there is underlying cardiac disease, such as ischaemia, but the level of the haemoglobin at which a normal T wave returns varies considerably. Sometimes definite improvement is apparent when the haemoglobin reaches 40 or 50 per cent, while in others only minimal improvement is seen until the haemoglobin reaches 70–80 per cent.

Clinical recovery approximates to the improvement in the cardiogram, but does not coincide with it. Congestive failure may disappear before a normal pattern is reached, or may still be present when the record is satisfactory. Sometimes oedema of the extremities increases as the anaemia improves.

In rare instances the electrocardiograph shows elevation of the ST segment suggestive of infarction, but which is not supported by the subsequent changes.

It is believed that the impact of pernicious anaemia on the heart is due to the anaemia and not to the direct effect of vitamin-B_{12} deficiency on the myocardium.

Symptoms due to involvement of the *central nervous system* other than the brain are relatively unusual, but occasionally are presenting features. Why some people are affected and not others is not known.

Peripheral neuritis, with paraesthesiae and patchy anaesthesia of the hands and feet, together with tenderness of the calves and diminution of limb reflexes, is the commonest finding.

These symptoms can be due to other causes. They are not unusual in the elderly and are often vaguely ascribed to the ageing process. Vascular insufficiency in the limbs and degenerative disk changes in the spine may confuse the issue.

Subacute combined degeneration of the cord with its demyelination of posterior and lateral columns is well documented. The incidence is decreasing and it is now a relatively rare complication. The sexes are equally affected.

Patients complain of bilateral paraesthesiae, progressive weakness, and unsteadiness of the legs. The onset is usually insidious though occasionally fairly rapid with mild pyrexia. There is tenderness of the calves, with diminution of knee- and ankle-jerks and absent vibration sense. 'Stocking' anaesthesia may be present. Later the muscles are paralysed and tender, with hypertonus in the arms. Flexor spasms may develop with signs of partial or complete cord transection, but sphincter involvement is late.

Megaloblastic anaemia is sometimes present, but may be mild, although the serum vitamin-B_{12} level is almost always below 50 pg. per ml. The diagnosis may be reasonably straightforward when advanced pernicious anaemia is present, but peripheral neuritis can occur without cord involvement, while diminution or absence of ankle-jerks and vibration and joint sense are not unusual in the later decades.

Mental confusion is often present and this makes it impossible to assess the central nervous system satisfactorily. The symptoms and signs resulting from cervical myelopathy may simulate those of subacute combined degeneration of the cord. Posterior infarction of the cord produces similar findings, although the onset is usually acute. Disseminated sclerosis, tabes dorsalis, and spinal tumours also enter the differential diagnosis.

Myelopathy.—Spinal cord involvement, not typical of subacute combined degeneration, can occur. The plantars may be extensor and the posterior columns unaffected. Discrimination of light touch, temperature, and pain may be greatly impaired and the lower limbs become spastic.

Cerebellar ataxia is occasionally a presenting feature.

Optic neuritis may develop and lead to bilateral optic atrophy. Though rare it can be the first manifestation. There is an overwhelming male preponderance and its development is not related to the degree of the anaemia, the duration of the disease, or to the presence of neurological involvement. Sometimes the pernicious anaemia is in the latent or early stage. Freeman and Heaton (1961) claimed that it occurred only in smokers, and presented evidence to show that 'tobacco amblyopia and retrobulbar neuritis in pernicious anaemia are one and the same condition'. The findings of Linnell and others (1968) supported the idea that a high cyanide intake (associated with smoking) could derange vitamin-B_{12} metabolism. The normal vitamin-B_{12} content of aqueous humour is of the same order as that of the C.S.F., the mean value being 21 pg. per ml. Ainley and others (1969) found that cyanocobalamin entered the aqueous humour from the blood much more readily than did hydroxocobalamin, possibly due to the latter's greater binding with plasma protein.

Impaired visual acuity and disturbance of colour vision may be present when the optic nerve and retina appear healthy.

Retinal haemorrhages are sometimes seen.

General symptoms, such as dyspnoea and oedema of the ankles, need no elaboration as they are common to all anaemias, but in the elderly their presence is variable because of diminished mobility, individual difference in reserve power of organs, the frequent coexistence of other abnormalities, and the fact that progression of the disease in its early stage is slow.

A *sore tongue* may be troublesome, but its presence probably indicates additional deficiencies, as of iron, thiamine, and riboflavine. Cheilosis, angular stomatitis, and glossitis—which may cause the tongue to be red and smooth, fissured with large fungiform papillae, or 'geographical' in that epithelium is shed in patches—are signs of malnutrition. Although the tongue may be normal, glossitis remains a valuable sign of vitamin-B_{12} and folate deficiency (Dawson, Ogston, and Fullerton, 1969).

Spontaneous bruising and even bleeding may be present if the associated thrombocytopenia is severe. Minot (1918) commented that: 'the development of purpura haemorrhagia in pernicious anaemia, even though it be manifested by only a slight oozing of the gums, is a serious phenomenon'. Two of the 9 cases described by Smith, Smith, and Fletcher (1962) were over 60 years of age, and the eldest, a female of 71 with epistaxis, petechiae, and bruises, developed uncontrollable bleeding from the site of intramuscular injection necessitating blood transfusion. Her platelet count was 14,000 per c.mm. Three of their cases had haematemesis and melaena, and in 2 there was also epistaxis and purpura.

Chronic dysphagia, as with iron deficiency in the Paterson-Kelly syndrome, is an occasional symptom, and in rare cases postcricoid carcinoma has developed (Jacobs, 1962).

Clinical Examination

This may not reveal any abnormal physical sign apart from pallor of the mucous membrane. Allowing for the preponderance of women in the later decades the incidence appears equal in the sexes.

Some have a 'biscuit coloration' of the skin or slight icterus. Diffuse or blotchy brownish pigmentation of the palms and soles is sometimes prominent.

Occasionally the tip of the spleen can be felt.

The tongue may be sore and neurological signs may be present. Optic neuritis is revealed by deterioration of vision beyond that expected from ophthalmoscopic examination, though papillitis may be noted and small retinal haemorrhages seen. Evidence of bruising is not unusual and ecchymoses may be prominent. Signs of congestive cardiac failure can dominate the picture. Unrelated diseases are often present and their clinical features may be the reason for referral or admission. In these patients pernicious anaemia may be but an incidental finding.

When following total or partial gastrectomy, associated deficiencies are more common. The incidence after partial gastrectomy is in the region of 5–6 per cent over a period of 8–12 years, though diminished absorption of the vitamin in the fasting state occurs in about 30 per cent. Absence or diminution of intrinsic factor can be demonstrated in these patients, and subacute combined degeneration of the cord has developed in isolated instances.

Latent Pernicious Anaemia

This was defined by Callender and Spray (1962) as a state in which 'the secretion of intrinsic factor is reduced and the stage is set for the full development of vitamin-B_{12} deficiency at any time, although the subject appears in excellent health and has no signs of anaemia or central nervous disorder'. Perhaps this accurate definition can be relaxed to include those who are not in excellent health but possess the other criteria. Serum vitamin-B_{12} levels may be low in these patients if the stores are depleted. When this stage is reached frank pernicious anaemia develops within a few months unless preventive measures are taken. These non-anaemic or mildly anaemic patients may be considered as having *early pernicious anaemia*, the dividing line between them and those in the latent stage being merely one of degree. Pederson, Lund, Ohlsen, and Kristensen (1957) studied 46 patients over 50 years of age with histamine-fast achlorhydria and mild anaemia. Seven were found to have 'partial megaloblastic erythropoiesis'. The stages associated with falling serum vitamin-B_{12} levels were: apparent normal health, achlorhydria with normoblastic erythropoiesis, partial megaloblastic erythropoiesis, and, finally, total megaloblastic erythropoiesis.

The incidence of low serum vitamin-B_{12} levels in patients with a haemoglobin above 80 per cent (11·6 g. per 100 ml.) is appreciable and does not differ greatly from that obtained in patients with a lower haemoglobin. *Table XIX* shows the result of an investigation comparing the incidence. Among 193 non-anaemic

Table XIX.—Comparison of Incidence of Low Serum Vitamin-B_{12} Levels with Haemoglobin Levels

Percentage Haemoglobin	Vitamin B_{12} (pg. per ml.)							
	0–20	21–50	51–80	81–110	111–150	151–300	301+	Total
<80 per cent	2	1	5	9	17	27	14	75
>80 per cent	1	7	7	18	27	91	42	193
Total	3	8	12	27	44	118	56	268

patients, 33 (17 per cent) had a serum level of vitamin B_{12} below 111 pg. per ml., whereas in the 75 anaemic patients the corresponding number was 17 (22 per cent). It is seen from *Table XIX* that 8 with a haemoglobin above 80 per cent had a serum level below 51 pg. per ml. The incidence was approximately equal in the sexes—among 114 non-anaemic females 20 were below 111 pg. per ml. (9 below 81 pg. per ml.), and in 79 non-anaemic males the corresponding numbers were 13 below 111 pg. per ml. and 6 below 81 pg. per ml. In the anaemic group the figures were: males 6 of 31 below 111 pg. per ml. (2 below 81 pg. per ml.); and females, 11 of 44 below 111 pg. per ml. (6 below 81 pg. per ml.).

It is apparent that the same low level of serum vitamin B_{12} may be obtained when there is no anaemia as when there is early or advanced disease. The difference is in the state of the body stores and probably in unknown factors governing vitamin-B_{12} utilization by the marrow. Not all patients with a low level become anaemic, but many do. Estimation of body stores would probably separate those who needed therapy from those who did not. The number could be considerable as the 50 patients with a serum level below 111 pg. per ml. occurred among 268 consecutive admissions over a period of 3 months. Furthermore, they suffered from other diseases that had to be investigated, in fact only 10 were admitted because of anaemia.

Aetiology

The cause of pernicious anaemia, as distinct from its mechanism, is not known. Discussion of possible factors includes racial, geographic, familial, and immunological influences. These various theories are not restated, but the importance of age is emphasized as pernicious anaemia is a disease of late adults and the elderly and its incidence increases with advancing age.

Whittingham, Ungar, Mackay, and Mathews (1969) studied 88 relatives of 13 patients with pernicious anaemia and 87 relatives of 13 patients with simple chronic atrophic gastritis. The relatives of cases of pernicious anaemia differed from the others in that they showed a significantly greater number with pernicious anaemia or 'linked conditions'—diabetes mellitus, Addison's disease, premature greying of hair, allergic disease, positive auto-immune serological reactions to gastric and thyroid antigens, and an increased mortality. They concluded that the gastric atrophy of pernicious anaemia differed from that of simple chronic gastritis, and that it influenced non-specifically various environmental agents, and indicated an inherited defect in immunological tolerance which prejudiced against survival to old age.

The disease is commonest in white people from temperate zones, and is rare in Negroes, Indians, and Chinese, although Jayaratnam, Cheng Siang, Da Costa, Kheng-Khoo, and O'Brien (1967) recorded 6 cases of pernicious anaemia (4 in Chinese and 2 in Indians) among 40 consecutive patients with megaloblastic anaemia admitted to hospital in Singapore. Four were over 60 years of age. Of the remaining 34, 30 had nutritional folic-acid deficiency, 2 were vegans and had nutritional vitamin-B_{12} deficiency, and 2 had a haemolytic anaemia complicated by secondary folic-acid deficiency. Experience in Jamaica has also shown that its rarity has been overemphasized (Stuart and McIver, 1961). Britt, Stranc, and Harper (1970) found 2 cases of Addisonian pernicious anaemia out of 15 of megaloblastic anaemia in Punjabi immigrants in London.

Familial Incidence

This has been long recognized. Castle and Minot (1936) gave an estimate of 18 per cent. Wangel, Callender, Spray, and Wright (1968) in an extensive study of the relatives of patients with pernicious anaemia found that serum vitamin-B_{12} levels were lower in first-degree relatives over the age of 70 years than in control subjects matched for age and sex. Hippe and Jensen (1969) classified 56 cases into hereditary and non-hereditary types on the presence or absence of a familial history and/or coexisting diabetes mellitus, thyroid disease, and vitiligo. The average age at onset was 51 years (S.D. 15·7) in the 29 cases with the hereditary form, and 66 years (S.D. 13·6) in the remaining 27. This latter group had higher serum concentrations of IgG, IgA, and IgM antibodies.

Prevalence Rate

The prevalence rate in this country varies from 0·60 per 1000 in Hertfordshire to 2·46 per 1000 in a part of Scotland (Banff and Elgin), being 1·53 in Wales (Scott, 1960), but in the elderly it is approximately 7 per 1000 and is higher still in those with thyroid disease, diabetes mellitus, and rheumatoid arthritis. Mosbech (1952) in Denmark found an incidence of 2 per 1000 between 40 and 60 years, and 3 per

1000 between 60 and 80 years. It was calculated that 1 case of pernicious anaemia occurred per annum among 10,000 female inhabitants and 1 among 15,000 male inhabitants.

VITAMIN-B_{12} DEFICIENCY FROM OTHER CAUSES

Malabsorption

Patients with malabsorption need not have diminution of intrinsic factor secretion as the fault is in the small intestine. Some have abdominal pain (which can be colicky) and also diarrhoea. Steatorrhoea may be present and the stools contain 10–20 g. of fat in 24 hours. Marked osteoporosis or osteomalacia can develop with pain in the bones and sometimes pseudo-fractures. Chronic ill health, anorexia, and loss of weight are usually present. The glucose-tolerance curve may be flat and the serum proteins low. Anaemia is not usually severe, a level of haemoglobin between 50 and 60 per cent being common. The blood-film may be hypochromic, normochromic, or macrocytic, but the sternal marrow usually contains a varying number of megaloblasts.

Low serum levels of iron, vitamin B_{12}, and folate are often obtained. Other vitamin-B complexes can also be deficient and glossitis marked. Radiological examination of the gastro-intestinal tract may show the presence of multiple diverticula in the jejunum.

The serum level of vitamin B_{12} is not usually as low as that obtained in classic pernicious anaemia, although there are many exceptions. A level below 40 pg. per ml. is unlikely and assay results of 60–70 pg. per ml. are common.

The full clinical picture is not often seen. It is more usual for the patient to be free from abdominal symptoms and to present with those of anaemia. Steatorrhoea may be minimal or absent, and there is often no evidence of malabsorption of glucose, minerals, protein, or electrolytes. Serum vitamin B_{12} is not grossly reduced, but is usually below 90 pg. per ml. and the levels of folate and iron are also low, although there are exceptions and one or other may be normal or raised. Urinary excretion of absorbed xylose is below the normal 20 per cent, but this test is so often positive in the elderly that its validity is doubtful. Quantitative estimation of blood xylose is probably more reliable, although it is debatable whether such detailed investigation is routinely necessary.

Satisfactory evaluation of the cause of the anaemia may be difficult. The patients are often ill from other disease and therapy cannot justifiably be delayed. Hydrochloric acid may be present in the stomach and the Schilling test indicate impaired absorption unaffected by the addition of intrinsic factor, but in others there is complete achlorhydria and partial improvement with intrinsic factor, so that it is difficult to decide whether they have early pernicious anaemia, a low-grade absorption defect, or a combination of both.

A Crosby-capsule biopsy of small intestine shows varying degrees of villous atrophy.

If barium studies show clumping, diverticula of the jejunum, or dilatation with delay in transit, a diagnosis of malabsorption is supported, but unfortunately it is sometimes extremely tedious or impossible to perform the investigations satisfactorily. Moreover, similar radiological findings are seen in patients who have no evidence of malabsorption. It is difficult to explain how lesions of the jejunum can cause a lowering of the serum vitamin B_{12}. There is possibly excess utilization by certain proliferating bacteria, irrespective of whether the vitamin is in the free state or bound to intrinsic factor.

Pigmentation of the skin is sometimes noted and the patient may have exfoliative dermatitis or widespread psoriasis. Other dermatological diseases have also been implicated.

Chronic pancreatitis and biliary cirrhosis rarely present with anaemia. Isolated examples of malabsorption due to Crohn's disease and the reticuloses have been seen.

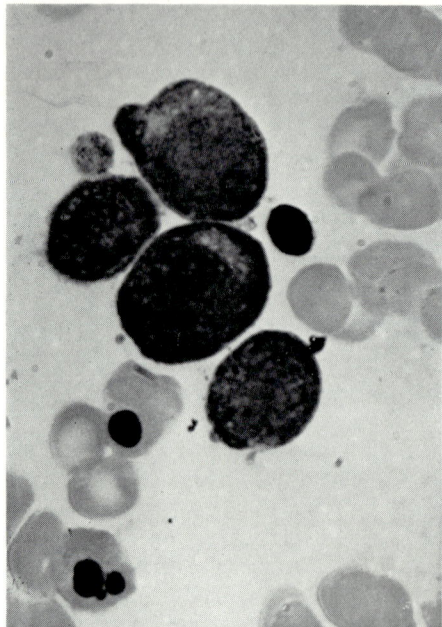

Fig. 23.—Case 2. Megaloblastic bone-marrow. ($\times 1100$.)

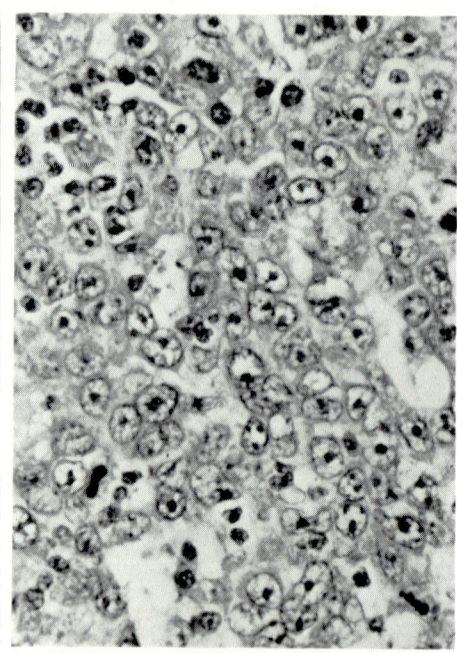

Fig. 24.—Case 2. Axillary lymph-node—reticulum-cell sarcoma. ($\times 400$.)

Case 2.—A 77-year-old man, who had been working as a credit draper until 6 weeks prior to admission in January, 1969, complained of increasing dyspnoea, cough, weakness, anorexia, and weight-loss. A chest X-ray showed several rounded opacities at the left base and in the upper half of the right lung. The Hb was 46 per cent (6·6 g. per 100 ml.), M.C.H.C. 30 per cent, and W.B.C. 7600 per c.mm. The red cells were macrocytic and the neutrophils showed a right nuclear shift. The sternal marrow was megaloblastic. No free gastric acid was secreted on peptavlon stimulation. Serum vitamin B_{12} was 60 pg. per ml., and serum folate 2·4 ng. per ml. Tests for parietal-cell and intrinsic factor antibodies were negative, but the R.A. latex fixation test was positive. His serum iron was 130 μg. per 100 ml.; T.I.B.C., 255 μg. per 100 ml. (saturation 51 per cent); and faecal fat, 3·3 g. per day.

The Schilling test gave 3·1 per cent excretion, which remained at 3·2 per cent after adding intrinsic factor.

An intestinal biopsy showed partial villous atrophy.

He remained feverish in hospital and enlarged nodes developed in the groins and axillae. One of these which was biopsied showed an anaplastic lymphoma, probably a reticulum-cell sarcoma (Figs. 23, 24).

A reticulocyte response of 18 per cent was obtained to cytamen, but the haemoglobin did not improve beyond 60 per cent (8·8 g. per 100 ml.). The reticulosis failed to respond to steroids or cytotoxic therapy and he died 3 months after admission.

This patient who died from reticulosis had malabsorption of vitamin B_{12} which could not be corrected by intrinsic factor. It was not established whether this was due to the villous atrophy that had been found or to direct neoplastic involvement of the intestine.

Association with General Disease

Serum vitamin-B_{12} levels may be raised in leukaemia and in liver disease characterized by necrosis, owing to release of tissue vitamin. Reference has been made to its reduction following gastrectomy and in ileal disorders interfering with absorption. The main problem, however, is the low serum level that often occurs in patients whose illnesses are unrelated to known alteration in vitamin-B_{12} metabolism. Presumably, the association is mainly due to chance, although this is not necessarily so, because general diseases can alter the mucosal cells of the small intestine.

A list of the diseases in which we have found low levels would be unwieldy and therefore classified groups of consecutive admissions are considered. Data are presented in *Table XX*.

Table XX.—Serum Vitamin-B_{12} Levels in Disease Categories

Clinical Diagnosis	Serum Vitamin-B_{12} Levels (pg. per ml.)							
	0–20	21–50	51–80	81–110	111–150	151–300	301+	Total
Blood-loss and gastro-intestinal disease	1	1	2	7	5	14	5	35
Infection and rheumatic disease	0	4	2	6	20	40	18	90
Neoplasm	0	0	1	2	0	9	7	19
Cardiovascular disease	0	3	3	9	20	49	26	110
Miscellaneous	1	0	5	6	10	27	12	61
Total	2	8	13	30	55	139	68	315

Auto-immune Disorders

There is an interrelationship between all the diseases thought to be due to, or associated with, auto-immune processes. These include auto-immune thyroiditis, rheumatoid arthritis, systemic lupus erythematosus, Sjögren's syndrome, pernicious anaemia, hepatic cirrhosis, Addison's disease, myasthenia gravis, haemolytic anaemia, and diabetes mellitus so that patients are occasionally seen in whom pernicious anaemia is part of a much wider disease complex.

Schiller, Spray, Wangel, and Wright (1968) found that among 300 patients with hyperthyroidism 6 had overt pernicious anaemia, 9 latent pernicious anaemia, and suspicious results were obtained in another 21. They suggested that if the gastric parietal-cell antibody test was used few cases of pernicious anaemia would be missed, but this is a crude test and serum vitamin-B_{12} levels would be more informative. Hypothyroidism—particularly when it develops spontaneously—is associated with pernicious anaemia fairly frequently. Tudhope and Wilson (1960) gave an incidence of 10 per cent. The relationship between these diseases is further supported by the fact that about 50 per cent of patients with pernicious anaemia have complement-fixing antibodies to thyroid (Irvine, Davies, Delamore, and Williams, 1962).

Ungar and others (1968) concluded that the latent phase was present in 4 per cent of insulin-dependent diabetics, but not in the others. This coexistence was ascribed to genetic and/or auto-immune relationship between the two disorders.

Partridge and Duthie (1963) reviewed 2544 patients with rheumatoid arthritis and noted that the incidence of macrocytic anaemia was 1·38 per cent as compared with 0·27 per cent in controls. Folic-acid absorption was normal. In 2 cases prednisolone corrected the anaemia and caused a return to normoblastic erythropoiesis.

Surgery

Special attention has to be given when *operative surgery* on the gastro-intestinal tract has been performed. Total gastrectomy always causes pernicious anaemia because intrinsic factor cannot then be secreted, and it has been mentioned that partial gastrectomy—particularly of the Polya type—may eventually result in a similar deficiency. Vagotomy and gastrojejunostomy can sometimes be associated with diminished absorption. Resection of the lower 2 feet or so of the ileum removes the absorptive area for vitamin B_{12}, as does jejunal resection for folic acid— although to a certain extent folates can be absorbed lower down the intestinal tract. Extensive resection of any portion of the small intestine reduces transit time and thereby causes malabsorption. Blind loops following side-to-side anastomosis or intestinal by-pass cause stagnation and altered bacterial flora (as with diverticula of duodenum and jejunum) which can interfere with absorption and sometimes cause steatorrhoea. Fistulae of the intestinal tract, due to disease or following surgery, are rare but potent causes of deficiency.

TREATMENT

Transfusion of whole blood or, preferably, packed red blood-cells may be required in extreme cases. It is essential that the transfusion rate is slow and that not more than 1 pint is given. The necessity of raising the oxygen-carrying capacity of the blood is of greater urgency in the elderly than in the young. Cardiac failure, mental confusion, and rapid progression of anaemia are special indications.

Specific treatment consists of regular and lifelong injections of vitamin B_{12}. There is little or no place for oral treatment in the elderly other than in the exceptional instance where hypersensitivity to injected vitamin B_{12} develops.

The choice lies between cyanocobalamin, hydroxocobalamin, or preparations combined with complexes to delay absorption.

Hydroxocobalamin is favoured because it is retained in the body far more efficiently than cyanocobalamin, it binds more strongly to serum proteins, reaches the liver in greater concentration, and its percentage loss in the urine is less.

Initial treatment aims at saturating the depleted body stores by giving four subcutaneous injections of 1000 μg. of hydroxocobalamin at weekly intervals. Maintenance therapy is more than adequately covered with 250 μg. monthly or 500 μg. every 2 months.

Side-effects.—These are very rare. Gillhespy (1955) described a patient who experienced generalized urticaria 12 hours after each injection. Bedford (1952) reported side-effects from preparations of vitamin B_{12} derived from *Streptomyces* but none when the preparation was derived from liver. Moderate anaphylactic shock occurred in an isolated instance (Beresford, 1960) and we have seen a patient in whom eczema was exacerbated.

RESPONSE TO TREATMENT

No patient should be treated without the response being measured. Pretreatment investigation with its array of tests has tended to produce a relative neglect of this aspect and as a result important diagnostic information may be missed. A suboptimal response is suggestive of a mistaken diagnosis, or the presence of intercurrent disease. The clinical response is evident within 2 days, but the peak reticulocyte response takes 5–7 days to develop and the level reached depends on the initial red-cell count:—

Initial Red-cell Count per c. mm.	Approximate Peak Reticulocyte per cent
$1 \cdot 0 \times 10^6$	40
$1 \cdot 5 \times 10^6$	30
$2 \cdot 0 \times 10^6$	20
$2 \cdot 5 \times 10^6$	15
$3 \cdot 0 \times 10^6$	10

The red-cell count response should exceed 3 million per c.mm. after 2 weeks.

A subsequent fall or delayed rise in haemoglobin may be due to iron and/or folate deficiency. A refractory state should also raise the possibility of carcinoma of the stomach or other disease.

ORAL THERAPY

Intramuscular injections of vitamin B_{12} may perhaps be difficult in exceptional circumstances, in which case oral therapy is feasible. Crystalline vitamin B_{12} alone can be given either in single massive doses of 3000–9000 μg. or in a daily dosage of 50–500 μg. Maintenance with 1000–3000 μg. every 1–4 weeks is possible.

Vitamin-B_{12} peptide is more effective than crystalline vitamin B_{12}, but a daily dosage of 200–500 μg. is necessary (Shinton, 1961) although Mooney and Heathcote (1966) used a much lower dose. They successfully treated 50 patients, 40 of whom were over 60 and the oldest 84, with a non-commercial preparation for periods of up to $3\frac{1}{2}$ years. The average daily vitamin B_{12} given was 19·5 μg., although in 22 per cent higher doses had to be given later, in 2 instances amounting to 100 μg. They considered low serum vitamin-B_{12} levels during therapy to be of doubtful significance, because 99·5 per cent of the vitamin resides in the liver and other tissues. No instance of true refractoriness occurred. These authors believe that the essential process in vitamin-B_{12} absorption is detachment from associated protein, rather than attachment to intrinsic factor, and that this is achieved by virtue of an endopeptidase, absence of which causes pernicious anaemia. They stated that their preparation was effective because it resembled the final form in which the vitamin was absorbed.

Various combinations of vitamin B_{12} and hog intrinsic factor, for example, hog IF 50 mg. with vitamin B_{12}, or 60 mg. IF with 15 μg. vitamin B_{12}, may be prescribed. Ellenbogen and Williams (1960) successfully maintained remission for 2–3 years without evidence of antibody effect—but this method is not generally favoured.

Steroids can give rise to a haematological response in patients with pernicious anaemia. The mode of action is not known, though perhaps they have an effect on the antibody mechanism. Obviously steroid therapy is not used for these patients, but it is possible that when given for some other reason the development of pernicious anaemia can be masked.

Associated Deficiencies

Hypochromia with M.C.H.C. below 30 usually indicates iron deficiency, but we prefer to estimate the serum iron, and if a transferrin saturation of 10 per cent or below is obtained to commence iron therapy. Administration is by the intramuscular route owing to absorptive difficulty in patients with atrophic gastritis. If a sternal puncture has been performed Perls's staining for haemosiderin will show whether there is associated iron deficiency. Even if there is no deficiency the position should be reviewed when the haemoglobin level is approaching normal. Another method is to observe the rise of haemoglobin and if this is not progressive to administer iron. Iron deficiency is so common that when full investigation cannot be carried out it is justifiable to supplement with iron on the assumption that a degree of deficiency is probably present.

Estimation of serum folate is also indicated and we repeat this after 2 weeks. When the level is unchanged and below 2·0 ng. per ml. it is our practice to add folate in a dosage of 5 mg. t.d.s.

Many patients have severe glossitis. If this persists despite adequate vitamin-B_{12} therapy then other vitamins of the B group—such as riboflavine—should be given.

Congestive cardiac failure and dysrhythmia may be present. Although they improve with treatment of the anaemia it is sometimes necessary to prescribe digitalis and a diuretic. Their future need should be reviewed later.

Neurological Complications

Patients with neurological complications are usually given a higher dosage—250 μg. or even 1000 μg.—of vitamin B_{12} weekly, for at least 6 months, but there is no definite evidence that this is necessary.

Mental confusion may make general management difficult unless a tranquillizing drug such as chlorpromazine is prescribed. A dosage of 25–50 mg. t.d.s. is usually sufficient.

Persistent *apathy* and *depression* may need treatment with antidepressant drugs, but usually they can be discontinued later.

Low Serum Vitamin B_{12} other than from Pernicious Anaemia

This is a common finding particularly when routine vitamin-B_{12} estimations are performed in patients with mental confusion, and it is difficult to decide whether

MEGALOBLASTIC ANAEMIAS

Table XXI.—Differential Diagnosis of Macrocytic Anaemias in the Elderly

	Aniso-poikilo-cytosis	Poly-chro-masia	Reticulo-cytes	Serum Bilirubin	Fragility	W.B.C.	Platelets	Marrow	Serum Vitamin B_{12}	Serum Folate
Pernicious anaemia	++	Sl.	Sl. ↑	<3·0	±	<5000 (right shift)	↓	Megalo-blastic	<50	N or ↓ or ↑
'Nutritional' megaloblastic	+	Sl.	Sl. ↑	0-3·0	±	<5000	↓	Megalo-blastic	<80	↓
Congenital haemolytic	+ (spherocytes)	+	↑	2·0-5·0	++	10,000-15,000	N or ↑	N/trans.	N	N or ↓
Acquired haemolytic	+ (spherocytes)	+	↑	2·0-5·0	++	10,000-15,000	N or ↑ or ↓	N/trans.	N	N or ↓
Leuco-erythro-blastic	+	++	↑	N	N	10,000<	N or ↓	Neoplastic	N	N or ↓
Aleukaemic leukaemia	+	+	+	N	N	N	↓	Leukae-mia	↑	N
Chronic liver disease	±	Sl.	±	+	→	<5000	N or ↓	N	↑	N or ↓
Hypothyroidism	±	Sl.	Sl.	N	N	N	N	N	N or ↓	N

N = Normal; Sl. = Slight; Trans. = Transitional.

vitamin B_{12} should be given for the remainder of the patient's life. They are often ill with a variety of diseases which require investigation and treatment, and frequently it is not justifiable to attend to side-issues. Nevertheless, if this attitude is allowed to prevail in all such cases many will be readmitted with pernicious anaemia.

The following should be considered:—

Deficient Ileal Absorption.—If the stools contain excess fat, vitamin B_{12} should be given for an indefinite period in the same dosage as that given for maintenance therapy in pernicious anaemia. Malabsorption can occur without steatorrhoea, but failure of vitamin-B_{12} absorption alone is rare. It can be demonstrated by performing the Schilling test with and without intrinsic factor. Should there be evidence of intestinal disease or that other constituents are not being absorbed satisfactorily, we consider that vitamin-B_{12} therapy is indicated.

Low Level because of Ageing or Disease.—Assuming there is no achlorhydria or steatorrhoea a serum level in the region of 110 pg. per ml. or even as low as 80 or 90 pg. per ml. may not be significant. A nutritional cause should be considered although it is often impossible to assess dietary intake. Sometimes the patient cannot swallow meat because of oesophageal narrowing. A previous gastrectomy should arouse suspicion that the level is pathological, particularly if there is associated sideropenia. In general, however, we believe that in the absence of an obvious cause specific therapy is not indicated, but follow-up is necessary and the level should be estimated at 3-monthly intervals, if possible, for about a year. The development of anaemia or further lowering of the serum level means that vitamin-B_{12} therapy has been wrongly withheld, but usually it remains stationary or becomes elevated as the patient's general condition improves.

If there is mental disturbance the cause of which is obscure, it is our practice to prescribe vitamin-B_{12} therapy and to continue only if the mental state improves. Otherwise therapy is discontinued, after 3 months or so, and progress observed.

Low Level associated with Deficiency of Iron and/or Folate.—This is considered further in Chapter 6.

Blind-loop Syndrome.—Antibiotic therapy is indicated in order to correct the abnormal bacterial flora that has developed. Tetracycline is usually prescribed. Neomycin should not be given, because it causes and increases steatorrhoea. Surgery to remove an isolated diverticulum or a blind loop from a previous operation may occasionally be feasible. But even when a functional deformity has been treated, either medically or surgically, vitamin B_{12} and/or folate therapy is usually necessary.

REFERENCES

ADAMS, J. F., and BODDY, K. (1968), *Lancet*, **2**, 328.
AINLEY, R. G., PHILLIPS, C. I., GIBBS, A., ACHESON, R. R., WATSON-WILLIAMS, E. J., and BOTTOMLEY, A. C. (1969), *Br. J. Ophthal.*, **53**, 854.
BEARD, M. E. J., and WEINTRAUB, L. R. (1969), *Br. J. Haemat.*, **16**, 161.
BEDFORD, P. D. (1952), *Lancet*, **1**, 690.
BELL, T. K., BRIDGES, J. M., and NELSON, M. G. (1965), *J. clin. Path.*, **18**, 611.
BERESFORD, R. (1960), personal communication.
BOOTH, C. C., and MOLLIN, D. L. (1959), *Lancet*, **1**, 18.
BRITT, R. P., STRANC, W., and HARPER, C. (1970), *Br. J. Haemat.*, **18**, 637.
BROZOVIĆ, M., HOFFBRAND, A. V., DIMITRIADOU, A., and MOLLIN, D. L. (1967), *Br. J. Haemat.*, **13**, 1021.

CALLENDER, S. T., and SPRAY, G. H. (1962), *Br. J. Haemat.*, **8**, 230.
CANTOR, A. M. (1963), *Geront. clin.*, **5**, 23.
CASTLE, W. B., and MINOT, G. R. (1936), *Pathological Physiology and Clinical Description of the Anaemias* (Ed. CHRISTIAN, H. A.). New York: Oxford Univ. Press (reprinted from Oxford Loose-leaf Medicine).
CHANARIN, I. (1968), *Gut*, **9**, 4, 373.
DAWSON, A. A., OGSTON, D., and FULLERTON, H. W. (1969), *Br. med. J.*, **3**, 436.
DELLER, D. J., GERMAR, H., and WITTS, L. J. (1961), *Lancet*, **1**, 574.
DROLLER, H., and DOSSETT, J. A. (1959), *Geront. clin.*, **1**, 96.
ELLENBOGEN, L., and WILLIAMS, W. L. (1960), *Br. med. J.*, **2**, 1066.
FREEMAN, A. G., and HEATON, J. M. (1961), *Lancet*, **1**, 908.
GILLHESPY, R. O. (1955), *Ibid.*, **1**, 1076.
GIRDWOOD, R. H. (1952), *Blood*, **7**, 77.
GREEN, A. E., and PEGRUM, G. D. (1968), *Br. med. J.*, **2** 591.
HERBERT, V. (1968), *Blood*, **32**, 305.
HIPPE, E. (1966), *Acta pediat. scand.*, **55**, 510.
— — and JENSEN, K. B. (1969), *Lancet*, **2**, 721.
IRVINE, W. J., DAVIES, S. H., DELAMORE, I. W., and WILLIAMS, A. W. (1962), *Br. med. J.*, **2**, 454.
— — — — HAYNES, R. C., and SCARTH, L. (1965), *Lancet*, **2**, 397.
JACOBS, A. (1962), *Ibid.*, **2**, 91.
JAYARATNAM, F. J., CHENG SIANG, S., DA COSTA, J. L., KHENG-KHOO, T., and O'BRIEN, W. (1967), *Br. med. J.*, **3**, 18.
KATZ, J. H., DIMASE, J., and DONALDSON, R. M. (1963), *J. Lab. clin. Med.*, **61**, 266.
KAY, A. W. (1953), *Br. med. J.*, **2**, 77.
LIE, J. T., UNGAR, B., and COWLING, D. C. (1969), *J. clin. Path.*, **22**, 554.
LINNELL, J. C., SMITH, A. D. M., SMITH, C. L., WILSON, J., and MATHEWS, D. M. (1968), *Br. med. J.*, **2**, 215.
MINOT, G. R. (1918), *Med. Clins N. Am.*, **1**, 1103.
MOONEY, F. S., and HEATHCOTE, J. G. (1966), *Br. med. J.*, **1**, 1149.
MOSBECH, J. (1952), *Acta med. scand.*, **141**, 433.
MULTICENTRE STUDY (1969), *Lancet*, **1**, 341.
PARTRIDGE, R. E. H., and DUTHIE, J. J. R. (1963), *Br. Med. J.*, **1**, 89.
PEDERSON, J., LUND, J., OHLSEN, A. S., and KRISTENSEN, H. P. Ø. (1957), *Lancet*, **1**, 448.
POWELL, D. E. B., THOMAS, J. H., MANDAL, A. R., and DIGNAM, C. T. (1969), *J. clin. Path.*, **22**, 672.
RETIEF, F. P., and HUSKISSON, G. J. (1969), *Br. med. J.*, **1**, 150.
SCHILLER, K., SPRAY, G., WANGEL, A., and WRIGHT, R. (1968), *Q. Jl Med.*, **37**, 451.
SCOTT, E. (1960), *J. Coll. gen. Practnrs Res. Newsl.*, **3**, 80.
SHINTON, N. K. (1961), *Br. med. J.*, **1**, 1579.
SHULMAN, R. (1967), *Ibid.*, **3**, 266.
SMITH, M. D., SMITH, D. A., and FLETCHER, M. (1962), *Ibid.*, **1**, 982.
STUART, K. L., and McIVER, J. E. (1961), *Ibid.*, **1**, 236.
TUDHOPE, G. R., and WILSON, G. M. (1960), *Q. Jl Med.*, **29**, 513.
UNGAR, B., STOCKS, A. E., MARTIN, F. I. R., WHITTINGHAM, S., and MACKAY, I. R. (1968), *Lancet*, **2**, 415.
WANGEL, A. G., CALLENDER, S. T., SPRAY, G. H., and WRIGHT, R. (1968), *Br. J. Haemat.*, **14**, 161, 183.
WHITTINGHAM, S., UNGAR, B., MACKAY, I. R., and MATHEWS, J. D. (1969), *Lancet*, **1**, 951.

5

FOLATE DEFICIENCY

FOLIC-ACID METABOLISM

'FOLIC acid' is the usual term for the synthetic product pteroylglutamic acid (PGA). It has a molecular weight of 441·21 and consists of pteridine, para-aminobenzoic acid, and glutamic acid (*Fig.* 25). Folic acid is necessary for cell division which is the reason why folic-acid antagonists, such as methotrexate, are sometimes useful in neoplastic disease.

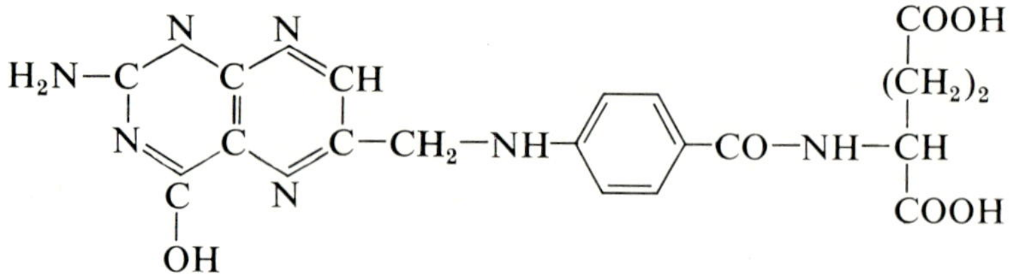

Fig. 25.—Pteroylglutamic acid ('folic acid').

PGA, and its conjugates, among which are pteroyltriglutamate and heptaglutamate, are found in fresh green vegetables, yeast, liver, and kidney, and synthesis by intestinal bacteria occurs. It is sparingly water soluble and insoluble in fat solvents, but the sodium salt is water soluble. The conjugates show a similar vitamin activity to PGA. Folinic acid (citrovorum factor) is derived from it.

Folic-acid antagonists prevent the conversion of PGA → folinic acid, and folinic acid inhibits the antagonistic effect of aminopterin. Folinic acid will convert the megaloblastic marrow of pernicious anaemia to normoblastic, whereas PGA may do so only partially.

The minimal adult daily requirement of folate is probably 50 μg. PGA (Herbert, 1962b), but approximately 75 per cent of ingested folates are excreted in the urine, which on a normal diet amounts to 1–4 mg. per 24 hours. This continues almost unchecked even in the presence of folate deficiency. Unlike vitamin B_{12}, folates are readily absorbed through the upper small intestine. Food folates are probably deconjugated enzymatically. There may be an active transport mechanism against a gradient.

The normal range for serum-folate levels is 6–21 ng. per ml. (using the *Lactobacillus casei* assay method), and the red-cell folate level is normally 150–650 ng. per ml. of packed red cells.

LABORATORY AND DIAGNOSTIC FEATURES

Folate deficiency can present either as anaemia, or as what is essentially a laboratory diagnosis.

BLOOD-PICTURE

Extreme degrees of anaemia in the elderly are usually due to pernicious anaemia or iron deficiency. Pure folate deficiency more commonly gives rise to moderate degrees of anaemia in the 6·0–10·0 g. per 100 ml. range. The anaemia may be normochromic, hypochromic, or dimorphic depending on whether there is coexistent iron deficiency. The M.C.V. is high normal or raised (96–110 c.μ). Examination of the blood-film is invaluable because it enables a more accurate interpretation when there are mixed states. Macrocytes and ovalocytes may be seen and occasional nucleated red blood-cells. Hypersegmentation of the neutrophils is a suggestive feature, although this can be seen in any megaloblastic anaemia, iron deficiency, or uraemia.

Leucopenia and thrombocytopenia often occur.

Although these features are a replica of those found in pernicious anaemia in our experience the florid peripheral blood-film associated with megaloblastic anaemia in the elderly is more often associated with vitamin-B_{12} deficiency than uncomplicated folate deficiency. The most common finding in folate deficiency has been a moderate or slight anaemia, possibly with hypersegmented neutrophils, and not clearly hypochromic or macrocytic.

BONE-MARROW

The abnormal bone-marrow features parallel the severity of the anaemia, and bone-marrow aspiration is not indicated in the non-anaemic elderly patient as a method of diagnosing folate deficiency. The earliest marrow changes are in the neutrophil series, viz. the appearance of macropolycytes and giant metamyelocytes. Frank megaloblastosis is a later development, although prior to this transitional forms may be seen. Perls's stain often shows an excess of haemosiderin unless there is also an iron-deficiency state.

SERUM FOLATE

A reduction in serum-folate levels is an early indication of folate deficiency. However, one of the chief difficulties lies in defining the normal range in the elderly. The serum-folate levels for healthy adults is given as 6–21 ng. per ml. (Wintrobe, 1967)—as measured by the *L. casei* method. Mavor and Spence (1968) indicated the frequency with which a large proportion of control subjects in reported series fell below the normal range. Values in the 3–6 ng. per ml. range are commonly found in the elderly, especially in the presence of complicating disease or other deficiency states. Markedly reduced levels (below 2 ng. per ml.) are not uncommon in elderly hospital patients and their significance can only be interpreted in the light of other clinical and laboratory findings.

Raised levels may be found in patients suffering from jejunal diverticulosis or other small-gut anatomical abnormalities probably due to excess synthesis by the altered bacterial flora. These patients usually develop vitamin-B_{12} deficiency. Acute renal failure gives raised levels, but these fall to below normal in chronic failure. Peritoneal dialysis lowers the serum folate (Sevitt and Hoffbrand, 1969).

Red-cell Folate

It is claimed that the folate content of the red cells provides a more accurate indication of the state of the body stores—the normal range being 160–640 ng. per ml. packed red cells. Values below 140 ng. indicate folate deficiency (Hoffbrand, Stewart, Booth, and Mollin, 1966). Low values may be obtained in pernicious anaemia even when the serum folate is normal or raised. Blood transfusion or reticulocytosis elevate the red-cell folate level.

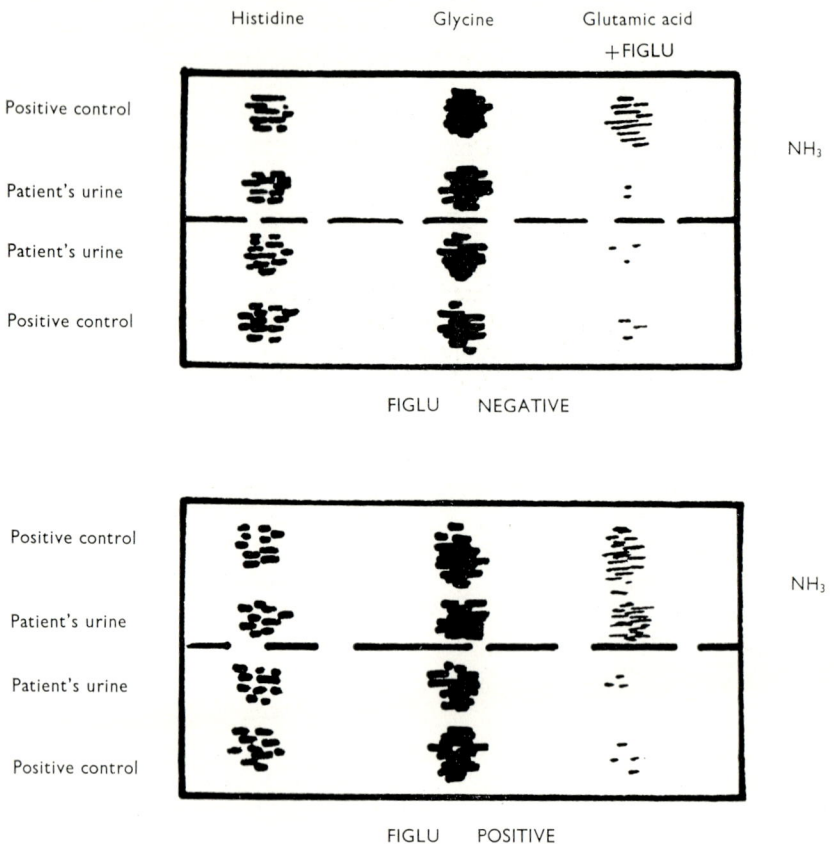

Fig. 26.—Diagrammatic representation of FIGLU test.

Histidine-loading Test (FIGLU)

Folate is required for the breakdown of formiminoglutamic acid (FIGLU) to glutamate and formiminotetrahydrofolate. In severe folate deficiency FIGLU and its precursor urocanic acid accumulate and appear in the urine (*Fig.* 26).

The FIGLU test consists of giving an oral dose of 15 g. L-histidine monohydrochloride mixed with water after an overnight fast. Urine is voided 3 hours later. This specimen is discarded but the next 5-hour sample is collected into 5 ml. of

N HCl. Cellulose acetate electrophoresis provides a convenient method of demonstrating FIGLU. The test may be made semiquantitative by comparing the FIGLU excretion with that of a control and the result given in mg. per hour. Chanarin and Bennett (1962) described a quantitative method using chick-liver enzyme. This gives a normal output of 1–17 mg., with a mean of 9 mg. Levels up to 1500 mg. may be obtained in folate deficiency.

This test should not be performed in hepatic failure because of the danger of precipitating mental symptoms or coma. It may also cause vasovagal collapse in post-gastrectomy patients.

Urocanic acid excretion may be excessive without an increase of FIGLU in liver disease, malnutrition, and following gastrectomy.

The FIGLU test can be used to screen for folate deficiency, but only in conjunction with other tests, because many cases of pernicious anaemia give a positive result.

Folic-acid absorption can be studied by measuring serum-folate levels following a standard oral dose (40 μg. per kg. body-weight) of folic acid, but where appropriate radio-isotope facilities exist, tritium-labelled (H^3FA) folic acid is preferable.

The folate-clearance test involves giving 15 μg. per kg. body-weight of folic acid intravenously. A sample of blood is taken 15 minutes later and the folate content assayed using *Streptococcus faecalis* (to measure injected PGA only). The normal 15-minute level is 20–80 ng. per ml. with a mean of 40. Very low levels are obtained in folate deficiency.

Hepatic Folate.—If a liver biopsy is available its folate content probably provides the best indication of deficiency. The normal content is 5·0–10·0 μg. of folate per gramme of wet liver.

THE CAUSES OF FOLATE DEFICIENCY

The factors concerned are:—

1. Insufficient intake.
2. Defective absorption.
3. Faulty formation.
4. Excess utilization.
5. Increased loss.

The body requires at least 50 μg. of folate daily and this is derived mainly from vegetables. A survey of elderly women living alone in London (Exton-Smith and Stanton, 1965) showed that of 60 who participated 7 took no green vegetables (raw or cooked leafy vegetables, fresh peas, beans, or cauliflower), 20 ate no root vegetables (carrots, onions, beetroot, swedes, parsnips, or marrow) while 8 excluded potatoes from their diet. Read, Gough, Pardoe, and Nicholas (1965) measured the folic-acid intake in 35 patients, ranging in age from 59 to 95 years, admitted to a welfare home. The mean intake in 11 men was 31·3 μg. per day and in 20 women 33·2 μg. per day while in 35 controls it was 52·6 for men (11 patients) and 52·7 for women (24 patients). It is evident that nutritional folate deficiency can be fairly common in those with decreased mobility, in those who are lonely, particularly if apathetic or depressed, and in those with financial worries. Occasionally, an elderly person pays more attention to his or her pets than to his or her own diet!

Absorption takes place in the upper small intestine so that disease and abnormality of this portion of the intestinal tract is often associated with deficiency.

Steatorrhoea is common and a low level of serum folate is almost invariable in these patients. Vague indigestion, upper abdominal pain, and loss of weight may be present. Diverticula of the jejunum are frequently visible on radiological examination. It is possible that mesenteric ischaemia occasionally plays a part. Intestinal hurry, blind loops, extensive resections, and altered bacterial flora within the intestinal lumen have also been implicated. The absorption of food folate may be defective when that of folic acid is normal, probably due to failure of deconjugation by an essential jejunal enzyme.

Defective formation is the favoured explanation for the folate deficiency that is sometimes associated with drug therapy of epilepsy. The fact that spontaneous haematological recovery occurs when the drugs are stopped and relapse when they are resumed suggests that the metabolic pathway is affected, perhaps because the anticonvulsants act as competitive inhibitors of enzymes involving folic acid. Serum vitamin-B_{12} levels may be low, though usually normal, and no malabsorption of synthetic folic acid can be demonstrated. The dietary intake is often inadequate and a full diet may afford some protection. Phenytoin and primidone are the main causative drugs but phenobarbitone has also been implicated. Many are receiving a combination of drugs and it is therefore difficult to be precise. In some cases a change of therapy, particularly the addition of another anticonvulsant, seems to precipitate the deficiency. Macrocytosis is reported to be far commoner than megaloblastic anaemia. In a randomly selected group of well-nourished epileptic patients on anticonvulsants Malpas, Spray, and Witts (1966) demonstrated macrocytosis in 11 per cent and a low serum folate in 37 per cent—despite the fact that only 2 of their 21 patients were elderly. The patients have often been on treatment for many years and usually have deteriorated mentally, with the result that it is difficult to evaluate their food intake. Although mental normality has sometimes returned with folate therapy we have not been convinced that a nutritional element was not present. Continuation of the drug has not resulted in relapse when folate has been added. An increase in fit frequency sometimes occurs when the deficiency is corrected.

Vitamin-C deficiency can interfere with folic-acid metabolism to such an extent that a megaloblastic anaemia results. Both folic acid and vitamin C are absorbed from the small intestine, so that when malabsorption is present a combined deficiency is common. Similarly, the diet may contain insufficient vitamin C and folate. But there are instances of folate deficiency occurring in patients with low levels of vitamin C in whom folate intake and absorption is satisfactory. Hyams and Ross (1963) described a female with scurvy, megaloblastic anaemia, and osteoporosis who was cured with vitamin-C therapy. They reviewed the literature and concluded that the vitamin-C–folic acid relationships were still far from clear.

Low serum folate is common in patients with lymphatic leukaemia, myelomatosis, and myelosclerosis. The cause is probably excess utilization by the rapidly dividing cells of the haemopoietic system leading to depletion of the folate stores. Compensatory increase of folate intake would presumably delay or prevent the deficiency, because folate therapy may correct the megaloblastic anaemia. Hoffbrand and others (1968) found marked megaloblastic erythropoiesis at some stage in 17 of 49 patients (33 over 60 years) with myelosclerosis.

Excess loss of folate will be considered later, in relation to dermatological disease.

CLINICAL FEATURES

These were demonstrated by Herbert (1962a) when a healthy male physician was placed on a diet of approximately 5 μg. of folate a day. The observations made are listed below in the order of appearance.

Fall of serum folate to below 3 μg. per ml.	3 weeks
Hypersegmentation of polymorphs	7 weeks
High urinary FIGLU	14 weeks
Sleeplessness and forgetfulness	16 weeks
Low erythrocyte folate activity	17 weeks
Macrocytosis, anaemia	18 weeks
Megaloblastic marrow	19 weeks
Irritability	20 weeks

The buccal mucosal cells became abnormal but no change occurred in gastric aspirate, in intrinsic factor secretion, in jejunal biopsy material, or in serum vitamin-B_{12} level, and no evidence of folate malabsorption was obtained. Leucopenia and thrombocytopenia did not occur. Within 24 hours of commencing therapy with 250 μg. pteroylglutamic acid the reticulocyte count began to rise and after 2 days the marrow was normoblastic. A fall in serum iron was noted.

It is clear that a fall in serum folate results from nutritional deprivation and precedes haematological changes, and that progressive alteration in behaviour and mental function are associated characteristics.

A similar pattern is seen in the elderly—except that mental changes are more pronounced—and the clinical features can be conveniently divided into three phases which, although interdependent, are sufficiently delineated for them to be described separately.

Low Serum Folate occurring alone

Serum folate levels below 6 ng. per ml. are found so often in the elderly that their significance is difficult to evaluate. Read and others (1965) found that it occurred in 80 per cent of 51 elderly patients admitted to a welfare home and most of them were not anaemic, although in general their haemoglobin levels were lower than in the control group. In 10 patients the serum-folate level was below 3 ng. per ml., and of these, 8 had normal haemoglobin levels. Increased urinary excretion of FIGLU occurred in 62 per cent of the total, but the relationship with a low serum-folate level was not absolute. After a stay in the home levels above 6 ng. per ml. were obtained in 7 of 23 that were followed up. Shulman (1967) reported levels below 6 ng. per ml. in 82 per cent of new admissions to a psychiatric hospital, and in 67 per cent of in-patients. There was no difference in serum-folate level between those living alone and those living with relatives, or receiving help with meals. Hurdle and Williams (1966) estimated serum folate in 72 hospital patients over 70 years of age and recorded that a level below 5 ng. per ml. was obtained in 28, 12 of whom were anaemic. FIGLU excretion test was positive in 50 per cent of them and hypersegmented neutrophils were present in 39 per cent. Two had folic-acid deficient megaloblastic anaemia.

Girdwood, Thomson, and Williamson (1967) compared the serum-folate levels of young controls (62 subjects) with patients over 65 living at home, and with 39 patients over 65 who had been in hospital for longer than 3 months. Values ranged as follows: young patients: 2·2–13·6 ng. per ml.; elderly at home: 2·0–25·0 ng. per ml; elderly patients in hospital: 1·6–9·1 ng per ml. They indicated that although overlap occurred between results in folic-acid deficient and in normal subjects, there was no reason to believe that levels, even as low as 2·2 ng. per ml., necessarily indicated folate depletion.

There are probably minor variations in the results obtained in different hospitals, but we consider levels above 2·5 ng. per ml. to be essentially normal. Serum-folate levels between 1·0 and 2·0 ng. per ml. usually indicate deficiency, and below 1·0 ng. per ml. deficiency is almost invariably present. The accepted range of 6–15 ng. per ml. appears to be too high.

Folate Deficiency with Symptoms and Signs other than Anaemia

Occasionally apathy, mild confusion, depression, and impaired intellect in patients with low serum folate improve markedly with folate therapy. Unfortunately the result is unpredictable and frequently disappointing. Strachan and Henderson (1967) described 2 patients in whom dementia responded to folate. Carney (1967), in an investigation of 423 psychiatric patients with a mean age of 54 years, found that values of 2 ng. per ml. or less were far commoner than in a control group. He decided there was no simple relationship between 'uncomplicated' low serum folate and a particular psycho-syndrome, but that association with affective disturbances and organic psychosis occurred 'with a precision which was unlikely to be coincidental'.

Peripheral neuropathy, with or without myelopathy, may be seen, and Grant, Hoffbrand, and Wells (1965) observed that megaloblastic haemopoiesis due to folate deficiency was remarkably common when the aetiology of the neurological disease was obscure. They suggested that a full investigation be carried out before the disorder was attributed to vitamin-B_{12} deficiency, as the features of folate deficiency could be clinically indistinguishable. The neuropathy sometimes improved with folate therapy. Isolated instances of subacute combined degeneration of the cord have been described (Anand, 1964) and also non-specific changes in the electroencephalogram.

It is still not clear whether the low serum folate in these patients is the result of the neurological disease or the cause. Perhaps an unknown factor in the vitamin-B_{12}–folate metabolic cycle is at fault. A low level of serum vitamin B_{12} probably indicates some diminution in the body stores, but this is not necessarily so with serum folate, because if intake is insufficient the amount entering the liver is small, and this in turn will displace little of the hepatic folate into the blood-stream. Consequently, the level of serum folate will be low but the amount in the liver normal—in one study over a third with a low serum folate had normal quantities in the liver. Coma can reduce the serum-folate level within a few days, long before the tissue stores can possibly be depleted.

Folate Deficiency with Anaemia

The anaemia is characteristically macrocytic in type and is often indistinguishable from that produced by vitamin-B_{12} deficiency. Mild icterus and splenomegaly are not usually present, but they are also frequently absent in Addisonian anaemia. Serum levels of vitamin B_{12} are usually normal, but sometimes the level is low though not in proportion to the degree of anaemia. A level of around 90 pg. per ml.

is common. Gastric assay may show the presence of acid, but achlorhydria even after gastric stimulation does not exclude folate deficiency.

When the deficiency is mild or has been present for a short period the anaemia is normochromic in type, though sternal puncture material may contain megaloblasts. As the anaemia progresses macrocytes appear in the peripheral blood. Hypersegmented polymorphs are seen and leucopenia and thrombocytopenia may occur.

The serum level is below 1·5 ng. per ml. and usually below 1·0 ng. per ml. Assay results of 0·6–0·8 ng. per ml. are often obtained. The patient may be receiving anticonvulsant drugs, or give a dietary history indicative of malnutrition. Intestinal hurry may be present, with or without steatorrhoea, and the clinical features may be consistent with malabsorption. Even when folate deficiency as a cause of the anaemia is suspected, serum for vitamin B_{12} and folate estimations should be obtained before therapy is commenced. If malabsorption is present ileal function should be investigated.

Anaemia due to folate deficiency is not rare in the elderly. Among 100 consecutive patients presenting with a haemoglobin level below 60 per cent (8·6 g. per 100 ml.) the anaemia was primarily due to folate deficiency in 7. The general incidence is difficult to estimate, but in our department it amounts to about a third of that caused by vitamin-B_{12} deficiency. In some areas the proportion is less, whereas in others it is greater particularly in the advanced elderly. Evans, Pathy, Sanerkin, and Deeble (1968) analysed 90 cases with megaloblastic anaemia. Only 1 was due to folic-acid deficiency alone, but 35 (40 per cent) had deficiencies of folic acid and iron. In patients with chronic neurological disease who develop megaloblastic anaemia deficiency of folate—presumably from reduced dietary intake—is commoner than that of vitamin B_{12}. Grant and his colleagues reported that of 10 such patients, 7 were folate deficient and 3 vitamin-B_{12} deficient.

There is a tendency to assume that megaloblastic anaemia nearly always indicates vitamin-B_{12} deficiency. This assumption is misplaced in the elderly and consequently serum levels of both vitamin B_{12} and folate should be ascertained.

Case 1.—A female, aged 83, was admitted in 1968 with mental confusion and burns. She had a long history of epilepsy and was living alone. The fits were controlled with phenobarbitone ½ gr. b.d. which had been prescribed for at least 30 years. On examination she was found to be pale with a very clear, slightly oedematous skin. Her Hb was 35 per cent (5·1 g. per 100 ml.) and the cells were hypochromic. E.S.R. was 55 mm. in the first hour; blood-urea, 22 mg. per 100 ml.; serum electrolytes, normal; serum iron, 42 µg. per 100 ml.; urine culture—scanty growth of proteus; chest X-ray—slight cardiac enlargement; and E.C.G. showed auricular extrasystoles and a right bundle-branch block. A silver-wire loop, which had been inserted in 1960 for control of a rectal prolapse, was protruding through the anus. There was obvious faecal blood-loss and a mild chest infection. Serum vitamin B_{12} was 470 pg. per ml. and serum folate 1·7 ng. per ml. Stainable iron was present in the marrow smear. There was no steatorrhoea. She was treated with ferrous sulphate and folate therapy. A month later, when her Hb was 66 per cent, she had a series of epileptic fits. Phenobarbitone, 15 mg. t.d.s., was supplemented with epanutin, 50 mg. t.d.s. Progress was thereafter uneventful and she was discharged 2 months after admission. Her blood-count was normal and she was mentally sound.

It is difficult to decide whether the folate deficiency was due to dietary insufficiency or to the phenobarbitone. The fits increased in frequency and severity as the anaemia responded. This could have been due to the folic acid reversing the anticonvulsant effect of the phenobarbitone, or perhaps to a direct stimulating effect on the brain. Such a possibility was suggested by Hunter, Barnes, Oakeley, and Mathews (1970). Folate concentration in the cerebrospinal fluid can be five to ten times that in the serum, and it is possible that excess concentration can alter the brain amines.

ASSOCIATION WITH OTHER DISEASES

A wide variety of diseases can be present and these may be the reason for the patient seeking medical advice. *Rheumatoid arthritis* has to be specifically mentioned. There are several references in the literature to their association. Deller and others (1966) studied 41 such patients and found a serum level of 2 ng. per ml. or less in 31·7 per cent. This was compared with the levels in 39 patients with joint and rheumatic conditions other than rheumatoid arthritis, as well as with 60 control subjects. In only 1 of these was a level below 2·3 ng. per ml. obtained. Gough, McCarthy, Read, and Mollin (1964) reported severe folate depletion in 33 per cent of the 46 patients they investigated. The explanation is speculative, but the role of increased utilization has to be considered. Anaemia is often present, but rarely is it due to folate deficiency.

Hoffbrand, Stewart, Booth, and Mollin (1968) studied 64 patients with *Crohn's disease*, ranging in age from 8 to 67 years, and found a high incidence of folate deficiency in the active stage, which they ascribed to inadequate intake, excess utilization, and/or malabsorption.

Among 25 patients with *cardiac failure*, 19 of whom were over 60, studied by Hyde and Loehry (1969), folate malabsorption was present in 7.

Roberts, Hoffbrand, and Mollin (1966) investigated 68 randomly selected *tuberculous patients* between 17 and 72 years of age, and found the serum-folate value to be below 3·0 ng per ml. in 35 per cent compared with none in their controls. The marrow was megaloblastic in 30 per cent. They discussed the cause and considered that general malnutrition, combined with increased demand because of the chronic inflammatory process, were probably important. None had vitamin-B_{12} deficiency.

Almost any severe systemic disease may be complicated by folate deficiency. This applies particularly to *neoplastic disease* even when there is no gastro-intestinal involvement. *Malignant lymphoma* is another disorder in which association with folate deficiency is often observed.

Case 2.—This lady was seen in 1965 when aged 64 years with a swelling on the right side of her neck. The peripheral blood-picture was normal. A biopsy of a neck lymph-node was diagnosed as reticulum-cell sarcoma. Radiotherapy was given with complete subsidence of the swelling.

In June 1966 she was seen again. Hb was 19 per cent; W.B.C., 2700 per c.mm.; and the red cells, macrocytic. Serum vitamin B_{12} was 260 pg. per ml.; serum folate, 0·5 ng. per ml.; and serum iron, 160 μg. per 100 ml. (38 per cent saturation). The marrow was fully megaloblastic. A reticulocyte response of 20 per cent was obtained with folic acid and the haemoglobin rose to 50 per cent. Thereafter it fell again and she died in September, 1966. Autopsy confirmed the presence of a reticulum-cell sarcoma in the spleen. The gastro-intestinal tract showed no abnormality.

Case 3.—This patient, aged 60, first attended hospital in June, 1969, suffering from eczema, and was admitted 1 month later with diarrhoea and weight-loss. He remained pyrexial, drowsy, and later developed chest pain. Hb on admission was 88 per cent (12·9 g. per 100 ml.); W.B.C., 7200 per c.mm.; E.S.R., 40 mm. in the first hour; and blood-urea 40 mg. per 100 ml. His serum vitamin B_{12} was 150 pg. per ml.; serum folate, 1·0 ng. per ml.; FIGLU test, positive; serum iron,

35 μg. per 100 ml.; T.I.B.C., 330 μg. per 100 ml.; and faecal fat, 23·5 g. per day. He died 2 months after admission. At post-mortem a dry scaling rash was noted on the face, fingers, and feet, and commencing gangrene of the left leg. Pulmonary embolism and femoral vein thrombosis were present. A smooth ill-defined swelling in the left paravertebral gutter was found to be a tumour mass which extended posteriorly and medially, destroying a portion of the body of the first lumbar vertebra and extending to reach the dura of the spinal cord. The intestine contained multiple sub-mucosal tumour deposits. The structure was that of undifferentiated sarcoma. No villous atrophy was found in the intestines (*Figs.* 27–30).

This patient had features of malabsorption and folate deficiency secondary to a retroperitoneal sarcoma which had metastasized to the intestines. The malabsorption was presumably due to direct involvement of the intestine rather than to villous atrophy,

Chronic Alcoholism.—Hines (1969) described a reversible type of sideroblastic anaemia in a group of severe alcoholic patients with liver disease. Ringed sideroblasts were found in 24 out of 35 patients, all of whom had low serum and red-cell folate in the presence of raised serum vitamin-B_{12} levels.

Case 4.—This lady, a widow, was first seen in 1956 at the age of 50 years with a severe depressive illness. She had been an alcoholic since the death of her husband 3 years previously. She lost weight and on admission to hospital in May, 1969, had extensive purpura. The haemoglobin was 31 per cent; reticulocytes, 10 per cent; platelets, 35,000 per c.mm.; bleeding time, 18 minutes; serum bilirubin, 3·1 mg. per 100 ml.; one-stage prothrombin ratio, 2·2; serum vitamin B_{12}, 1300 pg. per ml.; and serum folate, 0·8 ng. per ml. A sternal marrow showed normoblastic erythropoiesis and normal stainable iron. A needle biopsy of liver revealed severe portal cirrhosis. She died 1 month later. The liver findings were confirmed at autopsy.

This patient with severe anaemia and thrombocytopenia had chronic alcoholic liver cirrhosis. No sideroblasts could be demonstrated although folate deficiency was the likeliest cause of her anaemia.

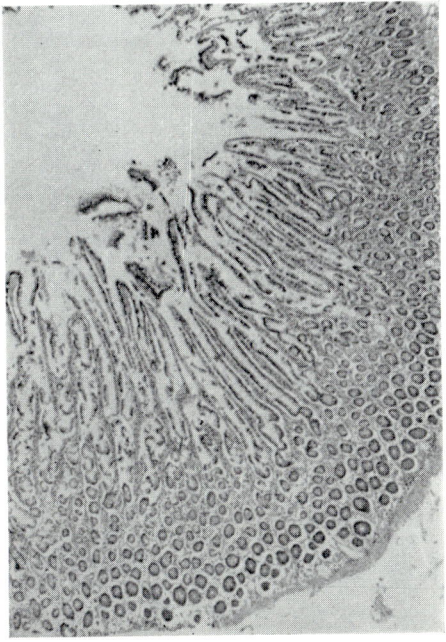
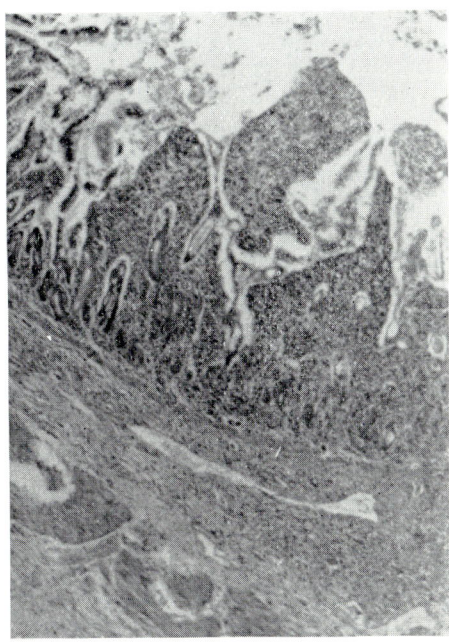

Fig. 27.—*Case* 3. Portion of small intestine with no evidence of villous atrophy. (×50.)

Fig. 28.—*Case* 3. Other portions of small intestine showing neoplastic infiltrate of mucosa. (×50.)

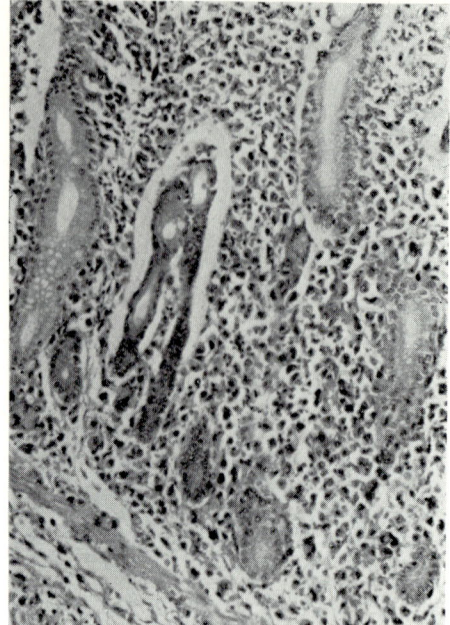 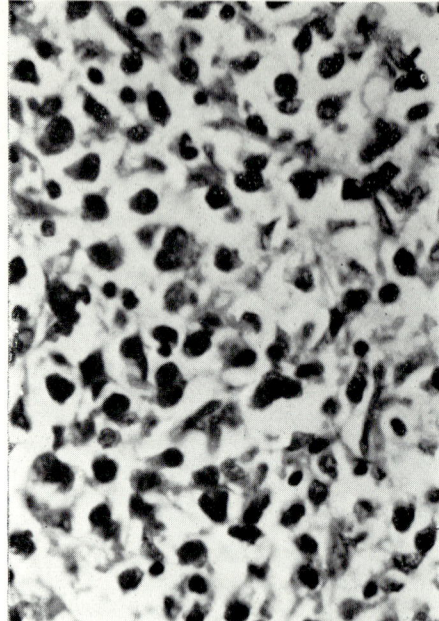

Fig. 29.—Case 3. Detail of neoplastic infiltrate in mucosa of small intestine. (×150.)

Fig. 30.—Case 3. Retroperitoneal sarcoma. (×400.)

Skin Disorders.—Folate deficiency can occur because of malnutrition, malabsorption, overutilization, excess loss, or the use of folic-acid antagonists.

The presence of skin pigmentation, dermatitis, and anaemia in patients with tropical sprue was noted by Manson-Bahr and Willoughby in 1930, and an association with idiopathic steatorrhoea was recognized soon afterwards. Of 100 such patients analysed by Cooke, Peeney, and Hawkins (1953), 20 had desquamative skin disease, and of 163 reported on by Badenoch (1960), 118 had glossitis, in 12 of whom it was a presenting feature, and 15 dermatitis (in 3 presenting). Exacerbation of both skin and intestinal disorder can occur together, and treatment of the intestinal lesion may improve that of the skin. On the other hand, patients with chronic eczema do not often exhibit definite malabsorption, although the presence of a dermatogenic enteropathy should be considered (Shuster and Marks, 1965). There may also be deficiency of vitamin B_{12}, iron, vitamin K, vitamin C, and/or pyridoxine.

In psoriasis, or exfoliating eczema, there is a continuous loss of protein, together with increased mitotic activity of the epidermal cells. The need for folic-acid substances, both in nucleic-acid synthesis and amino-acid metabolism, may mean that folates are used in excess (Wells, 1962).

The amount of folate—and of iron—lost in desquamated skin can be considerable.

Hild (1969) considered that this accounted for the low serum-folate levels obtained in patients with exfoliative dermatitis. He measured the folate content of the skin in 8 patients, 7 of whom had psoriasis, and found the daily loss to be 5–20 μg. Six had low levels of serum folate, but none had intestinal malabsorption. As the

FOLATE DEFICIENCY

condition had been present for many years, and hyperactive skin contains a higher level of folate (3·2–13·5 μg. per g.) as compared with normal skin which contains 0·11–2·00 μg. per g., the total loss must be considerable. Sweat also contains folate, and the 24-hour loss by this means, after maximal heat stimulation, has been estimated as 100 μg. (Johnson, Hamilton, and Mitchell, 1945).

When folic-acid antagonists, such as methotrexate, are prescribed, folic-acid deficiency often develops.

TREATMENT

Blood transfusion may be indicated, as with pernicious anaemia, when the anaemia is severe. A blood sample for estimation of vitamin B_{12}, folate, and preferably also iron, must be taken beforehand. When necessary we give all three haematinics intramuscularly until the result of the serum assays are available—and then decide what therapy should be continued. Many multivite preparations contain folic acid as do some iron preparations. They should not be prescribed to patients whose vitamin B_{12} state is not known.

Mild anaemia, or deficiency without anaemia, requires oral therapy with folic acid. If malabsorption is present the intramuscular route is used.

The main difficulty is to decide who requires treatment rather than how it should be carried out. We suggest the following should be treated:—

1. Those in whom the serum folate is below 1·0 ng. per ml.
2. Those with megaloblastic anaemia and a normal level of serum vitamin B_{12}.
3. Those on anticonvulsant drugs or in whom there is chronic neurological disease.
4. Those with steatorrhoea or malabsorption and low serum folate.
5. Those with iron deficiency, if there is macrocytosis, a dimorphic picture, or failure to improve on iron therapy, provided the folate is low and the serum level of vitamin B_{12} normal.

A low serum folate is often obtained in non-anaemic comatose patients but need not be due to deficiency. The same applies to patients with vomiting, dysphagia, or anorexia. The giving of vitamin B_{12} in pernicious anaemia can elevate a low folate level, but combined deficiencies also occur. We test for this by repeating the folate assay 2 or 3 weeks after commencing vitamin-B_{12} therapy, and if it remains low we prescribe folate.

The duration of treatment depends on the cause. If there is malabsorption it should be continued indefinitely, but if it is due to a deficient intake which can be corrected, further therapy is unnecessary. Whenever folate is given for a prolonged period the patient should be reviewed at 3- or 6-monthly intervals to detect possible incipient vitamin-B_{12} deficiency.

PREPARATIONS

Folic acid; acidum folicum; pteroylglutamic acid.

It is thought to be identical with the *Lactobacillus casei* factor of liver.

Folic Acid Tablets (5 mg. each).—The dosage is 10–20 mg. daily with 2·5–10 mg. daily for maintenance.

Folic Acid Injection.—The sodium salt can be given subcutaneously, intramuscularly, or intravenously. Parenteral therapy is indicated if the anaemia is severe or if intestinal absorption is known to be impaired.

The dosage is 15 mg. daily and maintenance 5–10 mg. daily.

Proprietary Preparations.—

Folvite   *Tablets*: 5 mg. *Soluble* 1 ml.–15 mg. Vials 10 ml.

Folvron   *Elixir*: 0·89 mg. folate per 5 ml. Ferrous gluconate also present. Dose 10 ml. t.d.s. *Tablets*: Ferrous sulphate with folate 1·7 mg. Dose 1 tablet t.d.s.

Other Preparations with Iron.—
Folaemin; Folex.

SIDE-EFFECTS

These are rare, but skin rashes and bronchospasm have been reported. 'Fit' escape may occur in epileptics. The most serious is the development of a neurological lesion, when folate is given to a patient who has vitamin-B_{12} deficiency.

REFERENCES

ANAND, M. P. (1964), *Scott. med. J.*, **9**, 388.
BADENOCH, J. (1960), *Br. med. J.*, **2**, 879.
CARNEY, M. W. P. (1967), *Ibid.*, **4**, 512.
CHANARIN, I., and BENNETT, M. C. (1962), *Ibid.*, **1**, 27.
COOKE, W. T., PEENEY, A. L. P., and HAWKINS, C. F. (1953), *Q. Jl Med.*, **22**, 59.
DELLER, D. J., URBAN, E., IBBOTSON, R. N., HORWOOD, J., MILAZZO, S., and ROBSON, H. N. (1966), *Br. med. J.*, **1**, 765.
EVANS, D. M. D., PATHY, M. S., SANERKIN, N. G., and DEEBLE, T. J. (1968), *Geront. clin.*, **10**, 228.
EXTON-SMITH, A. N., and STANTON, B. R. (1965), *Investigations into the Dietary of Elderly Women living alone.* King Edward's Hospital Fund for London.
GIRDWOOD, R. H., THOMSON, A. D., and WILLIAMSON, J. (1967), *Br. med. J.*, **1**, 670.
GOUGH, K. R., MCCARTHY, C., READ, A. E., and MOLLIN, D. L. (1964), *Ibid.*, **1**, 212.
GRANT, H. C., HOFFBRAND, A. V., and WELLS, D. G. (1965), *Lancet*, **2**, 763.
HERBERT, V. (1962a), *Trans. Ass. Am. Physns*, **35**, 307.
— — (1962b), *Archs intern. Med.*, **110**, 649.
HILD, D. H. (1969), *Ibid.*, **123**, 51.
HINES, J. D. (1969), *Br. J. Haemat.*, **16**, 87.
HOFFBRAND, A. V., STEWART, J. S., BOOTH, C. C., and MOLLIN, D. L. (1968), *Br. med. J.*, **1**, 71.
HUNTER, R., BARNES, J., OAKELEY, H. F., and MATHEWS, D. M. (1970), *Lancet*, **1**, 61.
HURDLE, A. D. F., and WILLIAMS PICTON, T. C. (1966), *Br. med. J.*, **2**, 202.
HYAMS, D. E., and ROSS, E. J. (1963), *Br. J. clin. Pract.*, **17**, 6, 332.
HYDE, R. D., and LOEHRY, C. A. E. (1969), *Gut*, **9**, 6, 717.
JOHNSON, B. C., HAMILTON, T. S., and MITCHELL, H. H. (1945), *J. biol. Chem.*, **159**, 425.
MALPAS, J. S., SPRAY, G. H., and WITTS, L. J. (1966), *Br. med. J.*, **1**, 955.
MANSON-BAHR, P. H., and WILLOUGHBY, H. (1930), *Q. Jl Med.*, **23**, 411.
MAVOR, W. O., and SPENCE, M. P. (1968), *Br. med. J.*, **1**, 430.
READ, A. E., GOUGH, K. R., PARDOE, J. L., and NICHOLAS, A. (1965), *Ibid.*, **2**, 843.
ROBERTS, P. D., HOFFBRAND, A. V., and MOLLIN, D. L. (1966), *Ibid.*, **2**, 198.
SEVITT, L. H., and HOFFBRAND, A. V. (1969), *Ibid.*, **2**, 18.
SHULMAN, R. (1967), *Ibid.*, **2**, 266.
SHUSTER, S., and MARKS, J. (1965), *Lancet*, **1**, 1367.
STRACHAN, R. W., and HENDERSON, J. G. (1967), *Q. Jl Med.*, **36**, 142, 189.
WELLS, G. C. (1962), *Br. med. J.*, **2**, 937.
WINTROBE, M. M. (1967), *Clinical Hematology*, 6th ed. London: Kimpton.

6

OTHER DEFICIENCY STATES GIVING RISE TO MACROCYTIC OR MEGALOBLASTIC ANAEMIA

VITAMIN DEFICIENCY

Vitamin C.—Subclinical vitamin-C deficiency is commoner in the elderly than in the lower age-group, although a picture of frank scurvy is not often seen. Usually there are other deficiencies also. The peripheral blood-picture may be that of normochromic, hypochromic, or frankly macrocytic anaemia. The bone-marrow is hypercellular with a macronormoblastic or a megaloblastic pattern. Some patients have shown diminished red-cell survival. There is no direct relationship between anaemia and the vitamin-C content of the body and its aetiology is obscure. Various theories have been postulated, such as decreased absorption of iron; failure of conversion of folic acid to its active state; decreased life span of erythrocytes; and increased usage in the presence of infection, rheumatoid arthritis and malignant disease, but none of these views is universally applicable. Nevertheless, anaemia is common in scorbutic states. Goldberg (1963) stated that almost 90 per cent had a haemoglobin level below 12 g. per 100 ml.

Scurvy may develop insidiously in the late spring among elderly men living alone. Perifollicular hyperkeratosis with petechiae on the back, outer aspects of the arms, buttock, thighs, shins, and ankles are characteristic features. Subcutaneous ecchymoses may be prominent. Ulceration and haemorrhage of the gums are often seen, except in edentulous patients. Minor trauma can cause haemarthrosis.

Treatment consists in the administration of 1 g. of ascorbic acid in four divided doses by mouth daily for 10 days, followed by 30 mg. or more per day (Anderson, 1967). Associated anaemia and other deficiency states also need correction.

In this country, as in Australia, Canada, and Norway, 30 mg. a day is considered sufficient for normal requirements, but in South Africa the recommended intake is 40 mg.; Central America, 45–50 mg.; the Netherlands, 50 mg.; Japan, 60–65 mg.; Russia, 70 mg.; and in the U.S.A. it is 75 mg.

Urinary excretion exceeds 20 mg. per 24 hours. The serum level is 0·6–1·5 mg. per 100 ml., but the amount in the red cells is almost twice this, and that in the leucocytes and platelets twenty to forty times.

Ascorbic acid aids the conversion of folic acid to folinic acid and by its reducing action maintains folic-acid coenzymes in their reduced active state. It is also involved in the absorption of ferrous iron and its incorporation with, and release from, ferritin. Therefore, not only are scorbutic diets often deficient in folates and iron, but deficiency of vitamin C may also further deplete the body's folate and iron stores. It may well be that some of the more striking haematological manifestations of vitamin-C deficiency are due to folate deficiency.

Low plasma ascorbate levels and rapid ascorbate clearance have been found in vitamin-B_{12}-deficient patients even when ingesting normal amounts of ascorbic acid (Cox, Meynell, Cooke, and Gaddie, 1958). Kahn and Brodsky (1968), using methyl malonate excretion as an index of vitamin-B_{12} deficiency, found that the abnormalities of ascorbate metabolism persisted during treatment of vitamin-B_{12} deficiency until the methyl malonate excretion ceased.

Vitamin B_6.—This is a class name for pyridoxine, pyridoxal, and pyridoxamine. It is involved in enzyme activities, particularly those concerned with the metabolism of amino-acids and nucleic acid, and is a coenzyme in the production of haemoglobin, acting at the porphyrin stage. When deficient there is failure of iron utilization and erythrocyte protoporphyrin is reduced.

Dietary deficiency in animals, particularly swine, has produced hypochromic anaemia with elevation of the serum iron, increased saturation of transferrin, irregular reticulocytosis, hyperplasia of the marrow, and excess tissue deposition of iron. This type of anaemia, manifested by failure of iron utilization when there is no true deficiency, is sometimes referred to as 'sidero-achrestic anaemia', but it is not specific to pyridoxine deficiency.

Man requires 2 mg. of pyridoxine daily and it is doubtful whether a diminished intake of pyridoxine alone can give rise to anaemia, but it may be precipitated by pyridoxine antagonists, such as isoniazid, penicillamine, and alcohol. A microcytic hypochromic type of picture develops with a normoblastic hyperplasia of the marrow, but frequently megaloblasts are present, possibly due to derangement of a common metabolic path with folate. The serum iron and transferrin saturation are usually normal or raised. Excess haemosiderin is present in the marrow. Red-cell survival may be impaired. Characteristic changes in the skin together with the clinical features of peripheral neuritis may be present, but it is in only half the patients that the tryptophan load test is positive. The serum level of pyridoxine, normally 5–25 μg. per 100 ml., is reduced. When all these findings are present it is disappointing that the anaemia is often not pyridoxine responsive, and even when a reticulocytosis is produced the haemoglobin level rarely returns to normal. Despite the use of large doses, in the region of 100–200 mg. daily, relapse can still occur when therapy is discontinued. Wintrobe (1967) suggested that there was possibly a genetic abnormality in some people leading to an increased requirement.

Jacobs and Cavill (1968) found reduced red-cell transaminase activity which could be stimulated by pyridoxal phosphate in patients aged 29–78 years (mean age 56·8 years) with the Paterson-Kelly syndrome. They also found an increased incidence of atrophic glossitis over the age of 40 years when the plasma level of pyridoxal phosphate was low.

Although anaemia due to pyridoxine deficiency alone is unusual, addition of the vitamin may stimulate or enhance erythropoiesis when an otherwise ordinary deficiency anaemia is seemingly refractory.

Other Vitamins.—

Nicotinic acid: The role of nicotinic acid in anaemia is obscure, but deficiency can lead to a hypochromic or a normochromic type of anaemia. Macrocytes may be present.

Riboflavine: Normocytic anaemia with a low reticulocyte count due to erythroid hypoplasia has been described.

Pantothenic acid: Although important in the biosynthesis of haemoglobin, deficiency does not appear to cause anaemia.

Generally speaking, isolated deficiencies of these vitamins are unlikely to occur so it is almost impossible to be precise about the type of anaemia, if any, that would result. Nevertheless, it is not uncommon in the elderly to find an anaemia which is neither clearly macrocytic nor hypochromic, when multiple deficiency states need correction.

SYSTEMIC DISEASES

Liver Disease.—Macrocytic anaemia may be found in hepatic cirrhosis, with or without an associated hepatoma. The erythrocytes are unusually thin in stained films, or appear as target cells, and the marrow is normoblastic or megaloblastic. An increase in plasma volume, when present, accentuates the anaemia. The red-cell survival time may be decreased.

The haematological changes in chronic liver disease are difficult to distinguish from those of folate deficiency, which often coexists.

Herbert (1968) suggested that an abnormal vitamin-B_{12}-binding globulin produced in chronic liver disease could hold vitamin B_{12} in the serum and not release it as required, so that vitamin-B_{12} deficiency could occur although the serum vitamin-B_{12} level was normal or raised. The liver stores of vitamin B_{12} are lowered.

Hypothyroidism.—There is an increased incidence of clinical or latent pernicious anaemia in these patients. But, apart from this, a macrocytic anaemia may be found. This differs from the macrocytic picture of pernicious anaemia by showing much less anisopoikilocytosis. The red cells are more uniformly enlarged and the bone-marrow is normal or hypoplastic. The anaemia responds slowly to thyroxine (*see* p. 54).

'REFRACTORY MEGALOBLASTIC ANAEMIA'

Refractory megaloblastic anaemia is encountered in the elderly as in others. It is unlikely that this constitutes a diagnostic group, as it probably includes unrecognized nutritional anaemia, drug reactions, or occult disease. Many patients with a megaloblastic or simple normochromic anaemia that respond tardily, if at all, to the customary haematinics subsequently manifest signs of a primary disease, such as gastro-intestinal neoplasia. Another possible finding in a non-responsive normochromic anaemia is a raised blood-urea due to chronic renal disease.

Dacie, Smith, White, and Mollin (1959) reported a study of 'refractory normoblastic anaemia' based on 7 patients, but there is probably no valid distinction to be made between these and the megaloblastic variety. In fact 1 patient had a megaloblastic marrow, and some of the others had features suggestive of megaloblastosis. Marrow smears showed excessive numbers of large siderotic granules. This study was before the routine estimation of serum folate or FIGLU was available, but only one responded (partially) to folic acid. There are undoubtedly refractory anaemias in the elderly which terminate in recognizable disorders such as leukaemia, myelosclerosis, or erythraemic myelosis.

HAEMOLYTIC ANAEMIA

Rarely, a prolonged haemolytic state may appear as a refractory or megaloblastic anaemia. Other haematological diseases that may be associated with some degree of megaloblastosis are the leukaemias and multiple myelomatosis. The underlying cause is folate deficiency, presumably from excessive utilization.

SIDEROBLASTIC ANAEMIA

A sideroblast is a nucleated red-cell precursor in which iron granules can be demonstrated by Perls's reaction. Three types are recognized. The first type may be seen in normal marrow, as erythroblasts sometimes contain scanty fine granules in their cytoplasm. The second variety is associated with an increased transferrin saturation, and the granules are larger and distributed throughout the cytoplasm. These are particularly associated with haemolytic anaemia, megaloblastic anaemia, and haemosiderosis. The third type shows large numerous granules arranged in a ring or crescent formation around the nucleus. These are found in dyshaemopoietic anaemias. A sideroblastic anaemia may then be defined as a dyshaemopoietic anaemia in which ringed sideroblasts are found in the marrow. It would avoid confusion if the term 'sideroblast' was confined to this ringed variety.

The sideroblastic anaemias include many inherited and acquired disorders. Several of these conditions have been described under such titles as 'sideroachrestic anaemia', 'refractory normoblastic anaemia', 'hypochromic anaemia with secondary iron loading', and others. They are broadly divided into hereditary and acquired types. The classification of MacGibbon and Mollin (1965) is as follows:—

HEREDITARY: Sex-linked hypochromic anaemia.

ACQUIRED:
Primary:
Refractory sideroblastic anaemia.
Secondary:
Malnutrition. Malabsorption.
Drugs (particularly antituberculous) and toxins.
Myeloproliferative conditions.
Malignant disease.
Haemolytic anaemia, etc.

Primary Acquired Sideroblastic Anaemia

This is predominantly a disease of the middle-aged and elderly. They commonly present as cases of megaloblastic anaemia that have proved refractory to vitamin-B_{12} and folic-acid therapy. Alternatively, they are first seen with chronic anaemia.

Blood examination shows hypochromic cells amongst a majority of normochromic cells. The M.C.H.C. is accordingly only slightly reduced. Macrocytes can usually be seen and the M.C.V. is above 100 c.μ.

The serum iron is often normal, as is the T.I.B.C., so that the percentage saturation is normal or at most slightly raised.

OTHER DEFICIENCY STATES

The diagnosis is made on marrow examination when most of the erythroblasts contain large siderotic granules, many of which show the ring formation. Megaloblastic features may be observed—indeed the smears may resemble those found in pernicious anaemia. Some of the late normoblasts have vacuolated cytoplasm.

Low serum and red-cell folate levels and a positive FIGLU test suggest folate deficiency, but only a minority of these patients respond to folic acid, and even then it is incomplete. However, a more satisfactory response is occasionally obtained, so that trial therapy is always justified.

There is nearly always excess iron in the stores due partly to prolonged iron therapy and multiple blood transfusions, but in addition iron absorption is increased. Haemosiderosis and, in advanced cases, features of haemochromatosis develop which may necessitate treatment by repeated venesection or chelation with desferrioxamine. Mollin and Hoffbrand (1968) referred to the possible development of a megaloblastic anaemia as the terminal manifestation of apparently typical primary acquired sideroblastic anaemia.

SECONDARY SIDEROBLASTIC ANAEMIA

A similar picture may be produced by many diseases and drugs. Numerous sideroblasts occur before anaemia is significant. Drugs that have been implicated include those used in antituberculous therapy (isoniazid, PAS, cycloserine), phenacetin, paracetamol, and lead. Disorders that may be responsible are: rheumatoid arthritis; myeloproliferative conditions such as leukaemia and myelofibrosis; malabsorption; chronic alcoholism; carcinoma; myeloma; partial gastrectomy; haemolytic anaemia; and myxoedema.

The drug-induced cases are usually cured if the drug is discontinued or pyridoxine given, but when part of a disease that produces increased cellular proliferation the change is often irreversible.

Damashek (1965) proposed that the first stage of the Di Guglielmo syndrome may be that of a sideroblastic anaemia.

Case 1.—In 1966 this lady, aged 50 years, was admitted as an emergency with intermittent, profuse vaginal bleeding of nearly 1 month's duration. The Hb fell to 36 per cent (5·2 g. per 100 ml.) and the presence of normochromic macrocytes was noted. She was transfused with 2 pints of blood and discharged. The curettings did not show any significant lesion.

In December, 1968, she had a haemoptysis. It then transpired that pulmonary tuberculosis had been diagnosed on an M.M.R. film in 1961, but no treatment given. Her sputum was positive for *Mycobacterium tuberculosis*, and streptomycin, PAS, and INAH were prescribed. The haemoglobin, initially 61 per cent, fell to 52 per cent.

In March, 1969, dizziness and paraesthesiae necessitated reduction of the streptomycin. Haemoptyses recurred. In April the Hb was 58 per cent, P.C.V. 26 per cent, and the peripheral blood showed a dimorphic picture. The sternal marrow was cellular and transitional megaloblasts and sideroblasts were present.

Serum vitamin B_{12} was 400 pg. per ml.; folate, 1·0 and 1·6 ng. per ml. on separate occasions; serum iron, 90 µg. per 100 ml.; and T.I.B.C. 300 µg. per 100 ml. (saturation 30 per cent). The red-cell saline fragility was slightly increased.

Folic acid was given and the reticulocytes rose to 20 per cent and the Hb to 80 per cent.

Case 2.—This lady was first investigated in 1951 when aged 59 and found to have a refractory anaemia for which repeated blood transfusions were subsequently given. In 1966 congestive cardiac failure developed and bruising was noted. The liver and spleen were enlarged. In 1967 the haemoglobin was 68 per cent (9·9 g. per 100 ml.); W.B.C., 6100 per c.mm.; E.S.R., 17 mm.; reticulocytes, 2·8 per cent; and platelets, 148,000 per c.mm. The peripheral blood contained occasional macrocytes, but was mostly hypochromic. There was increased iron in the marrow and sideroblasts were present. Serum iron was 200 and T.I.B.C., 285 µg. per 100 ml. The serum vitamin B_{12} was over 1000 pg. per ml., and FIGLU weakly positive, and a liver biopsy showed considerable haemosiderin.

She was seen next in 1969 because of dyspnoea. The haemoglobin was 60 per cent (8·7 g. per 100 ml.) and M.C.H.C., 30 per cent. Marrow smears again showed the presence of sideroblasts and siderocytes (*Fig.* 31). The red-cell fragility curve was normal. Serum iron was 210 µg. per

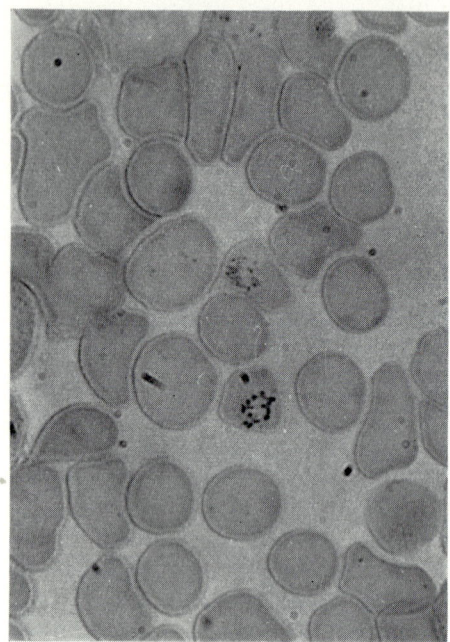

Fig. 31.—*Case* 2. Siderocytes in a case of sideroblastic anaemia of 21 years' duration. (Perls's stain × 1100.)

100 ml.; T.I.B.C., 255 µg. per 100 ml.; serum vitamin B_{12}, 400 pg. per ml.; and serum folate, 7·5 ng. per ml.

For 18 years this patient has been transfused at approximately yearly intervals. Features of a refractory sideroblastic anaemia are still present, although they cannot be entirely disentangled from complicating haemosiderosis.

THE INTERRELATION OF IRON, VITAMIN B_{12}, FOLIC ACID, AND ASCORBIC ACID (*Table XXII*)

The basic disorder in megaloblastic anaemia probably involves impaired production of folic-acid coenzymes. Vitamin-B_{12} participates in the production of these enzymes and in the control of their reduction. Ascorbic acid protects folic-acid reductase, and thereby preserves the coenzymes. Vitamin B_{12} also acts in the conversion of ribose to deoxyribose.

If pernicious anaemia patients are treated with folic acid there is initially a good reticulocyte and haemoglobin response, but when continued, central nervous complications arise, haematological relapse occurs, and the marrow becomes hypoplastic and partially megaloblastic. The picture is slowly reversed with vitamin B_{12}. However, when folic-acid treatment is coupled with small therapeutic doses of vitamin B_{12} the response is satisfactory although the serum vitamin-B_{12} level remains low. If, on the other hand, folic-acid deficiency megaloblastic anaemia is treated with vitamin B_{12} the reticulocyte and haemoglobin responses are well below the optimum. It would appear therefore that vitamin B_{12} plays an important role in the metabolism of folic acid (perhaps in the formation of folic-acid coenzymes), but that folic acid has little direct influence on vitamin-B_{12} metabolism (other than to aggravate a pre-existing deficiency).

Table XXII.—INTERRELATIONSHIPS BETWEEN IRON, ASCORBIC ACID, FOLIC ACID (FA), AND VITAMIN B_{12}

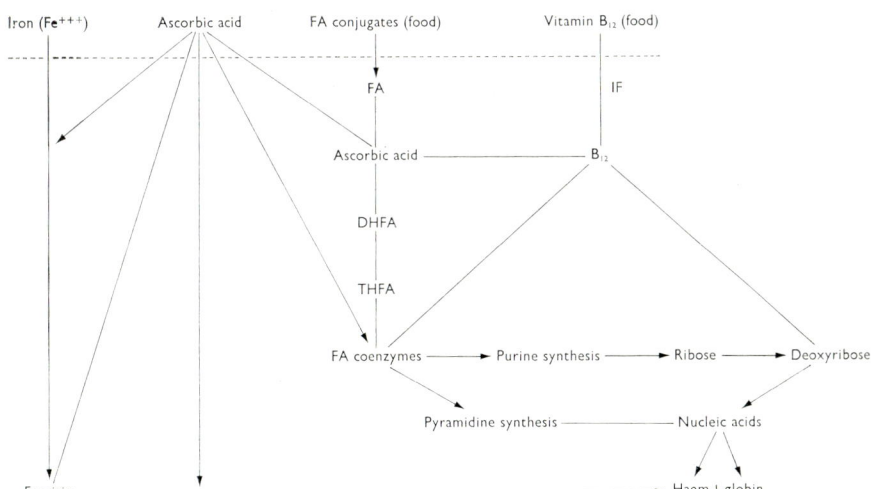

FA—Folic acid. DHFA—Dihydrofolic acid. THFA—Tetrahydrofolic acid. IF—Intrinsic factor.

Defective erythropoiesis from a deficiency of any of the haematinic factors often results in elevation of the serum level of one or more of the others. When the missing factor is given, and normal erythropoiesis returns, the other factors are utilized causing a fall in their serum level unless their intake is supplemented.

This inverse relationship is well seen in pure vitamin-B_{12} deficiency. Classically the serum-iron level is raised and saturation of transferrin increased. A level of serum iron above 150 μg. per 100 ml. and a saturation of more than 60 per cent may be obtained. The position is reversed with vitamin-B_{12} therapy.

Almost 50 per cent of the patients admitted to our unit are sideropenic. It is therefore not surprising that reciprocal changes in the levels of serum iron in vitamin B_{12} and folate deficiency are relatively unusual. This is illustrated in respect of iron and vitamin B_{12} in *Table XXIII.*

Sixty-eight per cent of those with a serum vitamin B_{12} below 111 pg. per ml. have a serum iron below 71 μg. per 100 ml. and 60·5 per cent of those with a level above 111 pg. per ml.

Of 176 patients with serum iron below 71 µg. per 100 ml., 34 (19 per cent) have a serum vitamin-B_{12} level below 111 pg. per ml.; whereas of 37 with a level of serum iron above 100 µg. per 100 ml., the corresponding number with a low serum vitamin B_{12} is 9 (24 per cent). In 11 patients with a serum vitamin B_{12} below 51 pg. per ml., 6 have a serum iron below 71 µg. per 100 ml. and only 1 above 150. Low

Table XXIII.—CHANGES IN SERUM VITAMIN-B_{12} LEVELS AND SERUM IRON

SERUM IRON (µg. per 100 ml.)	SERUM VITAMIN B_{12} (pg. per ml.)						
	0–20	21–50	51–80	81–110	111–150	151–300	301+
< 70	1	5	9	19	32	79	31
> 70	2	3	3	8	12	39	25
Total (268)	3	8	12	27	44	118	56

A further breakdown of this relationship is shown in *Table XXIV*.

Table XXIV.—RELATIONSHIP OF SERUM IRON AND VITAMIN-B_{12} LEVELS

SERUM VITAMIN B_{12} (pg. per ml.)	SERUM IRON (µg. per 100 ml.)							
	0–20	21–35	36–50	51–70	71–100	101–125	126–150	151+
0– 20	0	1	0	0	0	1	0	1
21– 50	0	1	1	3	2	1	0	0
51– 80	1	3	2	3	2	0	0	1
81–110	3	2	7	7	3	1	4	0
111–150	7	7	8	10	8	4	0	0
151–300	8	21	20	30	26	10	1	2
301+	4	4	7	16	14	6	3	2
Total (268)	23	39	45	69	55	23	8	6

serum levels of vitamin B_{12} are less significant in the elderly than similar levels in younger patients. Correlation analysis between serum vitamin B_{12} and serum iron in consecutive hospital admissions gave non-significant results in both sexes:—

	No.	r
Females	156	0·027
Males	29	−0·145

Folate deficiency anaemia shows a similar lack of relationship with iron.

When there is lone vitamin-B_{12} deficiency the serum-folate measurement may be 12–14 ng. per ml., but usually the level is below 3 ng. per ml. and the FIGLU excretion test often becomes positive. The giving of vitamin B_{12} may elevate the serum folate, possibly due to increased dietary intake from the improved appetite and general well-being.

When the anaemia is due to iron deficiency the interrelationship with vitamin B_{12} and folate depends on its aetiology. Defective absorption due to atrophic gastritis, whether primary or following partial gastrectomy, may later be associated with vitamin-B_{12} deficiency owing to loss of intrinsic factor. In these patients iron deficiency precedes the vitamin-B_{12} deficiency by a considerable period—perhaps 3 or 4 years or even longer. There is sometimes a low serum vitamin-B_{12} level that is corrected with iron therapy, suggesting that a failure of absorption has been reversed. Cox, Meynell, Gaddie, and Cooke (1959) compared 13 patients (4 over 60 years) who had iron-deficiency anaemia and a low serum vitamin B_{12}, with 12 whose vitamin-B_{12} levels were normal. All achieved satisfactory blood-levels on iron therapy alone, and the serum vitamin B_{12} returned to normal within 10 weeks, despite the fact that in 3 it was 30 pg. per ml. or less. Five patients with subnormal vitamin-B_{12} levels had had a partial gastrectomy. The haematological picture did not differ significantly in the two groups: the haemoglobin level was similar and all had hypochromia, but 2 patients with a low vitamin B_{12} had a macrocytic anaemia—they also responded to iron therapy.

Organ-specific antibody to gastric parietal cells is present in the serum of over 80 per cent of patients with pernicious anaemia and in 20 per cent of those with iron-deficiency anaemia, but in only 6 per cent of matched controls. This antibody nearly always indicates the presence of histamine-fast achlorhydria and if found in a patient with iron-deficiency anaemia, atrophic gastritis is invariably present. When iron-deficiency anaemia is associated with histamine-fast achlorhydria the chances of developing pernicious anaemia are 13 per cent and if, in addition, the antibody test is positive then the chances are 32 per cent (Dagg, Goldberg, Gibbs, and Anderson, 1966).

In folate-deficient megaloblastic anaemia folic-acid therapy may elevate the serum vitamin B_{12}. It has been noted (Cox and others, 1959) that where there is no depletion of vitamin B_{12}, its serum activity increases during blood regeneration induced by haemorrhage, folic acid, or iron therapy. Conversely, in uncomplicated pernicious anaemia the serum folate is normal or raised, but this does not exclude folate deficiency, because the red-cell folate level is often reduced and there may be increased excretion of FIGLU. The only entirely accurate way of diagnosing a combined vitamin-B_{12} and folate deficiency is by giving minimal therapeutic doses of both. Folate deficiency responds to 200 μg. of folic acid daily, whereas vitamin-B_{12} deficiency does not. A parenteral dose of 2–5 μg. of vitamin B_{12} daily will correct deficiency of this vitamin without any effect on folate deficiency. These therapeutic tests are seldom practicable in the elderly, although they remain the most accurate means of assessing combined deficiencies.

In elderly patients admitted to hospital a serum-iron level below 71 μg. per 100 ml. is obtained in 50 per cent, a serum vitamin B_{12} below 111 pg. per ml. in 20 per cent, and a folate below 6 ng. per ml. in 80 per cent so that various combinations of low levels can occur by chance. None of the levels is directly related to the presence or absence of anaemia, so care has to be taken to avoid overemphasizing the association between them when dealing with a particular patient.

REFERENCES

Anderson, F. W. (1967), *Practical Management of the Elderly*. Oxford: Blackwell.
Cox, E. V., Meynell, M. J., Cooke, W. T., and Gaddie, R. (1958), *Clin. Sci.*, **17**, 693.

Cox, E. V., Meynell, M. J., Gaddie, R., and Cooke, W. T. (1959), *Lancet*, **2**, 998.
Dacie, J. V., Smith, M. D., White, J. C., and Mollin, D. L. (1959), *Br. J. Haemat.*, **5**, 56.
Dagg, J. H., Goldberg, A., Gibbs, W. N., and Anderson, J. R. (1966), *Br. med. J.*, **2**, 619.
Damashek, W. (1965), *Br. J. Haemat.*, **11**, 52.
Goldberg, A. (1963), *Q. Jl Med.*, **32**, 51.
Herbert, V. (1968), *Blood*, **32**, 305.
Jacobs, A., and Cavill, I. (1968), *Br. J. Haemat.*, **14**, 291.
Kahn, S. B., and Brodsky, I. (1968), *Blood*, **31**, 55.
MacGibbon, B. H., and Mollin, D. L. (1965), *Br. J. Haemat.*, **11**, 59.
Mollin, D. L., and Hoffbrand, A. V. (1968), 'Sideroblastic Anaemia', in *Recent Advances in Clinical Pathology* (Ed. Dyke, S. C.), Ch. 17. London: Churchill.
Wintrobe, M. M. (1967), *Clinical Haematology*, 6th ed. London: Kimpton.

7

PREVENTION OF ANAEMIA

DEFICIENCY anaemias are largely preventable and if this could be achieved hospital admission would diminish, and a great deal of chronic ill health might be avoided.

The number and proportion of elderly people in the country is increasing; at present they comprise around 10–12 per cent of the general population, but in retirement areas and country districts the proportion is considerably higher, probably 25–30 per cent, whereas in newer industrial towns they amount to 8 per cent. Consequently, any preventive service must be based on the special requirements of the locality and be sufficiently elastic to allow variation in demand. An integrated service involves the participation of hospital doctors, local authority personnel, and family doctors, but a haphazard approach based on patient request is too erratic for any worth-while objective to be achieved. Preventive clinics would have to be supplemented by home visits to non-attenders, so that their general health and blood state could be ascertained. Further investigation could be performed either in the home, out-patients' department, or day unit of a hospital and appropriate therapy prescribed by the family doctor.

The prevalence of anaemia in general practice, hospitals, and localized communities has already been discussed (Chapter 1).

Many surveys have been carried out, but it is sometimes difficult to compare the findings because of the varying use of haematinics in different areas. Where the number of general practitioners is high relative to the population it is reasonable to assume that the prevalence of anaemia may be lower than in areas where the medical service is less satisfactory—other factors being equal. The frequency with which patients contact their doctor and the quality of the treatment given also vary. Some doctors prescribe vitamin-B_{12} injections and iron preparations as general tonics, and although unscientific it would be surprising if the onset of deficiency anaemia was not thereby prevented, or at least delayed. The higher incidence of anaemia in country districts compared with that in industrial towns could be related more to the doctor–patient relationship and the medical service given than to different dietary habits.

In a preventive programme it is necessary to pursue schemes of detection that can be widely applied. In the first instance it has to be decided whether all elderly persons should be assessed or only those with illnesses or symptoms; and then a method has to be formulated. Should they be seen at home? Is it feasible to request their attendance at a special clinic? What would be the refusal rate? Could other investigations be carried out simultaneously? In any programme it is obvious that the very old, the bedridden, and the immobile cannot be omitted.

These questions have been partly answered by the result of surveys carried out in South Wales and elsewhere.

Attendance at a *central clinic*: All female residents in an industrial area were visited and invited to attend (Elwood, Waters, Green, and Wood, 1967). Of 128 in the age-group 60–64, 19 (14·8 per cent) refused. All those with haemoglobin levels below 12 g. per 100 ml. were asked to supply three specimens of faeces for occult blood testing by the haematest method, but 17 per cent refused. The results of the tests were equivocal, and the authors felt that much work remained to be done to define positivity more clearly before relevance to a low haemoglobin level in the community could be accepted.

Assessment of *symptomatology* by *questionnaire*: Wood and Elwood (1966) studied the relationship between symptomatology and 'anaemia' in persons between the ages of 15 and 74 years living within a quarter of a mile of a local authority clinic. They were interviewed at home and invited to participate in a haematological investigation. Thirty per cent of those approached declined to take part, and home visits were necessary in 40 per cent of those who attended the clinic, either to retrieve questionnaires or to complete them. They concluded that a prevention programme should not be based on the presence or absence of symptoms. Dawson, Ogston, and Fullerton (1969) also demonstrated the unreliability of symptoms in assessing the severity or type of anaemia.

There are three principles inherent in any *preventive programme*:—

A. In the first instance it is essential that *prevention is worth while*. The deficiency anaemias lower vitality and when this occurs in an elderly person the impact can be considerable, not only on the patient but also on those whose services may then be required. The physical and mental health may deteriorate so gradually that anaemia of a severe degree may be present before medical attention is sought. By then it is possible that irreversible cellular changes have taken place. Frequently, there is accentuation or precipitation of organ weakness, so that congestive cardiac failure or uraemia may dominate the picture. Admission to hospital is often necessary and the preceding period of ill health may be extensive. The medicosocial problems that arise are troublesome. Financial outlay is considerable.

B. *The disease that is being prevented must be recognizable in its early stage.* Deviation from the normal should be distinct, but not necessarily abrupt. When we apply this reasoning to the deficiency anaemias we see that there is no clear-cut demarcation between blood normality and abnormality. It is still not known whether individual variation is of clinical significance. The difficulty lies in the fact that a slight lowering of the haemoglobin level need not be associated with specific symptoms although Beutler, Larsh, and Gurney (1960) suggested that fatigue and lack of concentration could result from insufficient iron at cellular level, and Stafford (1965) agreed. Nevertheless Wood and Elwood (1966) failed to find a statistical correlation with fatigue, faintness, palpitations, pain in the chest, swelling of ankles, breathlessness, pallor, lack of concentration, dizziness, headache, or irritability. Absence of symptoms, however, is not synonymous with absence of disease, because many illnesses are symptomless in their early stages. A haemoglobin level of 80 per cent could be normal for one person and abnormal for another, depending on its duration and on whether it could be elevated by therapy. Both persons may be symptom-free at the time, but it is possible for one to progress imperceptibly to frank anaemia and for the haemoglobin concentration of the other to remain stationary.

If therapy is prescribed it has to be accepted that either a normal state or one of early anaemia might be treated. Though unnecessary in one it would be beneficial in the other, as a more advanced stage would be prevented.

The doctor trained in clinical medicine is more inclined to ascertain the existence of definite anaemia before considering the need for treatment, but the discipline of preventive medicine considers it permissible, or preferable, to treat when there is a reasonable chance that early pathology exists. Fundamentally, the point at issue is what proportion of persons with a given haemoglobin level develops definite anaemia within a relatively short period. It appears from analysis of survey material that in general the lower limit of normality is around 85 per cent (12·5 g. per 100 ml.) If this is accepted, then in the average person a haemoglobin of 80 per cent (11·6 g. per 100 ml.) denotes early anaemia. Exceptional cases cannot easily be catered for in a programme of this kind, although it would be possible to apply different criteria where necessary.

The progress of the deficiency anaemias in their early stage may be so slow that subjective phenomena can be overlooked, particularly in the elderly, because so many of their disabilities are ascribed to the ageing process. We have frequently been impressed with the improvement that occurs in 'symptomless' persons when haematinics are prescribed. Iron depletion precedes iron-deficiency anaemia, and sideropenia may be present when the haemoglobin level is 100 per cent (14·5 g. per 100 ml.). There is evidence to suggest that iron therapy is still beneficial and when treatment is omitted several develop iron-deficiency anaemia within a few months.

The presence or absence of symptoms is of no particular importance, either in the detection of anaemia, or indeed in the decision regarding the need for treatment. Of greater relevance is the argument that perhaps all elderly persons should receive iron therapy intermittently, irrespective of their haemoglobin level, or, if this is not acceptable, that attention be given to the iron content of the body rather than to the blood state.

C. That the *method of detection is simple*, accurate, and generally applicable.

The simplest and the easiest method is the age-old examination of the mucous membrane, but it gives only an approximate estimate. Analysis of the clinical findings in 1000 consecutive home visits at the request of family doctors showed that pallor of the mucous membrane was present in 56 of 138 (40 per cent) persons living alone, and in 221 of 862 (25 per cent) of those living with husband, friend, or member of the family. There were 47 whose daily activities were severely limited although still living alone. Twenty-two of them (47 per cent) were clinically anaemic.

McAlpine and Douglas (1957) compared the clinical assessment of haemoglobin concentration with that obtained by estimation of capillary blood using a photo-electric colorimeter. Two hundred consecutive new patients were investigated, but their ages were not stated. They showed that when conjunctival estimates of 90 per cent haemoglobin was made, 29–36 per cent had a true haemoglobin value of 80 per cent or less, but when a clinical estimate of a haemoglobin value of 60 per cent was made, 94–95 per cent of patients did in fact have a true haemoglobin level of 80 per cent or less.

Parsons, Withey, and Kilpatrick (1965) came to a similar conclusion. Twenty-five of 38 pale subjects had a haemoglobin level of 80 per cent or over, while of 24 with a haemoglobin of less than 80 per cent, only 13 were considered to be pale.

It is thus apparent that if anaemia is to be detected in its early stage clinical assessment is relatively valueless.

The *method* whereby the haemoglobin level is measured has been simplified since battery-operated apparatus has become available. Accurate results can be obtained using a drop of whole blood. Repeated checking of such apparatus is necessary. Most pathology departments in the United Kingdom now have an 'open-door' policy to requests from family doctors. When convenient more use might be made of such facilities.

PRIMARY PREVENTION

A distinction should be made between prevention and treatment of the early case. The first depends on supplying haematinic factors when the blood state is normal, and the second on regular blood examination followed by treatment when anaemia first appears. One is based on the principle that a practice which benefits the majority is justified, and the other questions the wisdom of this, because in the minority the recognition of treatable conditions might be delayed.

In a survey of the diet of elderly women living alone by Exton-Smith and Stanton (1965) it was noted that the percentage fall in intake for subjects in their late seventies was as follows: calories, 19 per cent; proteins, 24 per cent; fat, 30 per cent; carbohydrates, 8 per cent; calcium, 18 per cent; iron, 29 per cent; and vitamin C, 31 per cent. Almost three-quarters of the women studied had no particular interest in either food or cooking. Kataria and Rao (1968) decided that of 105 elderly people living alone or with others, the food intake was 'poor' in 12·3 per cent and 'very poor' in 14·3 per cent. Davies, Jacobs, and Rivlin (1967) in a study of 187 healthy persons aged 20–69 years stated, 'the total amount of iron in the diet may be more important at levels of intake below 6 mg. daily, and in individuals with impaired absorption'. Townsend and Wedderbrun (1965) concluded that 600,000–700,000 old people were living below acceptable economic levels. Moreover, many are not aware of the domiciliary service and the financial aid that they are entitled to. In one area, for instance, '15 per cent of the pensioners in poverty were ignorant of their eligibility for a supplementary pension and 33 per cent of those who knew still failed to claim, often out of a mistaken sense of pride' (Thomas, 1969).

From these surveys, and others, it appears that a combination of sociological, physiological, and emotional factors have to be combated. They are all relevant in the prevention of anaemia. Extension of the 'meals-on-wheels' service is the most practical method of ensuring that the elderly receive an adequate intake of iron, vitamin B_{12}, and folate. Vitamin C and other vitamins are also required. People who live alone, or are depressed, or whose mobility is limited, need special attention.

It has been suggested that iron preparations, and vitamin-B_{12} injections at monthly intervals, could be given prophylactically. Perhaps the benefit to many would be considerable, but such a practice would complicate the management of anaemia and other illnesses. The diagnosis of neoplastic lesions could be delayed, many general diseases would not be treated, and, as the majority of people do not become anaemic, the drugs would be wasted.

Legislation specifies that white flour for the baking of bread contains 1·65 mg. of iron per 100 g. Normally the preparation used is ferrum redactum. Elwood (1963) indicated not only that this was poorly absorbed but that increasing it nearly forty-fold had little effect on its efficacy. There is no evidence as yet that iron-enriched bread exerts a measurable prophylactic influence on the development of anaemia.

Maddison (1963), in an account of his preventive medical clinic for elderly people at Teddington, Middlesex, stated that a third of those attending had a haemoglobin level below 85 per cent and because of this he added 35 mg. iron, 4 mg. of folic acid, 50 μg. vitamin B_{12}, and 50 mg. of ascorbic acid to a powder which he and his colleagues had devised. Medicaments were also included to combat other diseases of the elderly, such as osteoporosis, and the powder was dissolved if need be in maize oil and hot water and a flavouring agent added. All subjects were assessed clinically and it was claimed that improvement in general health was considerable. Hypochromic anaemia responded satisfactorily. The general preventive approach was universally applied and it was combined with as much investigation as was feasible.

There are possible objections to the inclusion of vitamin B_{12} and folic acid. In the absence of 'intrinsic factor', vitamin B_{12} would not be absorbed, in which case folic acid given alone could precipitate neurological disease. Measurement of the serum vitamin-B_{12} level at the first visit would not eliminate this risk. A more physiological quantity of folate would be preferable.

The addition of iron preparations would probably benefit about 50 per cent of those attending, but if the diet is adequate sufficient iron is already being supplied for normal erythropoiesis. If anaemia develops there must be another cause—the iron is being lost, is not being absorbed, or is not being utilized—and we believe that investigation is then necessary so that future management is clarified. When the intake is insufficient, due perhaps to apathy or disease, the addition of iron to ensure a normal daily intake of 10 to 12 mg. seems logical. The giving of a larger supplement is open to the objection that the patient is receiving 'blind' treatment. Supplementation with ascorbic acid is different, as many cooking procedures destroy the vitamin.

The incidence and the degree of malabsorption in the elderly are not known. Furthermore, the quantity of iron lost in the stool and urine may be greater than in young subjects. Perhaps the reserve absorptive power of the gastro-intestinal tract is diminished. Elucidation of these problems could well influence the general application of preventive measures.

EARLY DETECTION

There is increasing awareness that many diseases are being recognized too late for treatment to be successful. In others, early detection has little advantage with our present knowledge as the disease process can neither be arrested nor reversed. The deficiency anaemias are in a special category. Not only is treatment successful in the early stages, but the result is often satisfactory when the disorder is advanced. Moreover, correct treatment can prevent recurrence. But although mortality is relatively low the morbidity is high.

Early detection need not be unduly difficult. Nurses already visit the elderly in their homes and family doctors are consulted when illness supervenes. Moreover, registers are being compiled. Further machinery is unnecessary.

In the average healthy person yearly assessment would probably suffice, but special risk cases would need more attention. If these alone were supervised the impact could be considerable.

SPECIAL RISK CASES

A. SOCIAL DIFFICULTIES

Loneliness.—About 20 per cent of elderly women live alone and their social circumstances are often distressing. The number of men living on their own is less, but neglect is usually greater unless friends and neighbours help. Semmence (1959) found that women living alone had significantly lower haemoglobin levels than the others, and Hobson and Blackburn (1953) obtained similar results in men.

Decreased Mobility.—Difficulties in cooking and in shopping are almost insurmountable in some instances, despite denial by many who are inordinately independent. Not only may iron and vitamin-C intake be insufficient, but folic-acid deficiency may arise in those with physical disability, or illness and disinterest in food (Batata, Spray, Bolton, Higgins, and Wollner, 1967).

Incompatibility.—The nature of the sociological factors involved is irrelevant in the context of anaemia, because the end-result is the same. Disharmony leads to apathy, obstructive behaviour, antisocial habits, depression, and mental confusion. Meals are neglected and anaemia develops from malnutrition.

It is surprising how often anaemia is overlooked and allowed to progress when every effort is being made to cope with the social difficulties. The frequency with which anaemia and other treatable conditions are discovered when these patients are admitted to hospital emphasizes the close association that exists between clinical and social medicine. Repeated clinical assessment, including examination of the blood, is essential.

B. MENTAL DISORDER

Anaemia may cause or aggravate cerebral disturbance.

In a preventive programme it is visualized that persons loosely termed 'senile' or 'atherosclerotic' would be assessed periodically. Although these terms defy definition they are still commonly used. By and large they are people who are becoming forgetful, disinterested, garrulous, and sometimes confused. If such a programme were conscientiously pursued it is possible that the mental faculties of many would be preserved for longer than at present.

C. GENERAL DISEASE

Gastro-intestinal Disturbance and Surgery.—When symptoms suggest the presence of peptic ulceration or neoplasm hospital investigation is usually carried out, but long-term follow-up is necessary and this is not possible in hospital departments. Gastric herniation is in a similar category. Anaemia tends to develop or to recur. Edentulous persons have digestive problems and often dietary deficiency results. When partial gastrectomy, or ileal resection, has been performed malabsorption may cause anaemia many years later. Those who have undergone partial gastrectomy are particularly vulnerable and often need regular supplementation with iron, and sometimes vitamin B_{12}. However, gastro-enterostomy and vagotomy may also produce late effects (Wheldon, Venables, and Johnston 1970). According to Davies, Jacobs, and Rivlin (1967), 'it seems likely that in a normal population iron loss from the body is the most important determinant of iron status'.

In *chronic pulmonary disease* the haemoglobin level should be raised due to the erythropoietic effect of hypoxia. Anaemia that would be regarded as mild in a normal person could well be severe in a chronic bronchitic.

Congestive failure in the elderly poses a problem both in treatment and in management, but it is always beneficial to maintain a high haemoglobin level in order that the myocardium obtains sufficient oxygen. Anaemia, even of a mild degree, can precipitate failure when the cardiac reserve is low.

Neurological disease has a complex association with the anaemias. Vitamin-B_{12} deficiency can cause demyelination even when anaemia is minimal or absent, and Hodgkin's disease or leukaemia can present neurologically. The giving of anti-convulsant drugs in epileptics can lead to folate deficiency. When a patient with any chronic neurological disease is anaemic the cause is more likely to be a deficiency of iron/and or folate than of vitamin B_{12}. Long-term hemiplegics require special attention, particularly if they are becoming confused.

Patients with *rheumatoid arthritis* are prone to develop anaemia. Diminished mobility, resulting in malnutrition, is an important cause, but there are others, such as persistent occult blood loss in the stools from ingestion of aspirin, possibly decreased ileal absorption, and ill-understood alteration in iron metabolism. Anaemia causes fatigue which accentuates the disability, hampers rehabilitation, and reduces the desire and the ability to withstand the affliction.

Many *dermatological diseases* are associated with malabsorption. Psychological disturbances are common in these patients and the development of anaemia makes them more pronounced.

D. Previous Anaemia

Any patient who has been anaemic on a previous occasion—from whatever cause—requires regular supervision. Data from general practice, random surveys, and hospitals indicate that there is a tendency for anaemia to recur (Waters, Withey, Kilpatrick, Wood, and Abernethy, 1969).

Williamson (1967), in a discussion on the detection of disease in clinical geriatrics, suggested that it was logical to single out for special care: those living alone, those recently bereaved, those with significant locomotor difficulties, those showing evidence of mental impairment, and those recently discharged from hospital. He postulated that the most obvious person to screen the patients in such a programme was the health visitor, because of her nursing and social training.

MANAGEMENT

Having discovered a person with a haemoglobin level of 80 per cent or below the question of management arises. Presumably, in most instances, referral to the family doctor would be necessary and thereafter the treatment adopted would depend on the circumstances.

The following principles apply:—

1. A general history and examination should be augmented by inquiry into the diet and the social environment.

2. A report on a blood-film examination would be necessary.

3. If hypochromia is present iron therapy is indicated. The need for further investigation at this stage must be left to clinical judgement. Testing of the stools for occult blood should be practised more often than at present, but, on the other hand, too much reliance should not be routinely placed on the result as the test is very sensitive. If repeatedly positive, barium study of the gastro-intestinal tract is mandatory. Indiscriminate therapeutic use of iron should be guarded against (Jacobs, Kilpatrick, and Withey, 1965).

4. When the blood-picture is normochromic or macrocytic, serum levels of iron, vitamin B_{12}, and folate should be obtained.

5. A better liaison should develop between family and hospital doctors in the management of the early stages of anaemia, and local arrangements modified accordingly. Advice from physicians, pathologists, and haematologists should be freely available and perhaps special out-patients' clinics held.

6. The present attitude that mild anaemia need not be treated has to be changed if severe anaemia is to be prevented.

There are two aspects which merit further discussion.

Presence of a Neoplasm

Occult disease and multiple pathology are common in the elderly with the result that numerous investigations may be necessary. Many are time consuming and, moreover, may have to be repeated, because negative findings do not exclude the presence of disease. Carcinoma is primarily a disease of the elderly and the gastro-intestinal tract is a frequent site. McKeown (1965) in an analysis of 1500 autopsy results in patients over the age of 70 years reported an incidence of 3·6 per cent for carcinoma of the stomach: one-third had not been diagnosed prior to death. Carcinoma of the colon was slightly more common (5·5 per cent).

The fear that routine treatment of mild iron-deficiency anaemia might delay the diagnosis of neoplastic disease, particularly of the colon, is justified, but the danger could be minimized if more attention were given to occult blood testing of the stools, to follow-up of the haemoglobin level, to weight-loss, and to the development or persistence of symptoms.

Routine periodic health check-ups are important in the wider concept of preventive medicine, but become more complex and difficult to perform as age advances. Thorough check-ups would almost certainly reveal the need for increasing the number of investigations required rather than reducing them. Such an approach is not feasible at present, other than in those who are becoming incapacitated or who require considerable social support to remain in the community.

Measurement of Serum Levels

Knowledge of the serum levels of the major haematinic factors is invaluable in the management of anaemia, as reduction occurs before anaemia appears. Therefore, if the information were available and correct medication given, deficiency anaemia would not develop—provided follow-up was adequate. Unfortunately, interpretation is often difficult because of the interrelationship between the factors. Venous blood is required and a considerable expansion of laboratory facilities would be necessary for these to be done routinely, but it is possible that new methods may be discovered that will be more easily applicable. Until then estimation of serum levels should be reserved for special cases. When early anaemia is present—particularly if iron resistant—serum levels should be measured if it is intended to prescribe vitamin B_{12} or folate; but at this stage clinical judgement may indicate that other investigations, such as E.S.R., blood-urea, or barium meal, may be more appropriate. The health of the individual as a whole remains the main concern.

REFERENCES

BATATA, M., SPRAY, G. H., BOLTON, F. G., HIGGINS, G., and WOLLNER, C. (1967), *Br. med. J.*, **2**, 667.
BEUTLER, E., LARSH, S. E., and GURNEY, C. W. (1960), *Ann. intern. Med.*, **52**, 378.
DAVIES, R. H., JACOBS, A., and RIVLIN, R. (1967), *Br. med. J.*, **2**, 711.
DAWSON, A. A., OGSTON, D., and FULLERTON, H. W. (1969), *Ibid.*, **3**, 436.
ELWOOD, P. C. (1963), *Ibid.*, **1**, 224.
— — WATERS, W. E., GREEN, W. J., and WOOD, M. M. (1967), *Ibid.*, **4**, 714.
EXTON-SMITH, A. N., and STANTON, B. R. (1965), *Investigations into the Dietary of Elderly Women living alone*. King Edward's Hospital Fund for London.
HOBSON, W., and BLACKBURN, E. K. (1953), *Br. med. J.*, **1**, 647.
JACOBS, A., KILPATRICK, G. S., and WITHEY, J. L. (1965), *Post-grad. med. J.*, **41**, 418.
KATARIA, M. S., and RAO, D. B. (1968), *Br. J. geront. Pract.*, **5**, 1, 235.
McALPINE, S. G., and DOUGLAS, A. S. (1957), *Br. med. J.*, **2**, 983.
McKEOWN, F. (1965), *Pathology of the Aged*. London: Butterworths.
MADDISON, J. (1963), *How to Keep Old Folks Young*. County Council Teddington, Middlesex.
PARSONS, P. L., WITHEY, J. L., and KILPATRICK, G. S. (1965), *Practitioner*, **195**, 656.
SEMMENCE, A. (1959), *Br. med. J.*, **2**, 1153.
STAFFORD, J. L. (1965), *Ann. R. Coll. Surg.*, **36**, 280.
THOMAS, R. G. (1969), *Geront. clin.*, **11**, 321.
TOWNSEND, P., and WEDDERBRUN, D. (1965), *The Aged in the Welfare State*. London: Bell.
WATERS, W. W., WITHEY, J. L., KILPATRICK, G. S., WOOD, P. H. N., and ABERNETHY, M. (1969), *Br. med. J.*, **4**, 761.
WHELDON, E. J., VENABLES, C. W., and JOHNSTON, I. D. A. (1970), *Lancet*, **1**, 437.
WILLIAMSON, J. (1967), *Geront. clin.*, **9**, 236.
WOOD, M. M., and ELWOOD, P. C. (1966), *Br. J. prev. soc. Med.*, **20**, 117.

8

TUMOURS OF LYMPHOID TISSUES

CLASSIFICATION

THERE are many classifications of lymphoid tumours, but in complicated schemes the fact that intermediate forms are common and that a variety of histological patterns may be seen within the same tumour is ignored. Therefore, the following simple scheme is proposed and further subdivisions discussed later.

Cell Type.—
    Lymphocyte
        Lymphosarcoma
        Follicular lymphoma
    Reticulum cell or histiocyte
        Reticulum-cell sarcoma
        Histiocytosis
        Eosinophilic granuloma
    Mixed
        Hodgkin's disease
        Reticular lymphoma
    Anaplastic
        Sarcoma

INCIDENCE

Primary lymphoid tissue tumours (excluding multiple myeloma) showed a registration rate of 100 per million population in South Wales during 1961–4. This compared with 106 for leukaemia. Robb-Smith (1947) made a 6-year survey of lymphoid tumours in Oxfordshire and found an incidence of 47·5 per million as against 36·3 for all types of leukaemia.

Lumb (1954), from a total of 410 cases at the Westminster Hospital, gave the following relative proportions:—

	Per cent
Hodgkin's disease	46·1
Lymphosarcoma	19·2
Anaplastic sarcoma	16·9
Follicular lymphoma	7·1
Reticulum-cell sarcoma	5·6
Reticular lymphoma	5·1

MacMahon (1966) pointed out that in view of the long survival of some patients with Hodgkin's disease the incidence rates were higher than mortality-rates. The annual death-rate in the United States between 1958 and 1962 was 23 per million for white males, and 13 per million for white females. A 10-cities' survey in the United States in 1947 gave incidence rates of 35 per million and 26 per million, respectively.

Between 1923–7 and 1948–51 there was a considerable increase in the mortality-rates attributed to Hodgkin's disease in the United States (Shimkin, 1955). The figures for England and Wales show a steadily rising rate since 1911:—

Average Annual Death-rates per Million Population England and Wales

Years	> 50 Years of Age		All Ages	
	Male	Female	Male	Female
1911–15	20·8	11·2	11·3	5·8
1926–30	29·0	17·4	15·6	8·0
1941–5	32·5	17·9	17·1	8·8
1956–60	43·0	24·0	21·8	11·2

The rate in the 0–14-year age-group showed a decline in the United States as well as in England and Wales, so that the increase in the adult and elderly was disproportionate.

AGE DISTRIBUTION

The incidence of lymphoid tissue tumours increases with age. The South Wales rate of registration per million population for 1961–5 is shown in *Table XXV*.

Table XXV.—Rate of Registration of Lymphoid-tissue Tumours in South Wales—per Million Population per Annum

Age (years)	0–14		15–24		25–34		35–44		45–54		55–64		65–74		75+	
Sex	M.	F.	M.	F.	M.	F.	M.	F.	M.	F.	M.	F.	M.	F.	M.	F.
Lymphosarcoma reticulo-sarcoma	12	9	7	11	11	9	18	10	23	18	60	52	112	50	135	35
Hodgkin's disease	10	2	22	22	37	11	32	10	27	12	58	25	39	35	71	50
Other forms	—	1	3	1	5	1	1	1	7	7	12	6	3	10	26	8
Multiple myeloma	—	—	—	1	1	—	8	—	18	12	53	45	34	56	39	38

Most series show a steadily increasing incidence of lymphosarcoma with age. Thus, in Lumb's series, 54·4 per cent were over 50 years. Hodgkin's disease is often claimed to be different in that the peak incidence lies between 20 and 40 years. Lumb, for instance, found 38·9 per cent to be between 20 and 30 years. The South Wales figures do not agree. They showed a rising registration rate above 50 years with the maximum over 75 years. There was also an earlier peak at 25–35 years although the incidence was only half that seen in persons over 75 years (*Fig.* 32).

Several series have shown that age-incidence curves of Hodgkin's disease are bimodal (Dorken, 1960, Clemmeson, 1965). MacMahon (1957) showed that age might help in distinguishing two forms of the disease. He suggested that in the elderly it behaved as a neoplasm, whereas in young adults there were several features which were more suggestive of an inflammatory process. MacMahon summarized the age incidence in five series (a total of 1992 patients) and found that the age at onset was 40 or above in 64·5 per cent. He also found that reticulum-cell sarcoma did not show the bimodality which he found in Hodgkin's disease, but rather a progressive rise with age. In fact both conditions resemble each other in many respects in the elderly (*Fig.* 33).

Follicular lymphoma has a peak incidence between 25 and 40 years, but is not uncommon in the elderly. Indeed, contrary to the generally held view, Lumb's 1954 series showed an increasing incidence in the older age-groups.

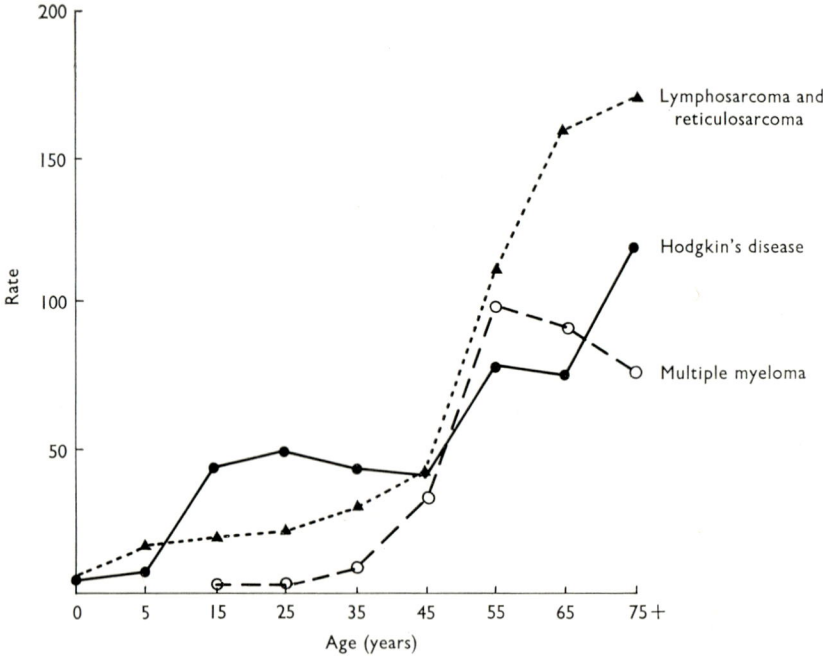

Fig. 32.—South Wales registration rates per million of population, 1961–5 (both sexes).

Cole, MacMahon, and Aisenberg (1968) studied the regional variation of mortality by age within the United States. They found that the mortality among the middle-aged and elderly showed no regional variation, but that of young adults in eleven contiguous southern states was half that in the remainder of the country. They suggested that these findings supported a 'two-disease' hypothesis. The mortality-rate in the elderly was higher than in any other country, but the rates in young adults were lower than those found elsewhere. Japan has the expected peak in the elderly, but the disease is almost never found in young adults.

SEX INCIDENCE

Lymphoid tumours are in general twice as common in males as in females, although this varies depending on the type of tumour and age distribution. MacMahon (1957) found that the male preponderance in Hodgkin's disease in Brooklyn increased with age, but he also suggested that the interpretation was complicated by the fact that the life expectancy for females with Hodgkin's disease was longer than that in males. There is also a sex difference in the distribution of the various histological types. The South Wales figures do not show an increasing incidence in elderly men, but rather the reverse. They resemble the data given by Shimkin (1955) from the United States who found the greatest male preponderance to be in the age-group 5–14 years, with a lesser peak at 45–54 years. Of the last 30

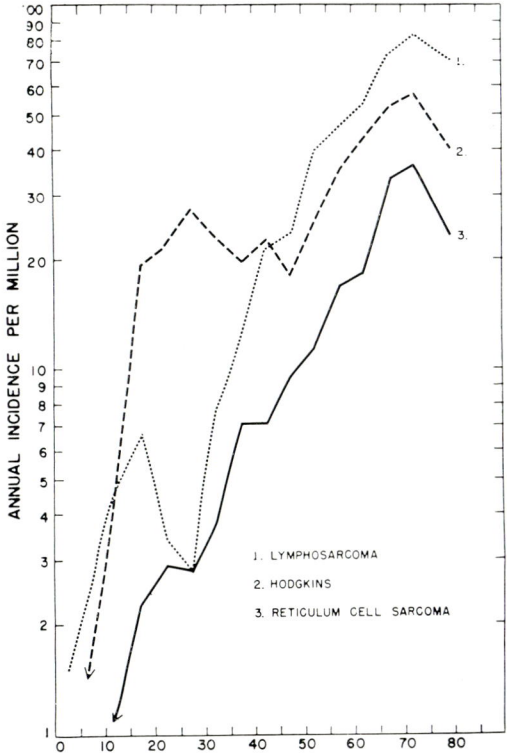

Fig. 33.—Age-specific incidence rates of Hodgkin's disease, lymphosarcoma, and reticulum-cell sarcoma, Brooklyn, 1943–52. (*With acknowledgements to MacMahon and the Editor, 'Cancer Research'.*)

patients with histologically confirmed malignant lymphoma in our hospital 23 were men.

Keller, Kaplan, Lukes, and Rappaport (1968) noted that the nodular sclerosing variety of Hodgkin's disease was twice as common in females as in males, whereas the mixed cellular type was seen twice as often in males.

LYMPHOSARCOMA

Any group of lymph-nodes may be involved in lymphosarcoma. The retroperitoneal and mesenteric groups are most commonly affected, although the superficial nodes usually attract attention. The disease is multicentric.

An affected node shows a loss of the normal follicular pattern and replacement by a sheet of lymphocytic cells. Occasionally the follicular pattern is partially preserved, so that this feature should not eliminate the diagnosis. Connective tissue is scanty.

Two main types of lymphosarcoma occur. In one the neoplastic lymphocytes are of the small-cell variety differing little from normal lymphocytes (lymphocytic lymphosarcoma), and in the other they appear large and immature (lymphoblastic lymphosarcoma). The former is the characteristic type found in the elderly. In the latter there is a greater degree of pleomorphism, with multinucleate cells and frequent mitoses.

Lymphosarcomatous infiltration may be found in many organs other than lymph-nodes, for example, gastro-intestinal tract, spleen, liver, testis, breast, tonsil, pharynx, and ovary. Cutaneous infiltration produces one type of mycosis fungoides. A more localized form of the disease can occur in the rectum.

Lymphosarcoma and chronic lymphatic leukaemia can be regarded as different manifestations of lymphocytic neoplasm. In fact lymphatic leukaemia develops in 30–40 per cent of cases. The histological appearances in the viscera in chronic lymphatic leukaemia and lymphosarcoma are identical.

CLINICAL FEATURES

The patient is usually ill with loss of weight and lassitude, but sometimes the sole complaint is of the presence of an enlarging node or group of nodes, which are often painful. The cervical, supraclavicular, axillary, and inguinal regions are common sites, but involvement of the mediastinal and intra-abdominal nodes often coexists. There may be splenomegaly and hepatomegaly with ascites or jaundice. Fever may be present and usually the patient becomes cachectic within a few months. The glands rapidly coalesce and become adherent to adjacent tissues.

Occasionally the course is slower and there is no apparent progression for several years. These are often instances of lymphosarcoma arising in a follicular lymphoma, but in others the initial histological picture is that of classic lymphosarcoma.

The blood-picture may be normal, although usually there is moderate anaemia. Frequently this is associated with chronic lymphatic leukaemia.

Case 1.—A female, aged 75, was admitted with congestive failure of 2 months' duration. On examination she was found to have generalized lymphadenopathy, ascites, hepatomegaly (7 cm.), and splenomegaly (10 cm.). X-ray of chest showed no evidence of mediastinal involvement. Her Hb was 70 per cent; W.B.C., 12,000 (polymorphs, 27 per cent; lymphocytes, 64 per cent; eosinophils, 7 per cent; smear, 2 per cent) and many of the lymphocytes appeared abnormal. Her E.S.R. was 10 mm. in the first hour and platelets, 135,000 c.cm. Examination of the marrow smear showed that 65 per cent of the cells were of lymphocytic origin (mainly immature lymphocytes). Lymph-node histology was that of a lymphosarcoma. Her serum proteins were 5·9 g. per 100 ml., and there were no paraproteins. Her Hb fell to 59 per cent and W.B.C. to 4600 (abnormal lymphocytes < 58 per cent). Temperature was 99° F.

Cyclophosphamide, 50 mg. t.d.s., was given and 2 months later her Hb was 72 per cent and W.B.C., 9000 (polymorphs, 54 per cent; lymphocytes, 39 per cent; monocytes, 6 per cent; eosinophils, 1 per cent). E.S.R. was now 4 mm. in the first hour. There were no enlarged nodes in axillae or right groin, although a few small ones were still palpable in the left groin. These were treated with X-ray therapy. She became symptom free and was discharged 3 months after admission. Liver and spleen were no longer palpable.

Seven months later she was readmitted with generalized painful lymphadenopathy and severe intractable pruritus. Both spleen and liver were enlarged. Her Hb was 59 per cent and W.B.C.,

21,600 (polymorphs, 22 per cent; lymphocytes, 54 per cent; smear, 18 per cent; monocytes, 3 per cent; myelocytes, 2 per cent; myeloblasts, 1 per cent). There was no response to cyclophosphamide therapy and she died 2 months after admission. The known duration of her illness was 12 months.

TREATMENT

There is no cure and the most that can be claimed is that some of the symptoms can be relieved, and that occasionally life is extended from a few months to a year or two. Surgical excision of a localized group of nodes is rarely beneficial. X-ray therapy of nodes and spleen may cause rapid regression, but recurrence is usual with diminution of effectiveness with the second application. Chemotherapy is often the only means whereby any worth-while improvement can be achieved, and in some patients the initial response is surprisingly good. Unfortunately, the disease then appears elsewhere or returns in a generalized form. Corticosteroids may control the anaemia and are sometimes indicated even when there is no evidence of overt haemolysis. Folate or iron deficiency may respond to appropriate therapy. Pruritus can be intractable, although tranquillizers may be partially effective. Pain is sometimes severe enough to cause insomnia.

Associated lymphatic leukaemia, when present, often responds temporarily to chemotherapy, but the blood abnormality is a secondary phenomenon and the underlying disease is not greatly affected.

RETICULUM-CELL SARCOMA

The diagnosis of reticulum-cell sarcoma is often more difficult than it is with other types of malignant lymphoma, due to the unsolved debate on the nature and origin of the neoplastic reticulum cell, and the interpretation of the varying histological pattern. However, this type is frequently seen in the elderly although it may be described as lymphosarcoma, reticulum-cell sarcoma, or merely anaplastic sarcoma.

Lymph-nodes, and almost any other site, may be involved. It does, however, show an unusual predilection for bone. Lumb in his series of 20 patients found a primary bone tumour in 3 (15 per cent). They all subsequently developed widespread reticulum-cell sarcoma.

The neoplastic cells are large (12–20 μ diameter) with large nuclei containing well-defined nucleoli. Silver impregnation methods show numerous reticulin fibres between the cells. However, this feature, as Willis (1967) emphasized, is not specific, as 'reticulin' is merely a form of collagen and may be found in other neoplastic or non-neoplastic conditions.

Sometimes it spreads in stages from a primary site, but in others dissemination is so rapid that it is probably multicentric.

CLINICAL FEATURES

It resembles Hodgkin's disease when superficial lymph-nodes are involved. Indeed, on rare occasions reticulum-cell sarcoma can develop in Hodgkin's disease tissue. Widespread dissemination gives rise to a picture similar to lymphosarcoma, except that the peripheral blood may show a monocytic rather than a lymphocytic leukaemia.

FOLLICULAR LYMPHOMA
(*Brill-Symmers Disease*)

This disease is largely confined initially to the lymph-nodes and spleen, which is palpable in approximately 40 per cent of cases.

The lymph-nodes are discrete and may be greatly enlarged. Naked-eye examination of stained sections with a hand lens may almost suffice to make the diagnosis. Large irregular follicles can be seen. These consist of closely packed lymphocytes and lymphoblasts. The surrounding lymph-node structures are compressed, and frequently there is an intervening 'split' in the tissue section. Reticulin stains help to show the follicular pattern and adjacent connective-tissue compression. Large, pale cells occur in the follicular centres. Mitoses are infrequent, unlike reactive Flemming centres, where mitoses are numerous. A similar appearance is found in the spleen.

As the disease progresses it metastasizes, for example, to the lung, kidney, liver, and bone. The same histological picture may be reproduced, but more commonly the picture becomes more anaplastic and pleomorphic so that the end-result is indistinguishable from lymphosarcoma, Hodgkin's disease, or simply anaplastic sarcoma.

CLINICAL FEATURES

Localized superficial adenopathy or splenomegaly may be discovered during routine examination of a patient with unrelated symptoms. Sometimes there is generalized weakness or abdominal discomfort. Occasionally an enlarged lymph-node presses on neighbouring structures causing appropriate symptoms and signs, but diagnosis is often difficult largely because the condition is unsuspected or is confused with a neoplasm or another reticulosis.

Case 2.—A female, aged 78, who was crippled with rheumatoid arthritis for 10 years, developed bilateral progressive pitting oedema of the legs, consistent with inferior vena cava thrombosis. There was no adenopathy or splenomegaly. Mild, intermittent iron-deficiency anaemia had been noted. The W.B.C. and platelets were normal, but E.S.R. had been elevated for 2 years (90–100 mm. in the first hour—Westergren). The Rose-Waaler was positive. No L.E. phenomenon was demonstrated. Her arthritis was clinically inactive and no abnormal serum proteins were detected. No abdominal mass was felt and there was no loss of weight. She had occasional mild pyrexia which was thought to be due to urinary infection.

At necropsy she had a follicular lymphoma adjacent to the descending aorta pressing on the inferior vena cava. There was no evidence of dissemination.

The disease may be confined to one group of lymph-nodes for months or even years, but eventually spreads throughout the lymphoreticular system. The involved nodes are generally discrete and often smaller and softer than in Hodgkin's disease.

Lymphosarcomatous transformation is almost invariable if the patient lives long enough, and occasionally lymphatic leukaemia develops. Whether it is a benign condition which becomes malignant or whether it should be regarded as malignant from its onset has no particular practical significance.

Although lymph-nodes, spleen, and marrow are the most common sites other organs such as the liver, lungs, tonsils, and intestine may be involved.

An important subgroup is that in which there is gross splenomegaly. Hickling (1964) described 5 cases and referred to the condition as 'giant follicular lymphoma of the spleen'. Two of his patients were over the age of 65 years. The characteristics he listed were: (1) Massive splenomegaly without superficial adenopathy; (2) Lymphocytosis with abnormal and immature cells, but no gross leucocytosis in bone-marrow aspirate; (3) Excellent clinical result of splenectomy with gradual return of a normal blood-picture. In 2 patients histology of the spleen showed large follicles with well-defined germinal centres. The other 3 spleens had a histological picture more like that of lymphatic leukaemia—the follicles were not well defined and the pulp contained a large number of abnormal lymphocytes.

Although follicular lymphoma has to be accepted as a rare cause of massive splenomegaly it is clinically very difficult to separate it from lymphosarcoma of the spleen.

HODGKIN'S DISEASE

The features which help in differentiating Hodgkin's disease from the other malignant lymphomata are: loss of normal lymph-node architecture, fibrosis, Reed-Sternberg cells, and eosinophilia.

Any group of lymph-nodes may be involved. The cervical chain accounts for approximately 60 per cent. Affected nodes are often considerably enlarged and tend to be more discrete than in lymphosarcoma. They are of firm consistency. Examination of stained sections by means of a hand lens shows destruction of the normal follicular pattern with replacement by irregular bands of fibrous tissue alternating with cellular areas. Fibrosis may cause lobulation. The neoplastic proliferation consists of reticulum cells and lymphocytic stem cells. Mononuclear and multinucleate reticulum cells occur indiscriminately throughout the tumour as isolated, small groups, or even sheets of cells. The Reed-Sternberg cells, containing two to five nuclei, are characteristic of the disease. Cellular areas intermingle with areas of fibrosis and necrosis, and the variation seen in one lymph-node is a striking feature when compared with the monotonous picture in lymphosarcoma.

The spleen is enlarged in approximately 50 per cent of cases, and the liver nearly as frequently. Other viscera are often invaded, such as the lungs, kidneys, bone-marrow, and gastro-intestinal tract.

Many attempts have been made to subdivide Hogkin's disease, and these appear justified on epidemiological and prognostic grounds. Broadly three groups can be considered:—

a. Paragranuloma (relatively benign).
b. Granuloma (ordinary).
c. Sarcoma (highly malignant).

Over 80 per cent fall into the granuloma group. Paragranuloma comprises about 12 per cent, but its frequency is less in the elderly. The follicular pattern is mostly destroyed and replaced with masses of lymphocytes resembling lymphosarcoma but containing scattered Reed-Sternberg cells. Similar in its relatively benign clinical behaviour is the type described as nodular sclerosing Hodgkin's disease, but in histological contrast large masses of fibrous tissue subdivide the lymph-node into irregular nodules. The cellular portions may show fields which are identical with the paragranuloma variant.

Another classification based on the work of Lukes (1966) consists of four groups:—

   a. Lymphocyte predominance (paragranuloma and some granuloma).
   b. Nodular sclerosis (subdivision of granuloma).
   c. Mixed cellularity (granuloma without collagenous bands).
   d. Lymphocyte depletion (sarcoma and some granuloma).

Keller, Kaplan, Lukes, and Rappaport (1968) showed how these groups are differently distributed according to age (*Fig.* 34).

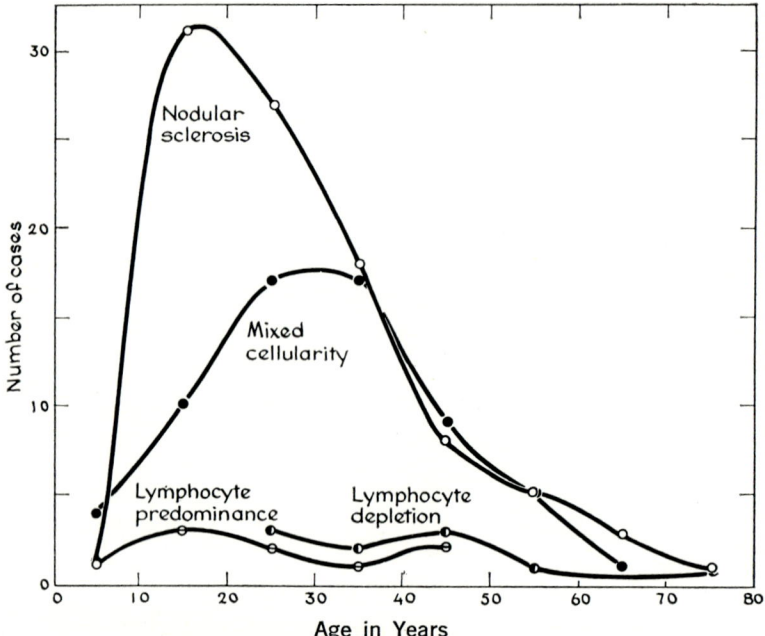

Fig. 34.—Age distribution of Hodgkin's disease patients by histological type. (*Reproduced by permission of Keller and others and the Editor, 'Cancer'.*)

CLINICAL FEATURES

When painless, enlarged, and discrete rubbery lymph-nodes are palpable in the posterior triangle of the neck, and observation shows a Pel-Ebstein type of fever, the diagnosis of Hodgkin's disease can be made with reasonable certainty, although histological proof is still necessary. But the mode of presentation is variable and symptoms may not appear until long after the true onset of the disease. On the other hand, constitutional symptoms such as lassitude, loss of weight, pruritus, fever, and sweats may be present months before the diagnosis is made.

The temperature may remain normal thoughout the course of the illness, although usually it is elevated in the terminal stages. In others, there is continuous, intermittent, or periodic fever and sometimes the only characteristic is an evening rise. An elevation for 4–14 days up to 100–104° F. (37·7–40° C.) followed by apyrexia lasting weeks or months and then recurrence in a similar pattern is termed Pel-Ebstein fever. The cause is obscure, but it occurs in approximately 16 per cent.

Primary or secondary mediastinal involvement is not unusual. A lobulated opacity in the hilum due to glandular enlargement may be seen radiologically. Sometimes both hila are involved and also the right paratracheal region. All the signs and symptoms of a mediastinal tumour may be present. Sarcoidosis, presenting in this manner, is extremely rare in the elderly, but carcinoma of the lung is relatively common and can be entirely intrabronchial, so that a definite diagnosis of Hodgkin's disease can seldom be made until an accessible lymph-node becomes available for biopsy. By then the disease has disseminated, with consequent reduction in survival time following treatment. Thoracotomy is rarely justified and trephine aspiration of lymphoid material is not a procedure to be undertaken lightly. In such instances it is reasonable to institute treatment despite the fact that a firm diagnosis has not been made. A high index of suspicion is enough.

Abdominal nodes are often difficult to palpate until greatly enlarged and patients may have gastro-intestinal symptoms for weeks or months before any abnormality is detected. Vomiting, anorexia, and loss of weight are usually prominent features when the coeliac nodes are affected. Carcinoma of the stomach may be simulated, and also carcinoma of the pancreas when pain radiates to the back and is associated with steatorrhoea. Enlargement in the lower abdomen can cause oedema of the legs.

Splenomegaly usually denotes dissemination, but is often present when the patient is first seen together with enlarged cervical and axillary nodes. Differentiation from lymphosarcoma is not possible without histological examination. Primary involvement of the spleen has been recorded. Enlarged cervical nodes may mat together and sometimes there is secondary infection leading to ulceration.

The liver may be enlarged and the patient jaundiced. Nodes in the porta hepatis can obstruct the bile-duct. Haemolysis can be present and sometimes there is an intrahepatic obstructive type of jaundice the cause of which is obscure. Occasionally, chlorpromazine is given for troublesome pruritus and jaundice can develop as a toxic side-effect. Only rarely is the liver sufficiently infiltrated for it to be the primary cause.

Anaemia is usually present at some stage and can be incapacitating. It may be of the myelophthisic or leucoerythroblastic type due to infiltration of the marrow, but in others there is hypochromia or macrocytosis and care has to be taken that deficiency of iron, vitamin B_{12}, or folate is not allowed to aggravate the illness. Auto-immune haemolysis is rare but the incidence of a non-immune haemolytic process may be as high as 40 per cent in the later stages (Bowdler and Prankerd, 1962). 'Latent' haemolysis, when the red-cell life span is reduced, but not sufficiently to cause anaemia, can also occur. Other possible reasons are marrow depression and hypersplenism. More than one mechanism may operate simultaneously. The blood sedimentation rate is usually elevated when the disease is spreading, but it may otherwise be normal.

Amyloidosis is a well-recognized complication and its onset is perhaps accelerated by the use of cytotoxic drugs. The presence of gross proteinuria should make one suspect the condition, although urogenital bacterial infection is a more common cause, and there may be infiltration of the kidney with Hodgkin's tissue.

Skeletal pain from infiltration and destruction is sometimes encountered, and when the vertebral column is affected root pains may occur and the spinal cord compressed. Spontaneous fractures may be seen. Peripheral neuropathy sometimes develops, due possibly to an unknown toxic factor.

A dermatological presentation is reasonably common. There may be non-specific manifestations such as brownish pigmentation, pruritus, exfoliative dermatitis, or erythrodermia, and specific lesions due to infiltration. They are usually nodular, circumscribed, and brownish in colour. These can remain localized for long periods without treatment (Szur, Harrison, Levene, and Saaman, 1970).

Any viscus can be involved as, for example, the lungs, where reticulation or nodulation may be present and sometimes a circumscribed tumour similar to a carcinoma. There may be atelectasis or a pleural effusion, which may be chylous due to blockage of lymphatics. An isolated tumour of the stomach or of the breast can be the presenting feature.

Steatorrhoea is sometimes present. Ehrlich, Staider, Geller, and Sherlock (1968) found that the bowel was involved in 30 per cent of a series of 323 necropsies and the small intestine in 23 per cent. Although steatorrhoea may be caused by reticulosis, in the majority this is unlikely, as the malabsorption has been present for too long a period. There is a possibility that in some patients the reticulosis can be a complication of the enteropathy (Gough, Read, and Naish, 1962).

Alcohol intolerance may be as high as 30 per cent—and higher in women—when specifically looked for. Violent pain may occur within a few minutes to half an hour of drinking alcohol, irrespective of the quantity. It may be located in an enlarged lymph-node, in the abdomen, in the chest, or in bone. A generalized body ache may occur. Sometimes there is acute distress of sudden onset, such as vomiting, sweating, headache, or shivering, and this may last half an hour or more. Usually there is no pre-existing pain, but if there is, it may be accentuated. Sometimes there is a lowering of threshold, and intoxication is more easily produced. The symptom is commoner in habitual drinkers than in the average person and may precede diagnosis by many months. In others it is an early manifestation, while occasionally the disease is already known to be present. With successful treatment the symptom disappears. Brewin (1966) investigated 155 cases of alcohol intolerance and found that in 84 a lymphoid tumour was present, Hodgkin's disease accounting for 60. He indicated that carcinomas—as of the cervix and lung—could also cause the symptom.

In the indolent type (paragranuloma) the disease may remain localized for 1–10 years or even longer. The presenting feature is nearly always cervical-node enlargement. Apparent regression may occur, but later there is transformation into ordinary Hodgkin's disease and occasionally into lymphosarcoma, reticulum-cell sarcoma, or lymphatic leukaemia.

In rare instances diseases of auto-immune origin develop, but as multiple pathology is so common in the elderly, it is difficult to be dogmatic about the association.

Another rare complication is multifocal leuco-encephalopathy, in which demyelination of the white matter of the brain occurs, particularly of the occipital lobes. Visual field defects, pyramidal signs, and dementia develop. The onset is variable and may be late. Similar spinal cord changes are also seen. Deterioration in these patients is invariably progressive.

The *course* of the disease is unpredictable. Anaemia, leucopenia, leucocytosis, neurological involvement, and skin infiltration are bad prognostic signs.

A useful guide is the stage of the disease when treatment is instituted.

a. Stage 1: The disease is localized to one main group of lymph-nodes. Survival of several years is common, particularly with treatment, but is not invariably so.

b. Stage 2: Two or more adjacent groups of lymph-nodes are involved; with or without symptoms. The prognosis has to be guarded, especially when there are severe constitutional features.

c. Stage 3: There is widespread disease with pyrexia and often anaemia. Although initial response to treatment may be reasonably satisfactory there is usually relapse within a few months.

Generally the course of the disease may be interrupted by periods of apparent inactivity or even regression.

TREATMENT

Supportive and symptomatic measures should not be neglected. Attention to the accompanying anaemia, if present, makes the patient's life more tolerable. Although frequently due to infiltration of the marrow there are instances when it is due to folate deficiency, blood-loss, or infiltration of the gastro-intestinal tract with resultant malabsorption. Sometimes it is truly incidental, as anaemia, particularly of the iron-deficiency type, is common at this age.

Pain due to bone involvement may be severe and require analgesics. The relief obtained by aspiration of a pleural effusion or abdominal paracentesis when ascites is present may be considerable.

Infections of the lungs, urogenital tract, or of the lymph-nodes themselves may be due to tubercle or other bacilli and usually respond to antibiotic therapy.

Three forms of treatment are currently practised:—

a. Surgical Excision.—This is appropriate when the disease is localized and the nodes accessible. In the cervical region excision is often reasonably satisfactory, but lymph-nodes in other sites are less amenable. Subsequent irradiation or chemotherapy is sometimes advised.

b. Irradiation.—X-ray therapy is more effective than radioactive substances, such as radiophosphorus. Each case has to be considered on its merits and the dosage modified accordingly. This form of treatment is indicated when the disease is localized to a group of nodes and also when it is generalized. Distress due to mediastinal involvement can often be relieved rapidly.

Although the initial response may be temporarily satisfactory it is usually less so when the disease relapses.

c. Chemotherapy.—This can be given both in the localized and generalized stages, particularly the latter. It is also useful as an adjunct to radiation or after radiation has lost its effect. One or more of three drugs are usually given.

i. *Mustine hydrochloride*: This is administered intravenously in a dosage of 0·1–0·3 mg. per kg. body-weight per injection each day. Up to 0·6 mg. per kg. body-weight can be given in each course. This is a rapidly acting drug. The incidence of nausea, vomiting, and insomnia may be lessened by giving concurrently an injection of chlorpromazine and a short-acting barbiturate.

The drug is particularly indicated for mediastinal obstruction and may be combined with radiotherapy.

ii. *Chlorambucil*: The oral dose is 0·2 mg. per kg. per day. The maintenance dose is 0·03–0·1 mg. per kg. per day, which can be given for protracted periods, provided a regular check is made on the neutrophil and platelet counts.

iii. *Cyclophosphamide*: Two hundred mg. can be given intravenously each day until a dosage of 4–6 g. has been attained. Alternatively 150–200 mg. taken orally is probably as effective. Therapy should be discontinued if the W.B.C. falls to 2000 or below but long-term maintenance treatment is sometimes possible.

This drug is a cyclic nitrogen mustard phosphamide ester and, unlike mustine, is stable in aqueous solution. Its activity is due to its ability to combine with nucleoprotein radicals—such as carboxyl, phosphoryl, or amino groups—at the site of the neoplasm. Apart from its marrow toxicity cyclophosphamide may produce alopecia or haemorrhagic cystitis.

Vinblastine sulphate: This is given by intravenous injections of 0·1–0·15 mg. per kg. per week. If the patient responds, weekly maintenance injections may be given. The toxic effects are neutropenia or peripheral neuritis.

Procarbazine hydrochloride: The starting oral dose is 50 mg. once daily with food, which is gradually increased to 200–300 mg. daily. The toxic effects are nausea, vomiting, drowsiness, confusion, leucopenia, and thrombocytopenia.

Combined Chemotherapy.—Mustine, vincristine, procarbazine, and prednisolone have been given together producing a remission rate of 90 per cent. A 2-week course of all four drugs is followed by 2–4 weeks without treatment.

When a haemolytic element is present corticosteroids are sometimes effective. Prednisolone 20–40 mg. daily is perhaps the most commonly prescribed form. If lymphosarcoma has developed this treatment seems to be occasionally beneficial even when there is no overt evidence of blood destruction.

Splenectomy may have to be considered when splenomegaly is associated with hypersplenism.

In general it may be said that although there is no specific remedy, treatment does appear to have an appreciable effect in delaying the final outcome (and even osteolytic bone lesions may calcify). Nevertheless, when the patient lives many years in apparent good health, it is likely that this is due more to the character of the disease than to the type of treatment.

LYMPHOMA OF THE GASTRO-INTESTINAL TRACT

The literature concerning primary lymphomatous involvement of the gastro-intestinal tract is considerable. Dawson, Cornes, and Morson (1961) presented 37 intestinal cases and considered 142 intestinal and 117 gastric from the literature. Ten of their patients were over 60 years of age and 1, with lymphosarcoma of the jejunum, was aged 89 years. From the recorded cases it appears that lymphosarcoma and reticulosarcoma involve the stomach almost twice as often as does ordinary Hodgkin's disease. Hodgkin's paragranuloma does not appear to present in this manner.

Lymphosarcoma is the most common lymphomatous tumour affecting the intestinal tract. Reticulosarcoma is about four times as common as Hodgkin's disease or follicular lymphoma. Males are affected approximately twice as often as females. The most frequent site of lymphomatous disease is the stomach followed by the ileum, caecum, and rectum.

The prognosis is better with follicular lymphoma and lymphosarcoma than with Hodgkin's disease or reticulosarcoma. Lesions in the duodenum are usually rapidly fatal.

Occasionally there are multiple primary tumours, but the prognosis following successful surgery is similar to that of single lesions. Involvement of regional lymph-nodes does not necessarily preclude long survival.

The presenting symptoms are in no way pathognomonic. Gastric involvement may be associated with nausea, vomiting, epigastric pain, loss of weight, or haematemesis, and a tumour may be palpable. Lesions of the small intestine present with acute abdominal pain, vomiting, and sometimes obstructive signs. Perforation is a recognized form of onset. When the large intestine is the primary site altered bowel habit, bleeding, malaise, and vague abdominal discomfort may occur. A mass may be found either on palpation or on rectal examination.

Malabsorption may be associated with lymphoid tumours of the small intestine. These tumours may arise as a complication but in others no association is apparent. Lee (1966) described the histopathology of the small intestine in 9 patients with a primary lymphoid tumour and compared it with that obtained in a closely matched series of small-bowel adenocarcinomata. The ages of the patients ranged from 32 to 70 years. There was a higher incidence of partial or subtotal villous atrophy in the lymphoid group and he considered that this could possibly be the result of immunological disturbances. Harries, Cooke, Thompson, and Waterhouse (1966) studied 202 patients with coeliac disease or idiopathic steatorrhoea. Nine males and 5 females were over 60 years of age; 5 of them developed reticulum-cell sarcoma and 1 Hodgkin's disease. They felt that there was no clear-cut evidence of an association and in a third the lymphoma did not infiltrate the intestinal wall.

Secondary involvement of the intestinal tract in patients with disseminated disease has received less attention. The largest series appears to be that by Ehrlich, Staider, Geiler, and Sherlock (1968). They studied a total of 323 patients with lymphoma at necropsy; 125 had reticulosarcoma, 123 Hodgkin's disease, and 75 lymphosarcoma. They were careful to distinguish between tumour and non-tumour disease, such as ulceration and fungus infection, and this differentiation was important when bleeding had been a feature, because the most common cause was a lesion other than the tumour. The oesophagus was directly involved in 24 cases, the stomach in 77, the duodenum in 14, jejunum in 34, ileum in 28, colon in 23, serosa and omentum in 61, the gall-bladder in 27, and the pancreas in 86. The overall survival period after the onset of abdominal symptoms was 24 months with Hodgkin's disease, 18 months with lymphosarcoma, and 6 months in reticulosarcoma. The most common causes of obstruction and perforation were reticulosarcoma and lymphosarcoma, rather than Hodgkin's disease or radiation damage.

Obstructive jaundice was a complication in 14 cases; in 6 there was common bile-duct invasion by a reticulosarcoma. The incidence of 2·4 per cent in Hodgkin's disease was less than half that seen in lymphosarcoma and reticulosarcoma. Jaundice occurs in about 12 per cent of patients with Hodgkin's disease but in only a small proportion is there true obstruction.

Treatment

The *treatment* of a primary lesion in the gastro-intestinal tract is surgical. Radiotherapy did not appear to influence the result in Dawson's series, although initially there may be marked clinical improvement with reduction in size of the abdominal mass. Follicular lymphoma has the best prognosis, but 1 patient, aged 65 years, with a single reticulosarcoma, survived 15 years and another, aged 48, with a lymphosarcoma, lived 16 years following surgical removal and subsequent radiotherapy. Both jejunum and ileum were involved. Even after this long interval there was local recurrence.

ANAPLASTIC SARCOMA

In Lumb's 1954 series of 68 cases, 40 per cent were over 50 years of age. The primary site is usually in the cervical and mediastinal lymph-nodes. Rapid enlargement occurs, although there are inexplicable exceptions. The neoplastic cells show marked pleomorphism with many abnormal mitotic figures. Necrosis and haemorrhage are common and any organ may be invaded.

GENERAL PROGNOSIS

It is difficult to prognosticate in an individual case of lymphoma. Series show statistical trends, but they include many variants.

Lumb's (1954) 5-year survival rates in 222 patients were:—

	No. of Cases	No. Surviving 5 years	Percentage Survival
Hodgkin's paragranuloma	10	8	80
Hodgkin's disease	123	43	35
Follicular lymphoma	8	5	62·5
Lymphosarcoma over 35 years	27	6	22·2
Lymphosarcoma under 35 years	8	1	12·5
Reticulum-cell sarcoma	8	1	12·5
Anaplastic sarcoma	38	2	5·3

Follicular Lymphoma

At first the disease is often symptomless, the only abnormality being enlargement of lymph-nodes, and, rarely, the course may remain benign. Usually it progresses slowly, but may terminate rapidly if the pattern changes to that of a more malignant type. Five-year survival rates vary from 30 to 75 per cent.

Hodgkin's Paragranuloma

This type probably merits its benign connotation, although it is only relative. Lukes (1963), who described 149 cases, found that there were twice as many 15-year survivors in his relatively benign group as in the ordinary type of Hodgkin's disease. Lumb and Newton (1957) had a 93 per cent 5-year survival. From a prognostic point of view Hodgkin's paragranuloma and nodular sclerosing Hodgkin's disease are similar.

Hodgkin's Disease

The ordinary type of Hodgkin's disease is ultimately progressive, but it must be emphasized that the course is not always relentless. Thus, enlarged lymph-nodes may show complete regression in the absence of specific treatment. This feature was noted in one case by Hodgkin himself.

The average survival is 3–5 years, although a significant number live 10 years or more (2·4 per cent in Lumb's series). The correlation between the histological appearance and survival is only approximate.

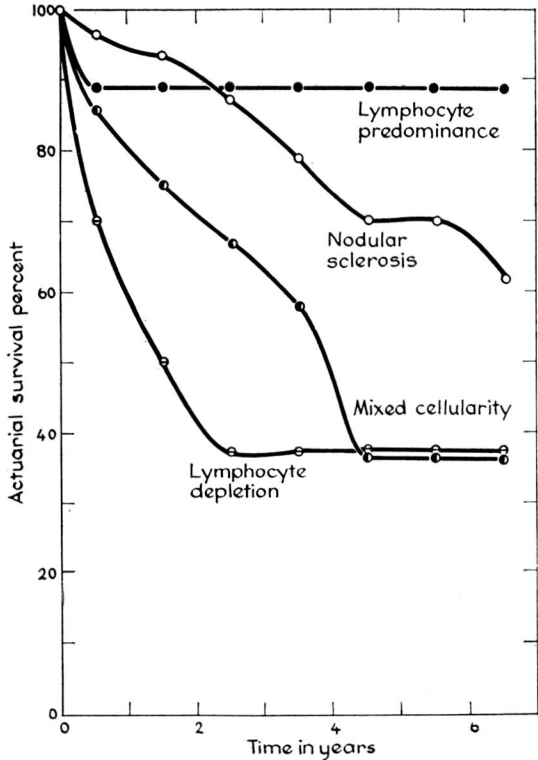

Fig. 35.—Actuarial survival in 176 cases of Hodgkin's disease according to histological types. The survival of the nodular sclerosis and mixed cellularity groups at 5 years is significantly different ($P < 0.02$). (*Reproduced by permission of Keller and others and the Editor, 'Cancer'.*)

Lumb (1954) found that age did not influence the prognosis. However, mortality-rates do show age differences, but these may well be related more to the different distribution of the various histological subtypes than to age itself (*Fig.* 35).

The histological appearances often show a progressive change to one of increasing anaplasia with time (MacMahon, 1966).

Overall survival rates are of limited value and may be excessively pessimistic. Several series (summarized by Hilton and Sutton, 1962) showed the value of clinical staging. Five-year survival rates for 'localized' disease have varied between

53 and 88 per cent. The same correlation is present when the absence of constitutional symptoms is taken as an index. However, this may simply reflect the association between extent and constitutional symptoms. Easson and Russell (1963) argued that Hodgkin's disease had acquired an over-sinister reputation. They claimed, on the basis of 10–15-year survival rates, that nearly 40 per cent of patients with Hodgkin's disease—and lymphosarcoma and reticulosarcoma—were curable. In both localized and generalized forms of the disease the prognosis is more favourable in women. Their 5-year survival in 545 cases of generalized Hodgkin's disease was 17·8 per cent, and in 277 localized cases 56·8 per cent. The 15-year survival in 127 generalized cases was 11·6 per cent, and in 64 where disease was localized, 39·7 per cent. No significant survival difference was found in cases of localized disease between those treated by irradiation alone and those who received irradiation combined with nitrogen mustard. This was adduced as further evidence against the presumed multifocal nature of the disease. The long-surviving cases were not exclusively of the paragranulomatous type, but no figures were given. Easson and Russell's work in this respect differs from that of Keller, Kaplan, Lukes, and Rappaport (1968). They found a clear association with age of the various histological patterns, and showed that unfavourable types were common in the elderly, particularly males. The other determining factor was the clinical stage. Keller and others concluded, 'Age, sex, and histological type taken together, approach the combination of clinical stage and histological type, as predictors of prognosis in Hodgkin's disease. However, age and sex contribute little additional prognostic information beyond that determined by histologic type and clinical stage.' They pointed out that the questions which remain to be answered are: why do older patients, especially men, tend to develop widespread disease of the mixed cellular type, and why are younger patients, especially women, more likely to have nodular sclerosis?

HAEMATOLOGICAL AND SYSTEMIC MANIFESTATIONS
Anaemia

Many patients are not anaemic at first. Rosenberg, Diamond, and Craver (1960) found haemoglobin levels of 12 g. per 100 ml. or over in 90 per cent of 1269 reported cases of lymphosarcoma. Wintrobe (1967) gave a figure of 70 per cent for his cases, and observed that anaemia is commoner in Hodgkin's disease where approximately one-third are anaemic when first seen. This is usually normochromic.

Occasionally severe haemolytic anaemia develops, especially in Hodgkin's disease, or lymphosarcoma with chronic lymphatic leukaemia. The anaemia is auto-immune with a positive direct Coombs's test. The peripheral blood-film shows microspherocytes, fragmented cells, and polychromasia.

Rarely, bone-marrow infiltration by a malignant lymphoma results in a leucoerythroblastic anaemia.

The condition of 'bone-marrow Hodgkin's disease' has been described (Krumbhaar, 1931; Isaacson, Spatt, and Grayzel, 1947); in these instances the spleen and marrow were involved without lymphatic enlargement. Wintrobe (1967) described another variant in which there was miliary involvement of the bone-marrow alone.

Case 3.—A woman, seen in 1964 at the age of 57, and known to have mitral stenosis, complained of weakness and abdominal discomfort for years. The spleen was greatly enlarged. The blood showed a Hb level of 66 per cent, with anisocytosis, polychromasia, numerous fragmented cells and tear drops, myelocytes, and nucleated red blood-cells. Reticulocytes were 7·5 per cent. Red-cell fragility was increased with 50 per cent haemolysis at 0·475 per cent saline. The bone-marrow aspirates were extremely hypocellular. An iliac crest biopsy showed a marked increase in fibrous tissue, so that a diagnosis of myelofibrosis was made (*Fig.* 36). No lymph-nodes were enlarged. Later in the year she died following mitral valvotomy. A post-mortem examination showed typical Hodgkin's granuloma of the spleen.

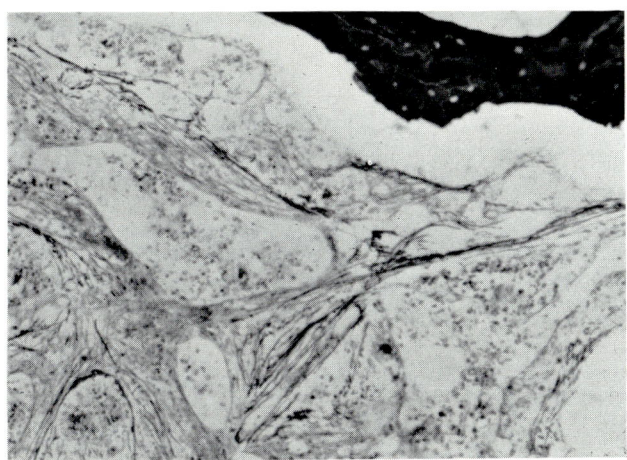

Fig. 36.—*Case* 3. Marrow fibrosis (reticulin preparation) in a woman aged 57 years who later showed evidence of Hodgkin's disease. (× 150.)

LEUCOCYTE COUNT

The total leucocyte count may be normal or raised in early Hodgkin's disease, although a relative and absolute lymphocytopenia can often be found even before treatment. Kaplan and Smithers (1959) suggested that a state of 'lymphatic depletion' can occur resembling that of homologous disease in animals.

Eosinophilia, of a mild degree, is present in approximately one-third of cases of Hodgkin's disease, but values up to 90 per cent have been found with elevated total leucocyte counts.

Reed-Sternberg cells are rarely seen in the routine preparations of peripheral blood. Bouronde (1966) examined blood from 135 patients by a silicone flotation technique and found that 37 per cent of those suffering from Hodgkin's disease had abnormal cells. Typical Reed-Sternberg cells were present in 18·5 per cent, in association with advanced disease.

Bennett, Nathanson, and Rutenburg (1968) studied the leucocyte alkaline phosphatase activity in Hodgkin's disease and suggested that raised scores were related to disease activity. If this is confirmed the test would provide a useful prognostic index.

Features of megaloblastic anaemia may be seen. This is usually due to folate deficiency.

Case 4.—This man, aged 61 years, had been diagnosed as a case of follicular lymphoma 10 years previously, and had been treated with radiotherapy.

He then reported with herpes zoster of the lower abdomen and penis. Hb was 61 per cent and the film showed numerous fragmented cells, macrocytes, and a right nuclear shift of the neutrophils. The marrow was highly cellular but normoblastic, although the serum folate was 0·5 ng. per ml. and vitamin B_{12} 100 pg. per ml. A repeat marrow showed giant metamyelocytes and macropolytes. He died within 1 year.

Platelet Count

This is usually normal but may be increased in Hodgkin's disease. Thrombocytopenia can occur in any of the malignant lymphomata as a result of marrow infiltration, but may be difficult to distinguish from that due to treatment.

Bone-Marrow

In typical cases of Hodgkin's disease the marrow usually shows myeloid and megakaryocytic hyperplasia. There may be depletion of lymphocytes and an increase of eosinophils. Local bone tenderness can indicate a focal lesion, and aspiration at such sites sometimes yields Hodgkin's disease tissue.

An increase in lymphocytes can occur in lymphosarcoma, and immature cells may be present.

Marrow aspirates should always be examined in section as well as smear preparations.

In general, bone-marrow examination is of greater value in excluding leukaemia than in making the diagnosis of a malignant lymphoma.

Serum Proteins

Hypogammaglobulinaemia is often found in chronic lymphatic leukaemia and lymphosarcoma. The degree of depletion correlates with the duration of the illness, and is a rare finding in Hodgkin's disease.

The formation of circulating antibodies is frequently impaired in malignant disease of the lymphoreticular tissue. Barr and Fairley (1961) discussed the variable results of many investigations and indicated the importance of distinguishing between the responses to primary immunization and reimmunization. They found that the formation of antitoxin (to tetanus toxoid) on primary immunization was depressed in all forms of reticulosis, especially in lymphosarcoma. This always occurred when the gamma-globulin was elevated or depressed (more usually the latter) and in about half when it was normal. The antibody responses on reimmunization (tetanus toxoid, anti-A agglutinins, and haemolysins) was grossly impaired in lymphosarcoma, but showed little or no impairment in the other reticuloses. Details of the patients' ages were not given, but in lymphosarcoma the range was up to 70 years, and in Hodgkin's disease up to 59 years. The ability to respond to antigenic stimulation may well be modified to a greater extent in the elderly, in whom acquired serum protein abnormalities are more frequent.

Aisenberg (1965) suggested that the anergy of early Hodgkin's disease was due to abnormal lymphocyte function. In the later stages a profound lymphocytopenia may contribute to more advanced immunological deficiencies, with a greater depression of delayed hypersensitivity, which may explain the tendency to severe mycotic and bacterial infections.

Paraproteinaemia.—Abnormal proteins, particularly of beta- and gamma-globulins, may be associated with any of the malignant lymphomata. They are considered further in Chapter 10, but it is important to recognize this feature because of the possibility of confusion with multiple myelomatosis in this age-group.

Associated Conditions

Infections.—Intercurrent infection is extremely common during the course of the illness and frequently causes death. This may be due to impaired antibody synthesis or marrow depression. The organisms may be common bacterial or viral pathogens. Alternatively 'opportunistic infections' due to normally non-pathogenic organisms may be found. A variety of exotic pathogens have been reported—moulds, yeasts, nocardia, herpes simplex, cytomegalovirus, pneumocystis, amoebae, toxoplasma, and histoplasma (Symmers, 1958).

Two illnesses have been particularly associated with Hodgkin's disease—namely tuberculosis and torulosis. In both there has been considerable discussion as to their possible aetiological significance. The position is complicated by the fact that the histological appearances, especially in tuberculous infection, may resemble those of Hodgkin's disease. Irrespective of this, it is important to recognize that elderly patients with Hodgkin's disease may also have tuberculosis.

Auto-immune Disease.—Kaplan and Smithers (1959) proposed that the tumour cells in Hodgkin's disease might be immunologically competent and capable of initiating a reaction against the host. Various investigations and case reports lend weight to this hypothesis—for example, the lupus erythematosus cell phenomenon, thyroglobulin antibody, and rheumatoid factor have been found in cases of reticulosis. Against this, Hoffbrand (1965) found no serological evidence of auto-immune phenomena in 39 cases of Hodgkin's disease—although one-third had raised gamma-globulin levels.

Case 5 (Powell and Thomas, 1968).—A man was first seen at the age of 57 years for a ventral hernia. Six years later he developed diabetes mellitus, and it was noted that he had an enlarged liver and spleen. Spinal cord compression with block developed, which responded partially to nitrogen mustard. Two slightly enlarged axillary nodes showed non-specific reactive changes only. After a further 2 years he was admitted in coma with hypertension and features of myxoedema. The TA latex thyroglobulin test was strongly positive. Response to thyroxine therapy was satisfactory but he was later readmitted and died. Post-mortem examination showed Hodgkin's disease, burnt-out chronic thyroiditis, and malignant renal arteriosclerosis.

This patient illustrates the difficulty that may arise in distinguishing between related disease syndromes from examples of multiple pathology in the elderly. His thyroid disease can be readily accepted as having an auto-immune basis, but the possibility of his Hodgkin's disease having a similar explanation remains an open question.

Hyperthyroidism.—Lymph-node enlargement and splenomegaly have often been noted in hyperthyroidism. Thyroxine has also been shown to produce lymphoid hyperplasia and tumours in animals. Ultman, Hyman, and Calder (1963) described 6 patients who developed a lymphoma subsequent to long-standing hyperthyroidism, and also referred to 3 additional cases. Their patients were aged 44, 54, 54, 57, 67, and 70 years. The histological diagnosis was lymphosarcoma in 4. One had Hodgkin's disease, and the other follicular lymphoma. Active hyperthyroidism had been present for periods ranging from 7 to 40 years.

Intestinal Malabsorption.—Lymphomatous involvement of the small intestine has long been recognized as a possible cause of steatorrhoea. However, the converse may also apply, and there is an appreciable incidence of small-bowel reticulosis in long-standing cases of idiopathic steatorrhoea with villus atrophy. This is a hazard of ageing in the patient with idiopathic steatorrhoea.

Leukaemia.—The association between lymphosarcoma and chronic lymphatic leukaemia is well known, although the picture of 'partial' leukaemia is more frequently encountered.

Reticulum-cell sarcoma may also terminate in leukaemia. Custer and Bernhard (1948) reviewed 1300 lymphatic tumours and suggested that the relationship between lymphosarcoma and chronic lymphatic leukaemia had its counterpart in reticulum-cell sarcoma and monocytic leukaemia. The conclusion has been disputed, but it is an undoubted fact that a minority of cases of reticulum-cell sarcoma do terminate in a leukaemic phase. Leukaemic reticulo-endotheliosis is characterized by circulating primitive reticulum cells in association with diffuse proliferation of such cells in the reticulo-endothelial system.

Diagnosis of Malignant Lymphoid Tumours

Routine investigation should include full blood-count, serum protein electrophoresis, and bone-marrow aspiration, although only rarely will the latter yield diagnostic information.

The diagnosis is nearly always made as a result of lymph-node biopsy. Whenever possible, the entire node or nodes should be excised and formalin-fixed before sectioning. Sampling of nodes that are not significantly enlarged is seldom worth while. Smears prepared from material obtained by needle aspiration may be satisfactory, but are more difficult to interpret than histological sections.

If there are no enlarged and accessible lymph-nodes the diagnosis may be made from needle biopsy of an enlarged liver or spleen, or by lymphography.

Occasionally a definite histological diagnosis cannot be made. If, however, the clinical features are highly suggestive and producing grave symptoms (such as mediastinal or spinal cord compression) a therapeutic trial is imperative. The result can be of diagnostic value.

The possibility of other causes of lymphadenopathy should always be considered. These include secondary neoplasia and a wide variety of infections. Drug reactions may also simulate a reticulosis. Hyman and Sommers (1966) reviewed 85 cases of 'pseudolymphoma' following anticonvulsant therapy. In these the histological appearances did not resemble a true lymphoma, but they also reported 6 patients with true Hodgkin's disease or lymphosarcoma. However, some case of 'pseudolymphoma' can mimic reticulosis histologically as well as clinically. Thus, Langlands, Maclean, Pearson, and Williamson (1967) described the case of a 71-year-old man who developed lymphadenopathy (and megaloblastic anaemia) after taking primidone for 4 years. A lymph-node biopsy was reported as a probable reticulum-cell sarcoma. The nodes regressed normally when primidone was withdrawn.

REFERENCES

AISENBERG, A. C. (1965), *Blood*, **25**, 1037.
BARR, M., and FAIRLEY, G. H. (1961), *Lancet*, **1**, 1305.
BENNETT, J. M., NATHANSON, L., and RUTENBURG, A. M. (1968), *Archs intern. med.*, **121**, 338.
BOURONDE, B. A. (1966), *Blood*, **27**, 544.

BOWDLER, A. J., and PRANKERD, J. A. T. (1962), *Br. med. J.*, **1**, 1169.
BREWIN, T. B. (1966), *Ibid.*, **2**, 437.
CLEMMESON, J. (1965), *Statistical Studies in Malignant Neoplasms. I, Review and Results.* Copenhagen: Munksgaard.
COLE, P., MACMAHON, B., and AISENBERG, A. (1968), *Lancet*, **2**, 1371.
CUSTER, R. P., and BERNHARD, W. G. (1948), *Am. J. med. Sci.*, **216**, 625.
DAWSON, I. M. P., CORNES, J. S., and MORSON, B. L. (1961), *Br. J. Surg.*, **49**, 80.
DORKEN, H. (1960), *Klin. Wschr.*, **38**, 944.
EASSON, E. C., and RUSSELL, M. H. (1963), *Br. med. J.*, **1**, 1704.
EHRLICH, A. N., STAIDER, G., GELLER, W., and SHERLOCK, P. (1968), *Gastroenterology*, **54**, 1115.
GOUGH, K. R., READ, A. E., and NAISH, J. M. (1962), *Gut*, **3**, 232.
HARRIES, O. D., COOKE, W. T., THOMPSON, H., and WATERHOUSE, J. A. H. (1966), *Am. J. Med.*, **42**, 899.
HICKLING, R. A. (1964), *Br. med. J.*, **2**, 787.
HILTON, G., and SUTTON, P. M. (1962), *Lancet*, **1**, 283.
HOFFBRAND, B. I. (1965), *Br. med. J.*, **1**, 1592.
HYMAN, G. A., and SOMMERS, S. C. (1966), *Blood*, **28**, 416.
ISAACSON, N. H., SPATT, S. D., and GRAYZEL, D. M. (1947), *Ann. intern. Med.*, **27**, 294.
KAPLAN, H. S., and SMITHERS, D. W. (1959), *Lancet*, **2**, 1.
KELLER, A. R., KAPLAN, H. S., LUKES, R. J., and RAPPAPORT, H. (1968), *Cancer, N.Y.*, **22**, 487.
KRUMBHAAR, E. B. (1931), *Am. J. med. Sci.*, **182**, 764.
LANGLANDS, A. O., MACLEAN, N., PEARSON, J. G., and WILLIAMSON, E. R. D. (1967), *Br. med. J.*, **1**, 217.
LEE, F. D. (1966), *Gut*, **7**, 361.
LUKES, R. J. (1963), *Am. J. Roent.*, **90**, 944.
— — (1966), *Cancer*, **19**, 317.
LUMB, G. (1954), *Tumours of Lymphoid Tissue.* London: Livingstone.
— — and NEWTON, K. A. (1957), *Cancer*, **10**, 976.
MACMAHON, B. (1957), *Cancer*, **10**, 1045.
— — (1966), *Cancer Res.*, **26**, 1189.
POWELL, D. E. B., and THOMAS, F. W. (1968), *Br. J. geriat. Pract.*, **5**, 235.
ROBB-SMITH, A. H. T. (1947), in *Recent Advances in Clinical Pathology*, p. 360 (Ed. DYKE, S. C.). London: Churchill.
ROSENBERG, S. A., DIAMOND, H. D., and CRAVER, L. F. (1960), *Ann. intern. Med.*, **53**, 877.
SHIMKIN, M. B. (1955), *Blood*, **10**, 1214.
SYMMERS, W. St. C. (1958), in *Cancer* (Ed. RAVEN, R. W.). London: Butterworths.
SZUR, L., HARRISON, C. V., LEVENE, G. M., and SAAMAN, P. D. (1970), *Lancet*, **1**, 1016.
ULTMAN, J. E., HYMAN, G. A., and CALDER, B. (1963), *Blood*, **21**, 282.
WILLIS, R. A. (1967), *Pathology of Tumours*, 4th ed. London: Butterworths.
WINTROBE, M. M. (1967), *Clinical Hematology.* London: Kimpton.

9

LEUKAEMIA

CLASSIFICATION

Acute
  Lymphoblastic
  Myeloblastic
  Promyelocytic
  Monocytic

Chronic
  Lymphatic
  Myeloid
  Histiocytic

Plasma-cell leukaemia
Megakaryocytic leukaemia
Erythraemic myelosis

INCIDENCE

Several surveys show that the incidence of deaths from leukaemia has increased over the past 40 years. The increase may be partly due to an extension of laboratory facilities, but this is unlikely to be the only explanation because the incidence has continued to rise in more sophisticated communities long after the establishment of the necessary diagnostic services.

Hewitt (1955) showed that the incidence increased by over two and a half times in England and Wales from 1931 to 1953. This rate of increase was exceeded only by carcinoma of the lung and coronary thrombosis. The incidence is higher in urban communities and where the standard of living is high. These findings do not reflect a higher proportion of elderly people because the differences for several populations standardized for age are even greater (Court Brown and Doll, 1959) (*Fig.* 37).

The distribution of the different types of leukaemia is difficult to assess accurately since diagnostic criteria vary widely. MacMahon and Clark's figures (1956) for Brooklyn are fairly representative: acute leukaemia, 53 per cent; chronic lymphatic leukaemia, 26 per cent; and chronic myeloid leukaemia, 21 per cent.

The number of patients registered as suffering from leukaemia in South Wales have been published by the Welsh Hospital Board. The registration rates for 1961–5 per 100,000 population per annum were:—

	Male	Female
Leukaemia and aleukaemia	5·92	4·69
Lymphatic	1·74	1·27
Myeloid	1·19	1·12
Monocytic	0·48	0·33
Acute	2·30	1·82
Unspecified	0·21	0·15

These rates can be compared with those for carcinoma of bronchus (75·06 in men, 8·48 in women), stomach (35·89 in men and 21·46 in women), and breast (0·79 in men and 55·78 in women).

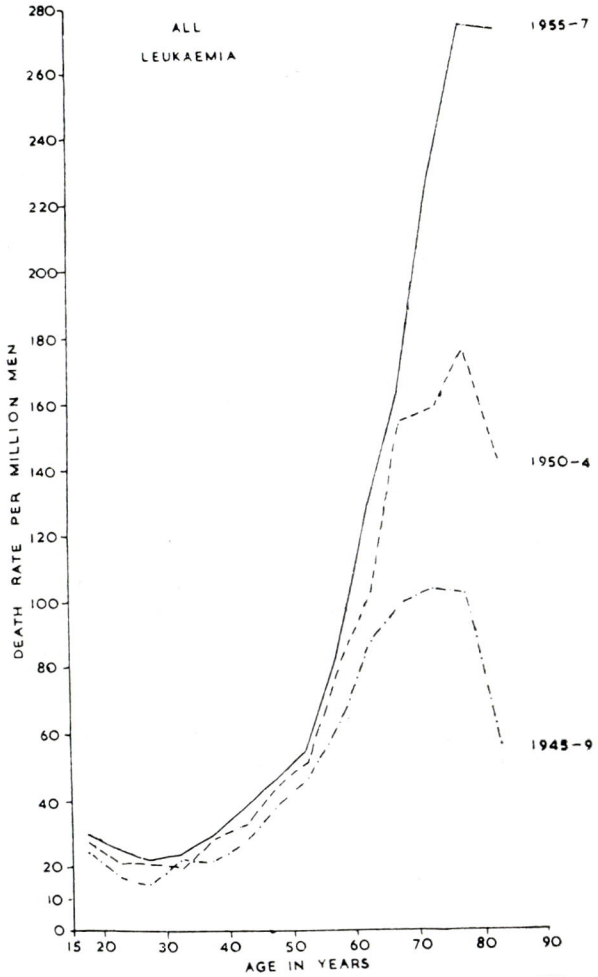

Fig. 37.—Mortality from all forms of leukaemia among men at different ages (from 15 years upwards) in England and Wales in 1945–9, 1950–4, and 1955–7. (*Reproduced by permission of Court Brown and Doll and the Editor, 'British Medical Journal'.*)

AGE DISTRIBUTION

The increase is mainly in the adult and elderly. Court Brown and Doll (1959) and Videbaek (1966) produced similar graphs that show this phenomenon clearly (*Fig.* 38).

The leukaemia registration rate in South Wales for 1961–5 per million male population was 57 for 0–5 years compared with 238 for those over 75 years. The rate for all ages was 59. Chronic lymphatic and myeloid leukaemias are almost restricted to adult years. Chronic lymphatic leukaemia is predominantly a disease of the elderly, showing a progressive rise with age. Chronic myeloid leukaemia shows an earlier adult onset with a maximal incidence around 50 years. This age-distribution pattern of chronic myeloid leukaemia has been noted since Bennet's description in 1845. Minot, Buckman, and Isaacs (1924) in the United States and Ward (1917) in Great Britain found that approximately 55 per cent of cases occur between 30 and 50 years of age. Conrad, Rappaport, and Crosby (1965) found that only 13 out of 69 patients with chronic myeloid leukaemia were over 60 years.

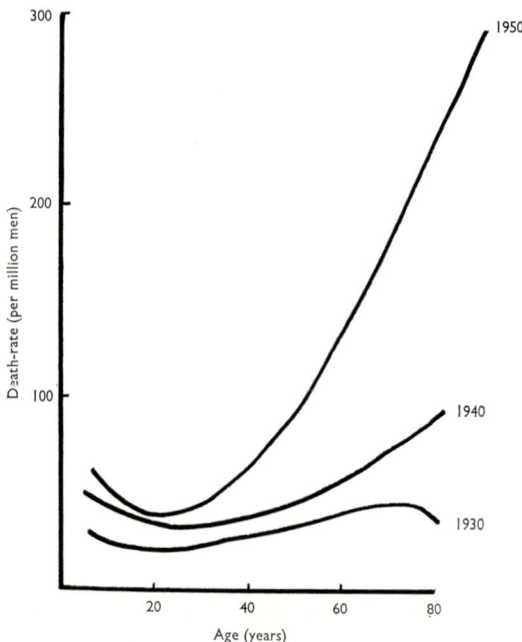

Fig. 38.—Schematic diagram showing increased incidence of leukaemia in the elderly in Denmark. (*After Videbaek, Aa.* (1966), '*Acta Haematol.*', **36**, 183).

The incidence of acute leukaemia shows a bimodal distribution. The first peak is below 10 years, with the lowest level between 15 and 35 years. Thereafter there is a steady rise with age, until the incidence in the elderly is significantly higher than that in childhood. Our experience confirms that acute leukaemia is encountered more frequently in the elderly than in children. The registration rate per million male population in South Wales (1961–5) was 71 above 75 years, compared with 45 below 5 years. It is possible, however, that cases of leukaemia in the elderly are designated as acute if the antecedent chronic phase has been missed (*Figs.* 39, 40).

SEX DISTRIBUTION

All types of leukaemia are commoner at all ages in males. The male to female ratio for all types is usually within the range 1·1–1·6.

LEUKAEMIA

AETIOLOGY AND PRECIPITATING FACTORS

The cause of leukaemia is unknown, and we do not propose to discuss the various theories and investigations other than to refer to the role of ageing and precipitating factors.

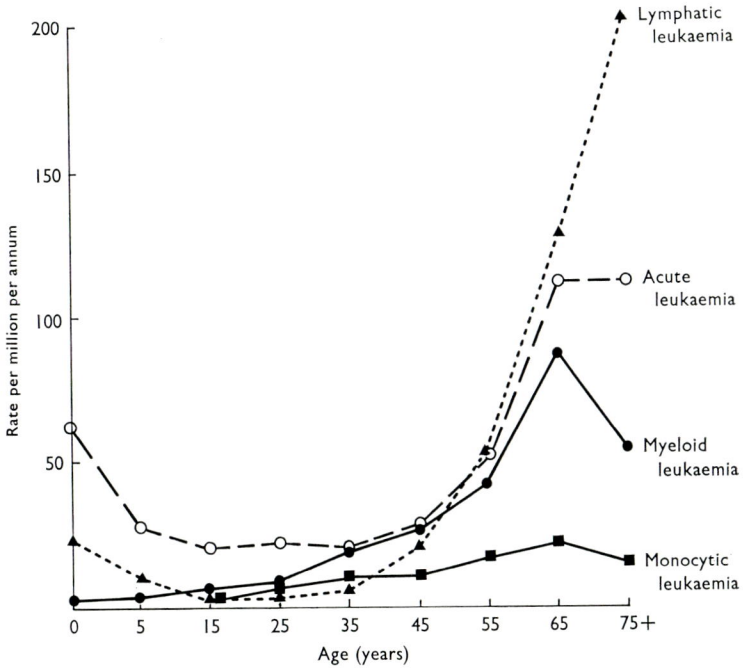

Fig. 39.—South Wales registration rates per million of population, 1961–5 (both series).

AGEING

Court Brown and Doll (1959) considered the possibility that the greater increase in the incidence of leukaemia in the elderly could be a cohort effect, due to the introduction of a leukaemogenic agent at a time when the present elderly population was susceptible. But they thought that improved diagnosis was a more likely explanation because a similar large increase in mortality had taken place from cancer of the lung and gastric ulcer, with a large decrease in the deaths attributed to senility. They also discounted the cohort effect because there had been no equivalent preceding increase at younger ages. However, this does not lessen the possibility that new leukaemogenic agents have been introduced, which require a long latent period to produce leukaemia.

The marked differences in incidence and mortality-rates with age suggest that the causes of acute, chronic myeloid, and chronic lymphatic leukaemia are distinct. Armitage and Doll (1954, 1957) found a straight-line relationship between the logarithm of the death-rate per million and the logarithm of the age in years $-2\frac{1}{2}$, for cancer of the stomach in men and chronic lymphatic leukaemia in men and women. This could be explained by a neoplastic stimulus which took place in two or more stages with a prolonged latent interval (*Fig.* 41).

Acute and chronic myeloid leukaemia do not behave in this way. This could be due to the shorter latent interval required for their induction—as for example by radiation.

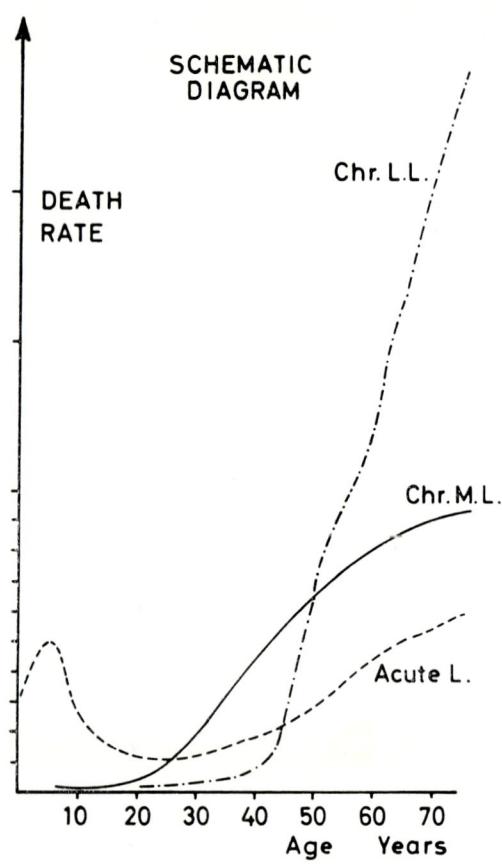

Fig. 40.—Schematic diagram showing relative frequency of three main types of leukaemia. Unlike the chronic types, acute leukaemia appears biphasic. (*After Videbaek, Aa.* (1966), '*Acta Haematol.*', **36**, 183.)

Hayhoe, Quaglino, and Doll (1964) divided their 140 cases of acute leukaemia into four groups, corresponding to lymphoblastic; monocytic and myelomonocytic; myeloblastic and promyelocytic; and erythraemic myelosis. When their incidences were plotted against age, the curve for the lymphoblastic group differed from the others in showing a steady fall after childhood except above 70 years. The other acute leukaemias showed a progressive rise with age (*Figs.* 42, 43).

PHENYLBUTAZONE

Bean (1960) reported 6 patients who developed leukaemia after recent phenylbutazone treatment. Woodliff and Dougan (1964), from Australia, found that

9 per cent of 55 cases of adult leukaemia had received phenylbutazone. This contrasted with a 1·2 per cent incidence of ingestion in 417 patients with chronic leukaemia, lymphoma, and allied disorders. Several other reports point to a relationship.

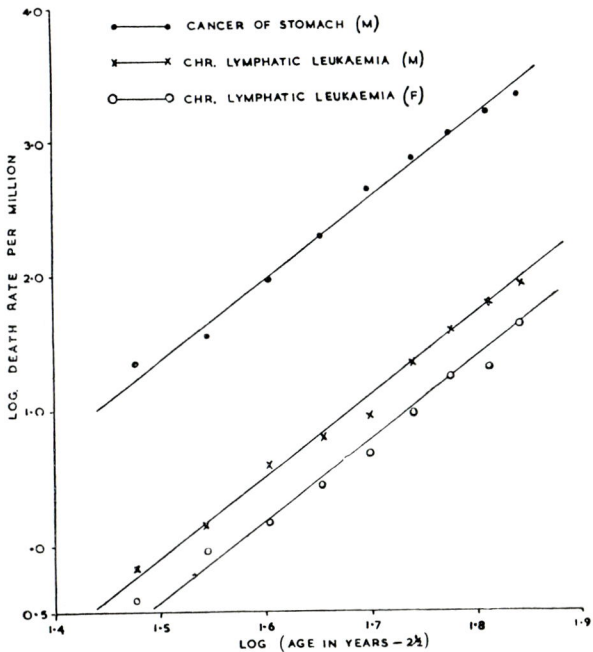

Fig. 41.—Relationship between age and estimated mortality from chronic lymphatic leukaemia in men and in women in 1955–7 compared with the relationship observed for cancer of the stomach in men in 1956. The logarithm of the death-rate per million persons is plotted against the logarithm of the age less 2½ years, for ages 30 years to 74 years. The straight line through the points has been drawn arbitrarily to give the best fit, subject to the gradient being 6 to 1. (*After Armitage and Doll*, 1954, 1957.)

Case 1.—A lady of 73 years had been treated for gout for 6 years. A variety of analgesics had been prescribed, including butazolidine. The blood was examined in 1963 and 1964 when the W.B.C. was normal and there was a mild hypochromic anaemia (Hb 70 per cent). She presented in June, 1965, with polyarthritis and lymphadenopathy. Hb was 58 per cent; W.B.C., 4900 per c.mm. with only 23 per cent neutrophil polymorphs, and nucleated red blood-cells and leucoblasts were present. Bone-marrow smears showed acute leukaemia. Blood transfusion and prednisolone were given with initial response, but in March, 1966, she became dyspnoeic when Hb was 39 per cent; W.B.C., 1900 per c.mm. (90 per cent lymphocytes); and platelets, 60,000 per c.mm. She died in May, 1966. The predominant terminal blood-picture was one of aplasia rather than uncontrolled leukaemia.

IRRADIATION

Exposure to radiation is a recognized factor in the onset of some instances of leukaemia. The survivors of the 1945 atomic bomb explosions in Japan showed a maximal incidence of leukaemia in 1951. The majority were examples of acute type (52) and chronic myeloid (39). Only 1 example of chronic lymphatic was seen in 92 cases of leukaemia. However, this type is very rare in the Far East. An increased incidence of leukaemia has also been found amongst radiologists; following X-ray treatment of ankylosing spondylitis, treatment of hyperthyroidism with radioactive iodine, X-ray irradiation of the thymus in children, and radioactive phosphorus treatment of polycythaemia vera. Patients suffering

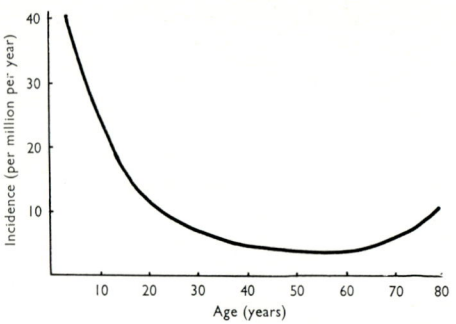

Fig. 42.—Incidence of acute lymphoblastic leukaemia by age. (*From Hayhoe, Quaglino, and Doll*, 1964.)

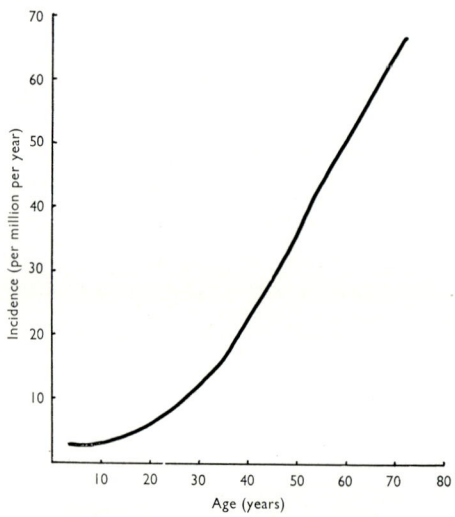

Fig. 43.—Incidence of non-lymphoblastic acute leukaemia by age. (*From Hayhoe, Quaglino, and Doll*, 1964.)

from chronic myeloid leukaemia give a history of greater exposure to radiotherapy and X-rays than do those who have chronic lymphatic leukaemia and lymphosarcoma. The role of ionizing radiations as a cause of the high incidence of leukaemia in the elderly is uncertain. One feature that discounts its possible significance is the clear relationship between chronic lymphatic leukaemia and ageing, whereas this is the one type of leukaemia which is least likely to be linked with radiation (Loutit, 1958). However, the possible link with acute and myeloid types remains an open question.

ACUTE LEUKAEMIA

Acute leukaemia is diagnosed clinically by its rapid progression and fatal outcome, and cytologically by the primitive nature of the white-cell proliferation. It may be difficult or impossible to differentiate the type of primitive leucocyte. Hitherto, this has made little or no difference in practice because the designation does not significantly influence treatment or prognosis. This may require modification with the most recently introduced drugs.

CLINICAL FEATURES

Acute leukaemia presents in many different ways, and this variability may be greater in the elderly. A period of vague ill health may give way to a rapid deterioration in the patient's condition. Various 'pre-leukaemic' states have been described, such as refractory anaemia, haemolytic anaemia, or thrombocytopenia. The relationship of leukaemia to the other manifestations of the myeloproliferative syndrome is discussed elsewhere (Chapter 11).

The patient suffering from acute leukaemia appears ill and is often febrile with a tachycardia. Symptoms are related to anaemia, thrombocytopenia, lymph-node enlargement, or visceral involvement. Marked pallor is usually present, and there are often scattered petechial haemorrhages of the skin and mucous membranes with extensive bruising. In the early case this can mimic senile purpura. Epistaxis is sometimes the first symptom. Bleeding may also take place into the alimentary tract, genito-urinary or central nervous systems. Sudden onset of visual impairment results from haemorrhage into the ocular fundus.

Enlargement of lymph-nodes may be noted externally or give rise to internal pressure symptoms. Hepatosplenomegaly is seldom gross in the acute case although this can be considerable if there has been an antecedent chronic phase.

Subcutaneous leukaemic infiltrates occur and these can ulcerate. Bone and joint infiltration or effusions will give rise to arthritic symptoms.

Abdominal pain and diarrhoea are usually related to alimentary deposits. Albuminuria is often present.

Gum swelling, gingivitis, oral ulceration, and bleeding may be troublesome.

Case 2.—This patient was aged 91 years and lived in an old peoples' home. He suddenly became confused and was admitted to hospital in a semiconscious state. Both plantar responses were extensor, but there were no localizing central nervous system signs.

Blood-urea was 70 mg. per 100 ml.; Hb, 88 per cent; W.B.C., 48,400 per c.mm.—these were largely atypical mononuclears, resembling those seen in monocytic leukaemia.

He died 5 days after admission. Autopsy showed a diffuse subarachnoid haemorrhage. There was an area of fibrocaseous pulmonary tuberculosis in the apex of the left upper lobe and extensive consolidation of the left lower lobe.

The spleen weighed 420 g. and was pale. There were tumour deposits in the ribs and enlargement of the paravertebral lymph-nodes.

Histological examination confirmed the presence of caseating pulmonary tuberculosis with tuberculous bronchopneumonia. The liver, spleen, marrow, and lymph-nodes showed leukaemic infiltration (*Figs.* 44–47).

This patient had therefore active tuberculosis at the age of 91 years which could have accounted for a leukaemoid reaction, but autopsy showed true leukaemic infiltration. Both these conditions would have been missed without investigation, and the death ascribed simply to cerebral haemorrhage.

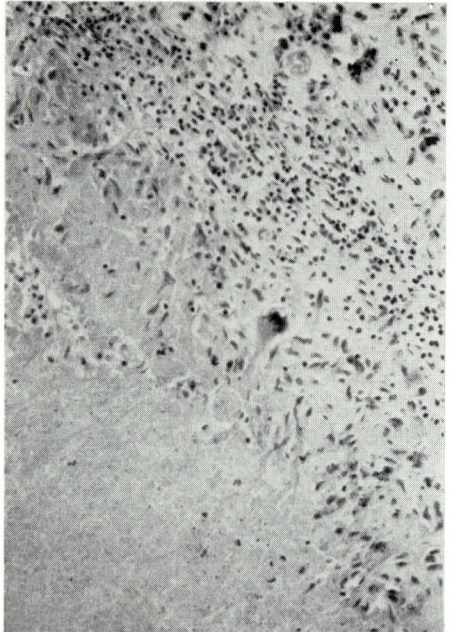

Fig. 44.—*Case* 2. Lung. Caseating pulmonary tuberculosis. (×150.)

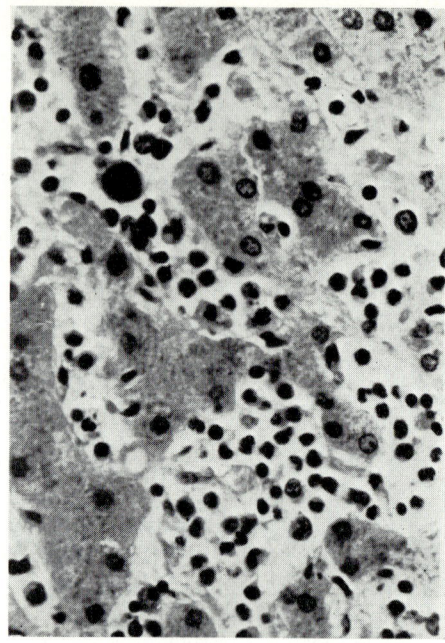

Fig. 45.—*Case* 2. Liver showing leukaemic infiltration. (×400.)

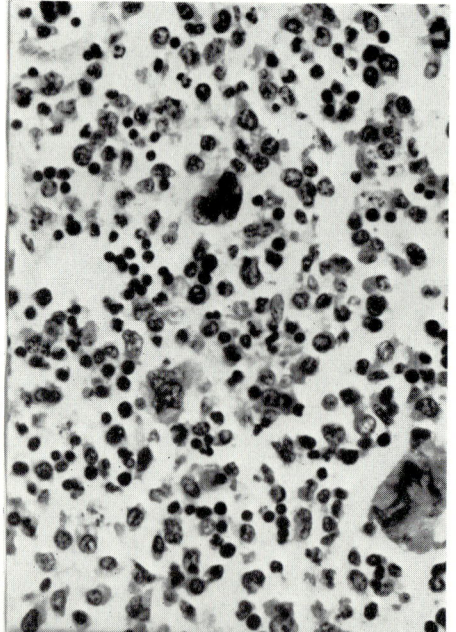

Fig. 46.—*Case* 2. Bone-marrow. Acute leukaemia. (×400.)

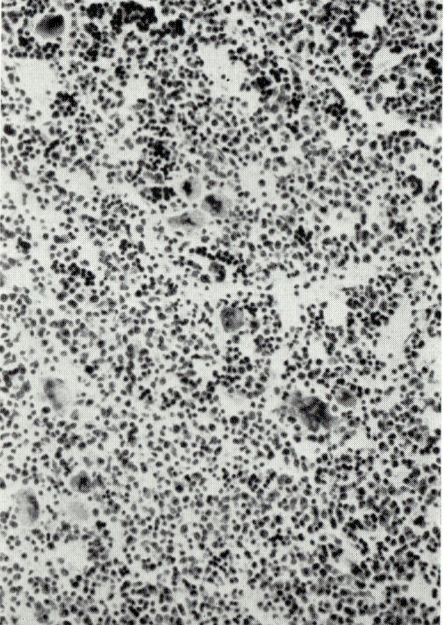

Fig. 47.—*Case* 2. Paravertebral node showing extramedullary haemopoiesis. (×150.)

LEUKAEMIA

DIAGNOSTIC LABORATORY FEATURES

Haemoglobin.—Most patients are anaemic when first seen, although this is by no means invariable, and acute leukaemia cannot be excluded on the basis of a normal haemoglobin (or normal white-cell count). However, even if not initially prominent, anaemia will soon develop and become severe. It is usually normochromic.

Erythrocytes.—The red cells show moderate anisocytosis, poikilocytosis, and polychromasia. Occasional macrocytes and nucleated red blood-cells may be found. The reticulocyte count is slightly elevated to approximately 5 per cent.

The E.S.R. is usually raised.

Leucocytes.—The total leucocyte count can be reduced, normal, or elevated. Approximately 30 per cent of patients have a count below 10,000 per c.mm. when first seen. The blood-film must be examined, when an abnormal differential count may be noted with a relative neutropenia and a left nuclear shift, or a preponderance of mononuclear cells. These mononuclears show the diagnostic features of primitive 'blast cells', but although they are usually characteristic of acute leukaemia it is often difficult to label them according to their original stem line (*Figs.* 48, 49).

Hayhoe, Quaglino, and Doll (1964) analysed the morphological and cytochemical data on blood and bone-marrow smears obtained from 140 consecutive cases of acute leukaemia. The following features were among those found helpful in distinguishing the cell type:—

	Lymphoblastic	*Myeloblastic*	*Monocytic*
Morphology	Regular nucleus	Regular cell outline	Indented twisted nuclei
Nuclear/cytoplasmic ratio	High	Not high	Not high
Auer rods	Absent	Often present	Often present
Accompanying cells	Lymphocytes >1 per cent of marrow cells	Promyelocytes	Promyelocytes
Neutrophil alkaline phosphatase	Normal	Low	Normal
Sudanophilia	Negative	Positive	Positive
P.A.S.	Positive	Negative or ±	Usually positive

Myeloblasts and monoblasts tended to have more nucleoli than lymphoblasts, but too many exceptions occurred in both directions for this to be diagnostically reliable.

Platelets.—The platelet count is almost always lowered and is frequently well below 50,000 per c.mm. Platelet morphology also may be abnormal with fragmented and giant forms. Marked thrombocytopenia is associated with a prolonged bleeding time and impaired clot retraction.

Bone-marrow.—This should be examined in all suspected cases, even if the peripheral blood-picture is unequivocal. In acute leukaemia the marrow is highly cellular and the dominant cell (95 per cent) is the leucoblast—the type conforms to that observed in the peripheral blood. There are also increased numbers of promyelocytes if the leukaemia is of myeloid type, but there may be a maturation arrest between this stage and the adult neutrophil polymorph. A gap in the representation of the intermediate white cells is frequently seen—the 'hiatus leukaemicus'.

Osgood (1969) claimed, however, that these are really examples of acute monocytic leukaemia—a condition which is underdiagnosed. As differentiating features, he emphasized the use of peroxidase which shows round black granules in granulocytes, but only a few scattered rod-shaped granules in promonocytes. There is also a complete absence of mature monocytes in monocytic leukaemia. In

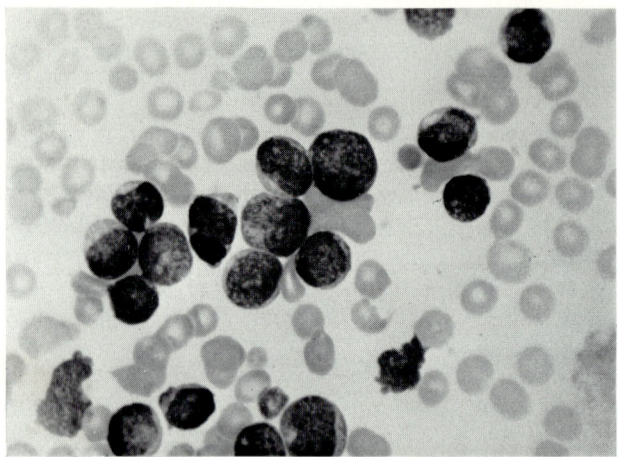

Fig. 48.—Blood. Terminal acute myelobastic leukaemia (male, 64 years). (×900.)

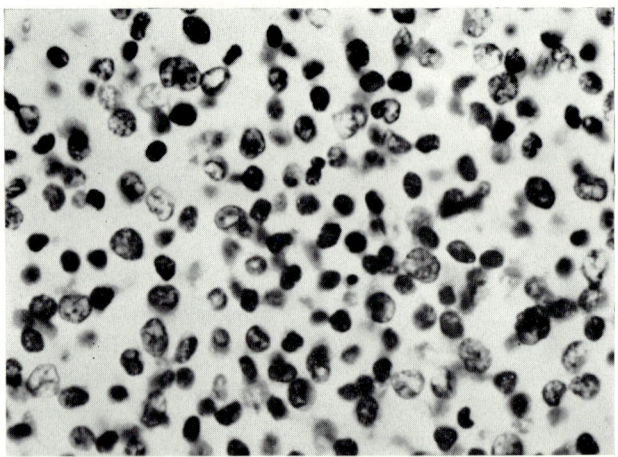

Fig. 49.—Section of leukaemic clot in post-mortem heart blood (male, 64 years). (×400.)

distinguishing from chronic myeloid leukaemia, thrombocytopenia is usual in monocytic leukaemia but the platelet count is normal or raised in the former. The leucocyte alkaline phosphatase activity does not appear to be a reliable index.

Erythropoiesis is depressed, and some of the red-cell precursors can show megaloblastic features. Megakaryocytes may be scanty or absent.

MONOCYTIC LEUKAEMIA

This usually pursues an acute or subacute course. The clinical picture may differ little, if at all, from that of the other types of acute leukaemia. Circumoral and gingival lesions are often prominent.

The circulating leucoblasts may be associated with an increased number of myelocytes (Naegeli) (*Fig.* 50) or a type more closely resembling the monocyte or reticulum cell is found in relative isolation (Schilling).

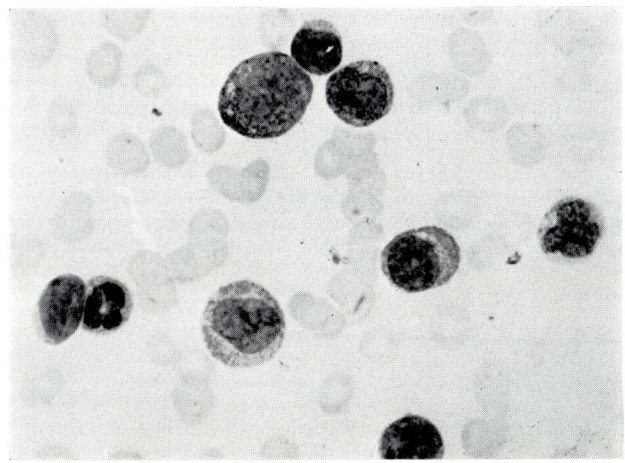

Fig. 50.—Female, aged 87 years, admitted as a 'social problem'. Hb, 52 per cent. W.B.C., 66,000 per c.mm. Acute myelomonocytic leukaemia. (×900.)

Case 3.— A woman, aged 67 years, was seen with a history of dyspnoea for 2 months; sudden attack of abdominal pain and vomiting 2 weeks before admission; and pain in the left hypochrondrium and left shoulder for 1 week. She was admitted to a surgical ward, where hepatosplenomegaly was found; Hb, 48 per cent; W.B.C., 39,000 per c.mm. The majority of the leucocytes were of myelomonocytic type, and similar cells were abundant in the bone-marrow smears. She died 3 weeks after admission.

Some examples of monocytic leukaemia follow a more chronic course with survival up to about 5 years.

ACUTE PROMYELOCYTIC LEUKAEMIA

This is another variant of acute leukaemia which is commoner in the elderly. The predominant cell is the promyelocyte, containing nucleoli and cytoplasmic granules. The presence of the latter may suggest a more chronic process than the condition warrants. Most of these patients die in less than a year from the time of diagnosis. There is often an associated coagulation defect, due to hypofibrinogenaemia and factor-V deficiency.

COURSE AND PROGNOSIS

Acute leukaemia usually pursues a more rapidly fatal course in the elderly, irrespective of treatment. In 1963 the M.R.C. Working Party found that in patients over 50 years the percentages who died within the first 4 weeks from the start of treatment were 90 per cent (on 6-mercaptopurine and high-dose prednisone), 54·5 per cent (on 6-mercaptopurine only), and 47·3 per cent (on 6-mercaptopurine and low-dose prednisone). The corresponding figures for the age-group 20–49 were 50 per cent, 31·5 per cent, and 18·2 per cent, respectively. It concluded that 'acute leukaemia in the adult is a rapidly fatal disease which is not greatly influenced by present methods of treatment'. The second Working Party in 1966 found the same shortening of survival time with age. The median survival time for the myeloid series varied from 21 to 70 days in the different treatment groups, and that for the lymphoblastic series from 53 to 235 days. The lymphoblastic type was more often found in the younger age-groups. A shortened survival was also correlated with a high initial blast-cell count. High neutrophil counts were associated with longer survival. Splenic enlargement in acute lymphoblastic leukaemia was associated with longer survival.

The use of new antileukaemic agents, such as rubidomycin and arabinosyl cytosine, whilst embodying justifiable attempts at improving the treatment, for practical purposes have not changed the course and prognosis of the disease in the elderly.

CHRONIC MYELOID LEUKAEMIA

CLINICAL FEATURES

The presenting features are usually related to anaemia, haemorrhage, thrombosis, intercurrent infection, hepatosplenomegaly, or enlarged lymph-nodes. Patients complain of increasing tiredness.

Anaemia may not be noticeable initially, but pallor follows as the general health deteriorates. The anaemia is refractory to the usual haematinics and may be aggravated by bleeding into the gastro-intestinal or genito-urinary tracts. This is not necessarily related to thrombocytopenia.

The spleen is practically always enlarged, and often this becomes extreme. It may be associated with dragging abdominal pain, and acute attacks due to perisplenitis or infarction can occur. The liver is less frequently enlarged (in approximately two-thirds).

Lymph-node enlargement is not such a prominent feature as it is in chronic lymphatic leukaemia, although most established cases show some degree of lymph-node involvement. Massive enlargement suggests that the condition is more likely to be Hodgkin's disease or lymphosarcoma.

Cutaneous involvement results from direct infiltration or non-specific leukaemoid reactions. Many types of skin reaction can be mimicked. Patients may present with herpes zoster. Subcutaneous nodules of myeloid tissue are firm, and grey to brown in colour. They usually presage rapid advancement of the disease and may ulcerate. Urticaria and pruritus can be troublesome, and are probably related to the basophilia that is often present.

Any of the viscera may be invaded, resulting in almost any symptom-complex, such as gastro-intestinal complaints, dyspnoea, bone pain, joint effusion, visual impairment, central nervous system disturbance, pericarditis, and obstructive jaundice. Priapism is more commonly found in chronic myeloid than in other types of leukaemia. Tonsillar enlargement in the elderly should suggest the possibility of leukaemia. The sudden appearance of a hernia or uterine prolapse may be due to increased intra-abdominal pressure.

Cachexia develops with progression of the disease, and the picture is complicated by the superimposition of infection and renal failure. Fever nearly always accompanies deterioration.

There is an increased incidence of peptic ulceration. Hyperuricaemia is common, but clinical gout is seldom seen in the absence of treatment.

LABORATORY FINDINGS

Chronic myeloid leukaemia is usually readily diagnosed, simply on the clinical picture and peripheral blood findings. Rare variants or the preleukaemic or acute terminal phase are more difficult.

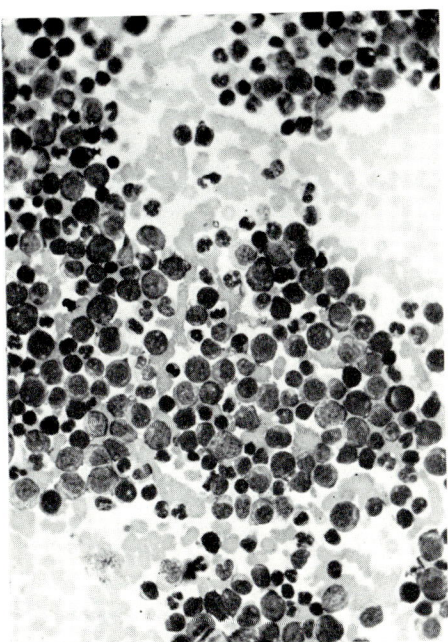

Fig. 51.—Peripheral blood. W.B.C., 790,000 per c.mm. Chronic myeloid leukaemia. ($\times$400.)

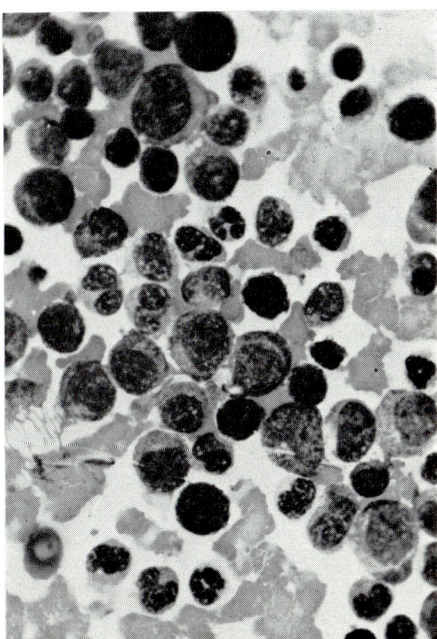

Fig. 52.—Peripheral blood. W.B.C., 790,000 per c.mm. Chronic myeloid leukaemia. ($\times$900.)

Haemoglobin.—The patient may not be anaemic at first—indeed there may be a preceding polycythaemic phase. However, anaemia develops sooner or later and is usually of normochromic type. The red cells show moderate anisocytosis and poikilocytosis. Nucleated red blood-cells are usually present.

White Blood-cells.—This is almost invariably markedly raised, with a total count of well over 100,000 per c.mm. made up predominantly of segmented neutrophils with a good admixture of metamyelocytes and myelocytes (*Figs.* 51, 52). A few promyelocytes and myeloblasts can usually be found. Basophils and to a lesser degree eosinophils are also increased.

Platelets.—The platelet count may be normal or raised. Irregular platelet fragments are often found in peripheral blood-films.

Marrow Findings.—The marrow, in the typical case, is practically indistinguishable from the peripheral blood-picture. The value of marrow aspiration lies not so much in its capacity to add to information obtained from the blood-picture, but rather to exclude other possible sources of confusion, such as myelofibrosis. It may help by giving an early indication of acute blast-cell transformation.

Leucocyte Alkaline Phosphatase Activity.—Leukaemic granulocytes show diminished alkaline phosphatase activity. The leucocyte enzyme content may be assayed quantitatively on concentrated leucocyte suspensions, but this is a time-consuming procedure and in routine work a cytochemical method is preferable. A substrate containing alpha-naphthyl-phosphate is used, and the liberated naphthol is coupled with a diazotized amine. Alkaline phosphatase activity shows as a reddish-brown precipitate. The intensity of staining is scored from 0 to 4. The total score is the sum of these ratings for 100 consecutive neutrophils. The normal range is 15–100, and there is a wide range of observer and technical error, but the demonstration of a marked reduction in activity provides useful confirmatory evidence of myeloid leukaemia.

The Philadelphia Chromosome.—Nowell and Hungerford (1960) described an abnormal extra minute chromosome in the blood-cultures of two men suffering from chronic myeloid leukaemia. This has been repeatedly confirmed as a reliable index of chronic myeloid leukaemia. However, a negative blood-culture result does not exclude the diagnosis, and in such cases direct examination of the marrow cells may show the presence of the abnormal chromosome. It has been shown (Rastrick, Fitzgerald, and Gunz, 1968) that erythroblasts, as well as myeloid cells, possess this chromosome.

The demonstration of the Philadelphia chromosome is seldom required for diagnostic purposes, other than in atypical cases. Krauss, Sokal, and Sandberg (1964) compared a group of 16 patients who showed the Philadelphia chromosome with a group of 12 who did not. The former conformed to classic chronic myeloid leukaemia in their clinical and haematological features, whilst the latter showed a marked male preponderance (11/12); they were older, had atypical haematological features, and responded poorly to therapy.

Diagnosis

The diagnosis of chronic myeloid leukaemia seldom poses difficulty in the established case. The clinical picture of splenomegaly, often with hepatomegaly and lymphadenopathy, and the peripheral blood findings are sufficient to make the diagnosis clear. Difficulty may arise, however, if the patient is seen early or late in the progress of the disease. Early presenting pictures may be those of polycythaemia, myelofibrosis, or refractory anaemia, and the late picture can be that of acute myeloid leukaemia.

Severe neutrophilia may resemble chronic myeloid leukaemia, although the white-cell count is seldom as high. Leucocyte alkaline phosphatase and chromosome studies can be helpful in such patients.

Conrad, Rappaport, and Crosby (1965) pointed out the difficulties that may arise in the diagnosis of chronic myeloid leukaemia in the elderly: other complicating diseases are often present; splenic and hepatic enlargement may be minimal or

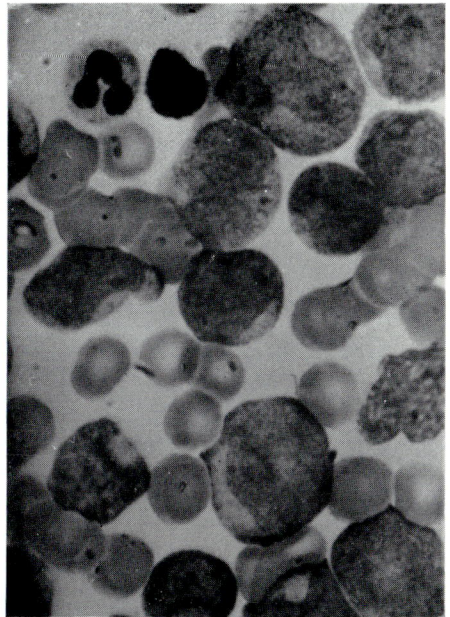

Fig. 53.—*Case* 4. Peripheral blood. Terminal acute blast-cell transformation in chronic myeloid leukaemia. (×1100.)

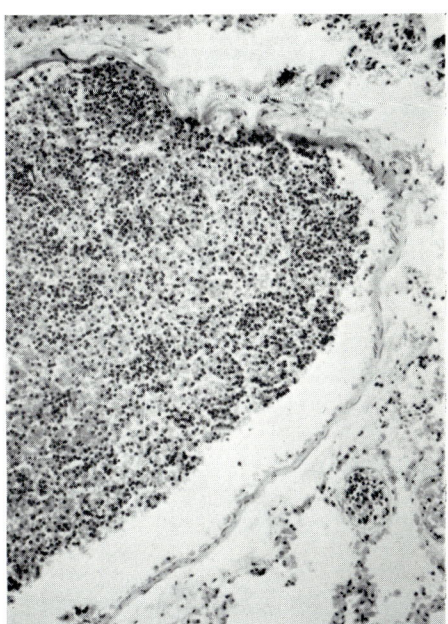

Fig. 54.—*Case* 4. Embolus in pulmonary artery, consisting of leukaemic cells. (×150.)

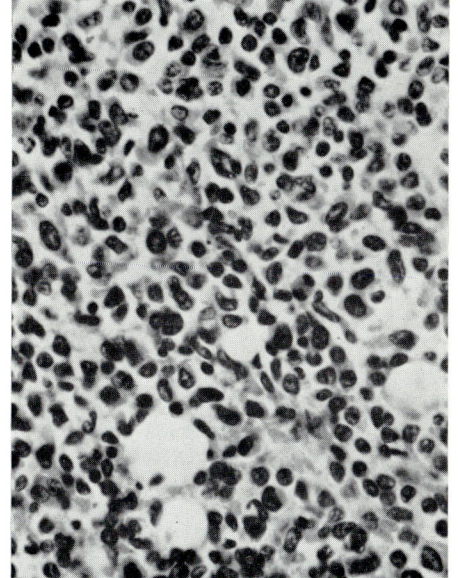

Fig. 55.—*Case* 4. Bone-marrow. Chronic myeloid leukaemia in acute blast-cell termination (section of post-mortem marrow). (×400.)

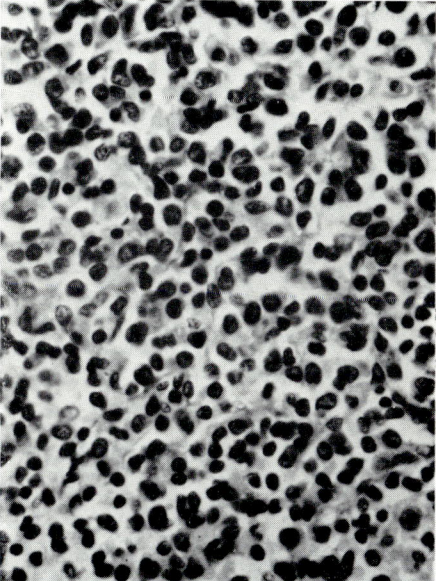

Fig. 56.—*Case* 4. Spleen. Myeloid leukaemia. (×400.)

absent; leucocytosis may be only moderate; thrombocythaemia is often prominent and alkaline phosphatase activity may be increased in mature granulocytes. The enzyme change is apparently not directly related to the chromosomal abnormality because the cases reported by Krauss and colleagues (1964) with a normal chromosomal pattern had a low leucocyte alkaline phosphatase activity.

PROGNOSIS

Acute myeloblastic transformation is a frequent mode of termination (*Figs.* 53–57). Intercurrent infection is common, although probably not as frequent as

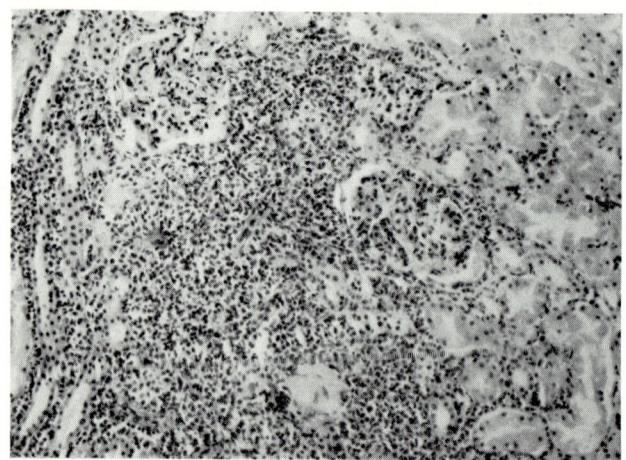

Fig. 57.—*Case* 4. Myeloid infiltration of kidney. (×150.)

in other forms of leukaemia. The survival time is shorter in the elderly. Bodley-Scott (1957) found a mean survival time of 39 months below 30 years, and 24 months over 60 years.

The 1968 M.R.C. Working Party found that 68/90 patients died from uncontrolled leukaemia. In 15 cases the cause of death bore no apparent relation to the leukaemia, which was well controlled. The median survival for busulphan-treated patients was $3\frac{1}{2}$ years, and $2\frac{1}{2}$ years for those treated with radiotherapy.

Case 4.—Female, aged 64 years. Admitted to hospital for social reasons with 'tonsillitis' of one week's duration. Deteriorated rapidly and died within 3 days. Hb, 92 per cent. W.B.C., 323,000 per c.mm. *Fig.* 53 shows peripheral blood—terminal acute blast-cell termination in chronic myeloid leukaemia. *Figs.* 54–57 show post-mortem findings—*Fig.* 54, embolus in pulmonary artery, consisting of leukaemia cells (this was the immediate cause of death); *Fig.* 55, section of post-mortem marrow, showing terminal phase of chronic myeloid leukaemia; *Fig.* 56, spleen (300 g.) showing myeloid leukaemia; *Fig.* 57, kidney showing myeloid infiltration.

CHRONIC LYMPHATIC LEUKAEMIA

Both principal forms of chronic leukaemia, namely myeloid and lymphatic, are distinct and in most instances readily classified. However, chronic lymphatic leukaemia shows a greater predilection for the aged, and also often illustrates the possible vagaries of the lymphoproliferative disorders.

LEUKAEMIA

CLINICAL FEATURES

The commonest presenting complaint is that of enlarged nodes. Splenomegaly is more likely to be symptomless than in chronic myeloid leukaemia.

General malaise, weight-loss, and dyspnoea usually bear some relationship to the severity of the anaemia. Angina pectoris may be unmasked.

Repeated intercurrent infections, especially of the tonsils, are a prominent feature of the progressive case.

Superficial skin infections and herpes zoster can occur. Skin, skeletal, or visceral infiltration may be found in any organ. The alimentary tract is noteworthy in this respect.

A significant proportion of patients are diagnosed as a result of a routine blood examination, and these have minimal or no symptoms referable to their leukaemia.

Serous effusions are not uncommon, particularly when the disease enters a more acute phase. The nephrotic syndrome has also been reported.

LABORATORY FINDINGS

The diagnosis of chronic lymphatic leukaemia is made essentially on the peripheral blood findings. The white-cell count is raised to 50,000–100,000 per c.mm. Mature lymphocytes comprise 90–99 per cent of the leucocytes. Smear cells are also numerous.

Anaemia, of normochromic type, may be present, but many early cases are not anaemic. The platelet count is usually normal.

Bone-marrow smears show a preponderance of lymphoid cells, although the general appearance is not as characteristic as it is in the peripheral blood, and this examination is not essential for diagnosis.

As the disease progresses anaemia becomes more severe, and, rarely, in the terminal phase partial blast-cell transformation occurs. However, too much significance should not be attached to the finding of occasional lymphoblasts in the peripheral blood because these may be found in the absence of any marked deterioration.

DIAGNOSIS

Chronic lymphatic leukaemia is usually diagnosed on the total white-cell count and peripheral blood film. The only theoretical source of confusion would be 'benign lymphocytosis', but in practice these are often variants of infectious mononucleosis—a condition which is almost never encountered in the elderly.

Other patients that present difficulty are those in whom the white-cell count is normal or slightly raised. The initial count is below 10,000 per c.mm. in approximately 10 per cent. The differential count may show only a partial preponderance of lymphocytes. These patients are usually either symptomless or the peripheral blood findings reflect a 'spilling over' from well-established lymphosarcoma. In the case of the latter the patient will show evidence of the neoplasm and will probably be anaemic. All gradations can be found between chronic lymphatic leukaemia and lymphosarcoma, the two diagnoses being merely the extremes of a continuous spectrum. If the 'partial' peripheral blood-picture is found in a symptomless person then the diagnosis of 'latent' chronic lymphatic leukaemia may be made without the necessity of either informing or treating the patient. The progress of such patients is considered below.

Associated Conditions

Intercurrent infections and pulmonary tuberculosis are not uncommon. The serum protein pattern can be abnormal, with an increase in gamma-globulin, or a paraprotein or cryoglobulin may be found. More commonly hypogammaglobulinaemia occurs which shows no correlation with age. Fairley and Scott (1961), in a study of 111 patients, found normal levels in 29 per cent, reduced in 67 per cent, raised in 3 per cent, and macroglobulinaemia in 1 per cent. The level fell as the disease progressed, and this could well be a factor in the increased susceptibility to intercurrent infection.

Auto-immune haemolytic anaemia is a possible complication. The degree of haemolysis may be slight, so that mild anaemia is attributed directly to the leukaemia. Alternatively, there may be a haemolytic crisis. The direct Coombs's test is positive; fragmented erythrocytes appear in the peripheral blood; while the reticulocyte count and the serum bilirubin level are raised. Thrombocytopenia can also develop due to a similar auto-immune mechanism.

Course and Prognosis

Chronic lymphatic leukaemia is the most benign of the various types of leukaemia. The diagnosis may remain a purely laboratory one for many years. Survival depends upon the rate of progression; the development of blast-cell transformation; the extent of visceral infiltration as in lymphosarcoma; the occurrence of intercurrent infection and associated complications such as haemolytic anaemia or thrombocytopenia.

The following patient illustrates the variable course of this disease, and the way in which it sometimes fails to pursue the relentless pattern one normally associates with the term 'leukaemia'. This applies particularly in the elderly, as they are more likely to die from unrelated disease before the leukaemia completes its natural history.

Case 5.—This man was seen in May, 1959, aged 60 years, with an acute myocardial infarction. Rubbery lymph-nodes were noted in the neck and groins. Biopsy showed lymphosarcoma and bone-marrow smears showed lymphocytosis. The white blood-cell count was 46,000 per c.mm. with approximately 50 per cent lymphocytes and very numerous smear cells. Hb was 100 per cent, and the platelet count, 510,000 per c.mm. He was later seen for acute bronchitis and a squamous carcinoma of the pinna and left temple. In March, 1965, the leucocyte count was 23,700 per c.mm., over 90 per cent of which were lymphocytes and smear cells. By December, 1965, this had fallen to 11,000 per c.mm. and the only abnormality noted was the presence of numerous smear cells. He was last seen in November, 1968 (age 69 years), complaining of palpable neck lymph-nodes. Biopsy showed an appearance of lymphosarcoma identical with that found in 1959, but now the peripheral blood-picture was entirely normal.

Case 6.—This man first attended in February, 1968, at the age of 67, with diarrhoea for 1 month and was found to have generalized lymph-node enlargement and hepatosplenomegaly. Rectal examination showed a nodular mass high up on the anterior rectal wall. At this time his Hb was 63 per cent (9·2 g. per 100 ml.); W.B.C., 39,900 per c.mm., over 95 per cent of which were lymphocytes and smear cells; and platelets, 91,000 per c.mm.

Rectal biopsy yielded fragments of a well-differentiated adenocarcinoma.

An abdominoperineal resection was performed. At operation the liver was noted to be diffusely enlarged and the spleen was four times its normal size. A generalized abdominal lymphadenopathy was present.

The resected specimen was of interest in that a fungating adenocarcinoma of the rectal wall, 9 cm. from the anus, was found, but adjacent mural lymph-nodes showed the appearances of lymphosarcoma. A lymph-node from the abdomen also showed lymphosarcoma.

The patient had a stormy postoperative time during which multiple infections developed. He died 1 month later.

Features of interest included the presentation with carcinoma of the rectum and the incidental finding of lymphatic leukaemia and lymphosarcoma.

OTHER VARIETIES OF LEUKAEMIA

Various types of leukaemia have been designated in accordance with the predominant cell type. Some of these are still the subject of dispute. Thus, eosinophilic leukaemia may be an exaggeration of the eosinophilia normally found in myeloid leukaemia, or part of the response to systemic disease such as polyarteritis nodosa, Hodgkin's disease, or Loeffler's syndrome. The same difficulty arises with the description of basophilic leukaemia. In mast-cell leukaemia the clinical picture is that of urticaria pigmentosa but pursuing an acute course with infiltration of several viscera.

PLASMA-CELL LEUKAEMIA

An excess of circulating plasma cells may be found in association with multiple myelomatosis. These patients usually succumb sooner than those without this type of 'spill-over'.

NEUTROPHILIC LEUKAEMIA

Occasionally, patients are seen in whom there is a high white-cell count, but the blood-film shows little apart from normal mature neutrophils. There may be associated splenomegaly. We have been able to follow several such patients in whom chronic myeloid leukaemia was suspected in spite of the absence of any significant increase in primitive leucocytes. They usually terminated as frank myeloid leukaemia.

ERYTHROLEUKAEMIA (DI GUGLIELMO'S DISEASE)

Di Guglielmo first described a rapidly fatal condition in which erythroblasts played a part comparable to that of the leucoblasts in acute leukaemia. Severe anaemia, hepatosplenomegaly, and fever develop. The peripheral blood contains many primitive nucleated red cells, but the leucocytes and platelets are usually reduced. The marrow shows a corresponding erythroblastic picture. Di Guglielmo pointed out that the spleen is greatly enlarged—much more than is found in acute leukaemia. Oral lesions are uncommon.

Subsequently it was recognized that there is also a chronic form of this disease—the erythroblastic counterpart to chronic myeloid leukaemia—chronic erythraemic myelosis.

The classic acute and chronic forms are readily recognized, but many examples of intermediate forms are encountered. Thus nucleated red cells can be very numerous in the peripheral blood in what is otherwise a typical example of chronic myeloid leukaemia. This state of *erythroleukaemia* is nearly always present to some extent.

ALEUKAEMIC LEUKAEMIA

This contradiction in terms describes those examples where the peripheral blood findings are either normal or in no way diagnostic, although the bone-marrow shows the presence of leukaemia. These patients are usually anaemic, and, as the anaemia can be normochromic or even macrocytic, pernicious anaemia may be mimicked. Examination of the buffy coat often shows primitive cells.

Aleukaemic leukaemia is chiefly a problem associated with acute leukaemia when the patient is first seen. It is seldom found in chronic myeloid leukaemia, other than in terminal cases. If a comparable situation is found in chronic lymphatic or histiocytic infiltrations then the preferable diagnosis is that of lymphosarcoma or medullary reticulosis respectively.

Case 7.—This lady presented with a 1-week history of tiredness and a punched-out ulcer on the outer aspect of her arm.

The peripheral blood-picture was: Hb, 26 per cent; W.B.C., 10,000 per c.mm. with nucleated red blood-cells, but no definite leucoblasts were seen. Platelets were 5000 per c.mm. The sternal marrow smears showed a picture indistinguishable from that of chronic myeloid leukaemia. Biopsy of the ulcer confirmed the presence of a leukaemic infiltrate. Thereafter, the disease progressed rapidly with a W.B.C. rising to 30,000 per c.mm. and containing numerous leucoblasts.

LEUKAEMOID REACTIONS

The presence of anaemia with primitive white and red blood-cells in the peripheral blood film is not sufficient for a diagnosis of leukaemia to be made. This caution is of great importance in the elderly in whom there are many other possible causes.

Anaemia, with neutrophils showing a left nuclear shift, myelocytes and occasional myeloblasts, polychromasia, and few or many normoblasts, constitutes *leucoerythroblastic anaemia*. This *may* denote marrow replacement by neoplastic tissue, but many other conditions can produce this picture—for example, haemorrhage, renal insufficiency, myelosclerosis, or haemolysis. However, apart from the necessity of recognizing the primary condition these should not be confused with leukaemia. The degree of polychromasia, reticulocytosis, and production of normoblasts usually overshadows that of the leucocyte series. Furthermore, marrow examination should exclude leukaemia.

Diagnosis is difficult when a leukaemoid reaction is more purely that of an overproduction of immature leucocytes, which shows in the marrow as well as the peripheral blood. Disseminated tuberculosis can give rise to this type of reaction, and this is readily overlooked in the elderly. The haematological distinction between this and true leukaemia is helped by noting the extent of marrow replacement with primitive white cells; whether the megakaryocytes are depressed, the leucocyte alkaline phosphatase activity, and in a few instances the demonstration of the Philadelphia chromosome may be diagnostic.

PATHOLOGICAL CHANGES

Acute Leukaemia

The lesions result from leukaemic infiltration, haemorrhage, thrombosis, and infection. Infiltration may be found in any viscera or musculoskeletal tissue. Meningeal infiltration is of particular importance, in that it can be present during an otherwise complete clinical and haematological remission.

Chronic Myeloid Leukaemia

Extreme bone-marrow hyperplasia is found, in which granulocytes predominate. A morphologically similar picture of myeloid metaplasia is found in other organs, especially the spleen, liver, and lymph-nodes. Splenic enlargement may be extreme. The organ is firm and has a thick capsule. Infarcts are often present. Sections of spleen show, in addition to accumulations of granulocytes, varying proportions of normoblasts and megakaryocytes. The follicular structure is relatively atrophied and diffuse fibrosis of the pulp takes place.

Chronic Lymphatic Leukaemia

The leucocytic infiltrate is much more pure than in other forms of leukaemia. Lymphocytes form almost the only cell seen. Enlarged lymph-nodes may show partial preservation of their follicular pattern, but more usually this is entirely replaced by sheets of lymphocytes. The picture is indistinguishable from that of lymphosarcoma. The hepatic infiltrate is more or less confined to the portal tracts. The degree of splenic enlargement may not be as great as that seen in chronic myeloid leukaemia, and infarction is less common.

TREATMENT (see Table XXVI)

Acute Leukaemia

It is justifiable to treat acute leukaemia in the elderly in view of the possibility of inducing remissions and alleviating symptoms. A variety of drugs is available.

Methotrexate is a folic-acid antagonist which can be given orally, intramuscularly, intravenously, or intrathecally. The side-effects include abdominal pain, diarrhoea, alopecia, and bone-marrow depression. Examples of hepatic necrosis and cirrhosis have been reported. It is particularly suitable for maintaining remissions.

6-Mercaptopurine is given orally and used for inducing remissions in addition to maintenance therapy. Its toxic effects are not usually troublesome, but it may give rise to bone-marrow depression and gastro-intestinal symptoms.

Drugs used especially for the induction of remissions are *cyclophosphamide, vincristine, corticosteroids, cytosine arabinoside,* and *rubidomycin*. The role of *asparaginase* is still uncertain. The advantage of combined therapy also is not as clear in adults as it is in children. The 1966 M.R.C. Trial found the longest survival in the myeloid series in those treated with steroid alone, followed by mercaptopurine, and the two combined showed the shortest median survival time. In the lymphoblastic series the longest survival again was with steroids alone, but the time with mercaptopurine alone was shorter than when it was combined with normal doses of steroid. The same working party noted a negative correlation between age and survival time in both types of acute leukaemia. Blood transfusion and antibiotics should be given when indicated.

Rubidomycin produced remission in 35 out of 64 patients with acute myelocytic leukaemia treated by Boiron and others (1969). The average total dose was 12 mg. per kg. Severe bone-marrow aplasia was a constant finding, and dosage was difficult to control. The other toxic effects included cardiotoxicity, stomatitis, gastro-intestinal disorders, alopecia, and local necrosis at the site of injection. These authors concluded that rubidomycin may be a useful drug for inducing remission, although its toxicity makes it less suitable for maintenance treatment. However, even this guarded assessment may be too optimistic in the elderly. Marmout, Damasio, and Rossi (1969) claimed that cardiotoxicity arises much more often in the adult and elderly in whom it is a very distressing condition. Furthermore, there

Table XXVI.—Drugs used in Treatment of Leukaemia

Drug	Dose	Route	Indication	Toxic Effects
Methotrexate	0·07–0·14 mg. per kg. per day or 3 mg. per m.^{2} per day	Oral	Acute leukaemia	Gastro-intestinal Alopecia. Bone-marrow aplasia Liver necrosis and fibrosis
	20–40 mg. per m.^{2}, twice weekly	I.M. or I.V.	Acute leukaemia	
	5–10 mg. daily	Intrathecal	C.N.S. leukaemia until blasts 10 per c.mm. C.S.F.	
6-Mercaptopurine	90 mg. per m.^{2} per day or 2·5 mg. per kg. per day	Oral	Remissions in all forms of leukaemia	Few gastro-intestinal with bone-marrow aplasia Hepatitis
Cyclophosphamide	100 mg. per m.^{2} per day or 3 mg. per kg. per day	Oral	Acute leukaemia	Bone-marrow aplasia Alopecia Haemorrhagic cystitis
	200 mg. per day 2–5 mg. per kg. per day	I.V. Oral	Chronic lymphatic leukaemia	
Vincristine	1 mg. per m.^{2} per week increasing to 2 mg. per m.^{2} per week	I.V.	Acute leukaemia	Neurotoxic Alopecia Constipation Myopathy
Cytosine arabinoside	2 mg. per kg. per day for 10 days	I.V.	Acute leukaemia	Bone-marrow aplasia Gastro-intestinal Hepatitis
	50 mg.	Intrathecal		
Rubidomycin	1–2 mg. per kg. per day	I.V. infusion	Acute leukaemia	Bone-marrow aplasia Cardiotoxicity
Busulphan	4–8 mg. per day to produce remission, then 0·5–4 mg. per day	Oral	Chronic myeloid leukaemia	Bone-marrow aplasia Adrenal failure Pulmonary fibrosis
Hydroxyurea	20–30 mg. per kg. per day	Oral	Chronic myeloid leukaemia	Gastro-intestinal Megaloblastic anaemia
Chlorambucil	0·2 mg. per kg. per day	Oral	Chronic lymphatic leukaemia	Bone-marrow aplasia Gastro-intestinal
Prednisone	40 mg. per day	Oral	Acute leukaemia Chronic leukaemia in blast phase Associated haemolytic anaemia	Psychosis Hypersteroidism Fluid retention, etc.
Asparaginase	200 I.U. per kg. per day	I.V.	Acute leukaemia	Defects in protein synthesis Hepatitis Pancreatitis

may be a toxic synergism between vincristine and rubidomycin. They found that fatal and non-fatal cardiotoxicity occurred after rubidomycin alone in 'safe' doses in the middle-aged and elderly.

Chronic Myeloid Leukaemia

It has been shown that *busulphan* is superior to radiotherapy in terms of survival time and maintenance of satisfactory haemoglobin levels (M.R.C. Working Party, 1966). The drug is used for inducing remissions and maintenance. The daily oral dose is 0·5–4 mg., but this must be carefully controlled otherwise profound marrow aplasia may occur. This may be permanent even after conventional doses have been given. Weatherall, Galton, and Kay (1969) reported 4 such cases, and recommended that the daily dosage should not exceed 4 mg.; white-cell counts should be done weekly as it approaches 20,000 per c.mm., and treatment stopped when it falls below this figure, or if the platelet count falls below 100,000 per c.mm. Thereafter the leucocyte count should be checked every fortnight and busulphan resumed at 2 mg. daily, aiming to stabilize the count at 10,000 per c.mm. On ordinary maintenance, counts should be done at least monthly. Other possible complications are adrenal insufficiency, cataract, and pulmonary interstitial fibrosis.

When the patient ceases to respond to busulphan or develops complications other drugs are available—such as *hydroxyurea* given orally 20–30 mg. per kg. per day. This drug may induce megaloblastic anaemia or give rise to gastro-intestinal symptoms.

Pipobroman (1·5–2·5 mg. per kg. per day) and *Piposulfan* (1·5–2·5 mg. per kg. per day) are other newer alkylating agents that may be given orally when busulphan is stopped. *Dibromomannitol* may also be substituted in the form of an initial course of 4–6 mg. per kg. per day for several days. Its principal danger is severe thrombocytopenia.

Chronic Lymphatic Leukaemia

This can be a purely laboratory diagnosis in a patient who is neither anaemic nor showing symptoms referable to his leukaemia. No treatment is indicated in such cases. Furthermore, the extent and rigour of any specific treatment that is given should be balanced against the clinical indications. These elderly patients may well live their normal span and die from other disease before the leukaemia has had time to run its course.

The two chief drugs used are *chlorambucil* and *cyclophosphamide*. Chlorambucil is given orally in doses of 0·2 mg. per kg. per day until the disease is controlled. Toxic effects include neutropenia, thrombocytopenia, and gastro-intestinal disturbances.

Cyclophosphamide is better given orally in chronic lymphatic leukaemia (2–5 mg. per kg. per day).

Auto-immune haemolytic anaemia should be treated with corticosteroids. Androgens may also help.

REFERENCES

Armitage, P., and Doll, R. (1954), *Br. J. Cancer*, **8**, 1.
— — — — (1957), *Ibid.*, **11**, 161.
Bean, R. H. D. (1960), *Br. med. J.*, **2**, 1552.

BENNET, J. H. (1845), *Edinb. M. and S. J.*, **64,** 413.
BODLEY-SCOTT, R. (1957), *Lancet*, **1,** 1053, 1099, 1162.
BOIRON, M., JACQUILLAT, C., WEIL, M., TANZER, J., LEVY, D., SULTAN, C., and BERNARD, J. (1969), *Lancet*, **1,** 330.
CONRAD, M. E., RAPPAPORT, H., and CROSBY, W. H. (1965), *Archs intern. Med.*, **116,** 765.
COURT BROWN, W. M., and DOLL, R. (1959), *Br. med. J.*, **1,** 1063.
FAIRLEY, G. H., and SCOTT, R. B. (1961), *Ibid.*, **2,** 920.
HAYHOE, F. G. J., QUAGLINO, D., and DOLL, R. (1964), *M.R.C. Spec. Rep. Series No.* 304. London: H.M.S.O.
HEWITT, D. (1955), *Br. J. prev. soc. Med.*, **9,** 81.
KRAUSS, S., SOKAL, J. E., and SANDBERG, A. A. (1964), *Ann. intern. Med.*, **61,** 625.
LOUTIT, J. F. (1958), *Practitioner*, **181,** 533.
MACMAHON, B., and CLARK, D. (1956), *Blood*, **11,** 871.
MARMOUT, A. M., DAMASIO, E., and ROSSI, F. (1969), *Lancet*, **1,** 837.
MEDICAL RESEARCH COUNCIL (1963), First Report, *Br. med. J.*, **1,** 7.
— — — (1966), Second Report, *Ibid.*, **1,** 1383.
— — — (1968), Third Report, *Ibid.*, **1,** 201.
MINOT, G. P., BUCKMAN, T. E., and ISAACS, R. (1924), *J. Am. med. Ass.*, **82,** 1489.
NOWELL, P. C., and HUNGERFORD, D. A. (1960), *J. natn. Cancer Inst.*, **25,** 85.
OSGOOD, E. E. (1969), *Blood*, **33,** 268.
RASTRICK, J. M., FITZGERALD, P. H., and GUNZ, F. W. (1968), *Br. med. J.*, **1,** 98.
SCOTT, R. B. (1957), *Lancet*, **1,** 1053, 1099, 1162.
VIDEBAEK, AA. (1966), *Acta haematol.*, **36,** 183.
WARD, G. R. (1917), *Br. J. Child. Dis.*, **14,** 10.
WEATHERALL, D. J., GALTON, D. A. G., and KAY, H. E. M. (1969), *Br. med. J.*, **1,** 638.
WOODLIFF, H. J., and DOUGAN, L. (1964), *Ibid.*, **1,** 744.

10

PROTEIN DISORDERS

PARAPROTEINS

ABNORMAL proteins or dysglobulins are found usually in the elderly, although they can occur at all ages, even infancy. Genetic factors are probably involved, as sometimes there is a familial pattern.

IMMUNOGLOBULINS

The immunoglobulins are those serum globulin fractions that may be associated with specific or non-specific lymphoreticular (including plasma-cell) proliferations. Their nomenclature was standardized by the World Health Organization (W.H.O., 1964):—

Name	Molecular Weight		Normal Serum Level (mg. per 100 ml.)
YM or IgM	1,000,000	(19S)	50–190
YA or IgA	170,000–500,000	(7S–12S)	100–400
YG or IgG	170,000	(7S)	800–1600
YD or IgD			0·5–40
YE or IgE			10–40

The complete immunoglobulin molecule contains a pair of light chains and a pair of heavy chains. Two principal types of light chains have been designated κ and λ, and five groups of heavy chains identified—α, δ, ϵ, μ, or γ. The chains are linked by disulphide bridges. Those between each light and heavy chain are near the carboxy terminal of the light chain. If the molecule is split at this point the two amino-acid terminals are termed the Fab fragments because they contain the antibody component. The residual carboxy terminal portion of two heavy chains is the Fc fragment (so termed because it is readily crystallized) (*Fig. 58*).

Normal immunoglobulins are made up of several types, but many diseases are associated with an excessive proliferation of one or a few types at the expense of the remaining normal ones—monoclonal proliferation. This must be distinguished from those in which there is hyperglobulinaemia and a generalized increase in immunoglobulins, as in chronic hepatitis, rheumatoid arthritis, hypersensitivity states, or acquired haemolytic anaemia.

Monoclonal immunoglobulins are usually detected as a well-defined band on the serum electrophoretic strip. They may be termed M proteins, MG proteins, or paraproteins, although Martin (1969) advocated that the last term should be abandoned in favour of a more specific identification of the abnormal protein with its associated clinical condition.

IgG Globulin

This constitutes approximately 75 per cent of the gamma-globulin fraction. It includes most of the antibacterial and antiviral antibodies. Although its Fc fragment contains no specific antibody it can fix complement and combine with rheumatoid factor. If an M protein is present in this fraction the level of normal IgG is lowered and the patient may have a diminished resistance to infection.

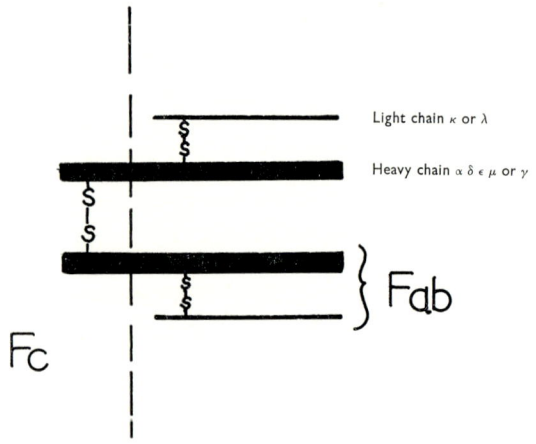

Fig. 58.—The immunoglobulin molecule.

IgA Globulin

This has a high carbohydrate content. It is found in colostrum, saliva, lacrimal glands, and intestinal mucosal glands and includes bacterial antitoxins.

IgM Globulins

These macroglobulins also have a high carbohydrate content. The type found in macroglobulinaemia consists of a pentamer linked by covalent bonds. The light chains are the same as in IgG, but the heavy chains vary.

These globulins include the isohaemagglutinins, saline Rh antibodies, cold agglutinins, heterophil antibodies, and the rheumatoid factor.

Bence Jones Protein

This is a polypeptide with a molecular weight of approximately 22,000 made up of light chains which may be one of two distinct antigenic types. Small concentrations can be demonstrated in normal serum and urine.

Detection of Paraproteins

Serum Electrophoresis

The majority of dysglobulinaemic states, including myelomatosis, can be detected on routine electrophoresis. The immunoglobulins migrate mostly in the gamma-globulin band, but some are found in the beta and alpha-2 zones. An abnormal immunoglobulin is initially distinguished from a simple hyperglobulinaemia by the sharp well-defined nature of its band (*Figs.* 59, 60).

Although this is a satisfactory screening procedure it does not exclude all cases, because the normal IgD level is between 0·5 and 40 mg. per 100 ml. and, therefore, it could be elevated tenfold without showing any obvious peak.

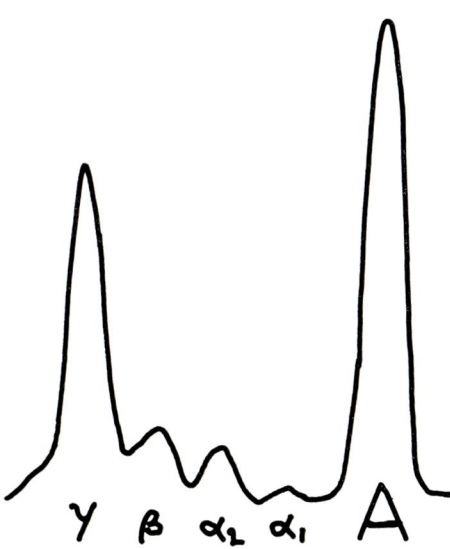

Fig. 59.—Serum-protein electrophoretic scan in myelomatosis (IgG). Male, aged 70 years. Albumin, 4·2 g. per 100 ml. Alpha-1-globulin, 0·24 g. per 100 ml. Alpha-2-globulin, 0·61 g. per 100 ml. Beta-globulin, 0·88 g. per 100 ml. Gamma-globulin, 3·0 g. per 100 ml. Total protein, 8·9 g. per 100 ml. A/G ratio, 0·9 : 1.

IMMUNOELECTROPHORESIS

Whenever an abnormal sharp peak is seen on the electrophoretic strip, or the clinical picture or urinary findings are strongly suggestive of myelomatosis, immunoelectrophoresis should be done. This basically involves exposing the fractions obtained on straight electrophoresis to the action of specific antisera.

OTHER SERUM TESTS

These range from simple screening tests, such as the formol-gel tests and the demonstration of cryoglobulins or pyroglobulins, to much more specialized procedures, such as ultracentrifugation. Fortunately, for clinical purposes serum electrophoresis coupled with immunoelectrophoresis is within the scope of routine laboratories and usually suffices.

URINE TESTS

Improved techniques have shown that a positive test for Bence Jones protein is quantitative as trace amounts of light-chain immunoglobulins are present in normal urine.

The routine screening for Bence Jones protein should include testing at different levels of pH, for example, placing a few ml. of urine (filtered if necessary) into each of three test-tubes, and after adding one or two drops of 33 per cent acetic acid to the second and third tubes respectively, warming all the tubes gently in a known temperature water-bath. Bence Jones protein precipitates between 40 and 60° C., and redissolves when heated to boiling point. Other proteins precipitate at a higher temperature and do not redissolve. If there is heavy albuminuria the boiling urine should be filtered hot prior to testing.

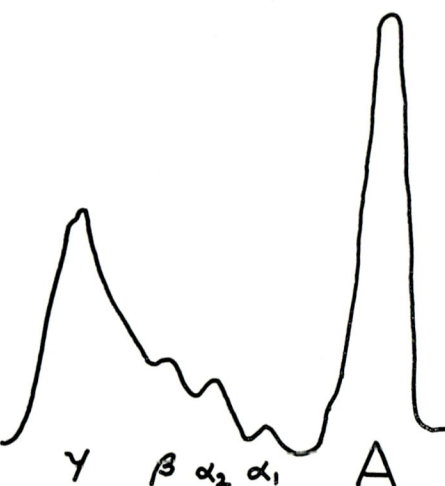

Fig. 60.—Serum-protein electrophoretic scan in hepatic cirrhosis. Male, aged 57 years. Albumin, 3·7 g. per 100 ml. Alpha-1-globulin, 0·2 g. per 100 ml. Alpha-2-globulin, 0·5 g. per 100 ml. Beta-globulin, 0·5 g. per 100 ml. Gamma-globulin, 2·9 g. per 100 ml. Total protein, 7·8 g. per 100 ml. A/G ratio, 0·9 : 1.

A negative result by this screening test does not exclude significant Bence Jones proteinuria. Repeated samples should be tested, and the urine concentrated by dialysis.

Final identification is by electrophoresis and immunoelectrophoresis—these distinguish between the diffuse bands that are present in normal urines or polyclonal hypergammaglobulinaemias from the well-defined band found in monoclonal gammopathies.

General Features

Although paraproteins have been intensively studied, their significance and the mechanism of their production have not been clearly defined. Once they develop they usually persist, but in some instances they disappear. The quantity in the serum may remain unchanged for many years, while in others a fairly rapid increase occurs, almost invariably denoting the presence of an associated disease.

Information regarding molecular size or immunological distribution is not of great diagnostic value in individual cases, because it is only when fairly large numbers are considered that a pattern appears. Similarly with the chemical characteristics of the paraprotein, such as precipitation in the cold, no particular disease can be diagnosed, although the pathogenesis of the clinical features may be clarified.

Case 1.—A female, aged 75 years, was admitted with ulceration of the legs for 2 years and blueness of the face, feet, and knees for 18 months precipitated by cold. Irregular pyrexia of 100–101° F. had been present for 18 months, and a mild ache in an interphalyngeal joint for 4 months. There was nothing else of note and she had no adenopathy, splenomegaly, or joint deformity. Her right kidney was palpable. The following results were obtained: Hb, 75 per cent; film, normal; W.B.C., 12,100 per c.mm. (polymorphs, 78 per cent; lymphocytes, 22 per cent); and E.S.R. (Westergren) varying between 98, 132, 18, and 118 mm. in the first hour. Laboratory testing showed the E.S.R. at 40° C. to be 30 mm. in the first hour; at 21° C. to be 98 mm. in the first hour; and at 37° C. to be 111 mm. in the first hour. The total protein was 6·7 g. per 100 ml. (albumin, 1·7 g.; alpha-1-globulin, 0·45 g.; alpha-2-globulin, 1·06 g.; beta-globulin, 0·90 g.; gamma-globulin, 2·0 g.; and cryoglobulin, 0·45 g.). The cryoglobulin had an electrophoretic mobility and antigenic property differing slightly from the normal IgG fraction. The Wassermann and Reiter's complement-fixation tests were negative. There were no cold agglutinins and the Coombs's test, both direct and indirect, was negative. The urine culture was sterile and there was no proteinuria. Her blood-urea was 21 mg. per 100 ml. Blood-culture was sterile, R.A. test negative, L.E. latex test negative, and no L.E. phenomenon could be demonstrated. Sternal marrow was normal, and so were X-rays of chest, skull, pelvis, and femora as well as I.V.P. The stools did not contain occult blood.

Half an hour after the I.V.P. her limbs and face became intensely cyanosed and 24 hours later her toes were cold and black. The temperature was 103° F. She recovered in 3 days. On the lateral surface of her upper thigh an area of blanching, surrounded by oedema and cyanosis, was present. There was no precipitation of cryoglobulin when urografin was tested against the patient's serum. In view of this it was thought that the precipitation was due to heat conduction from her thigh by contact with metal in the X-ray department.

She gradually improved and was symptom free and apyrexial for 6 weeks prior to discharge.

The cause of her paraproteinaemia was not ascertained. She had no evidence of myelomatosis or of malignancy. Her pyrexia was seemingly related to cryoglobulin precipitation and this probably explained her episodes of intense cyanosis with 'cold', and the variability of her blood-sedimentation rate.

Production

It is generally agreed that plasma cells produce the paraprotein, and if it disappears, presumably their activity has reverted to normal. When the protein persists there is often evidence of plasmacytosis and moreover the plasma cells frequently appear abnormal. It is possible that negative marrow findings merely indicate that the puncture has missed the pathological area, as multiple punctures of sternum, vertebral spine, and iliac crest give a higher positive yield than does puncture of a single site.

The plasma cells may be large with prominent nuclei and nucleoli. Their chromatin network may be more obvious and sometimes staining with eosinophilic reagents gives a flare appearance. Inclusion bodies have been described. On rare occasions the cells are smaller than normal (*Figs.* 61, 62).

An isolated, large, abnormal cell surrounded by apparently normal cells can be referred to as the 'rogue' plasma cell. It forms paraprotein, and later other abnormal cells appear which may aggregate together into a plasmacytoma or infiltrate throughout the marrow. Increase in plasma cells also occurs in other diseases—such as infections, neoplasms, and immune-body disorders (polyarteritis, systemic lupus erythematosus, and rheumatoid arthritis).

When the percentage of plasma cells in the marrow is considerably raised to 60 per cent or thereabouts, the diagnosis of a plasma-cell tumour or multiple myelomatosis is usually definite, but difficulty arises when the figure is below 20 per cent in a patient who has another disease which could be implicated. Nevertheless, proportions as low as 5–8 per cent may be associated with early myelomatosis, although repeated counts are often necessary before a diagnosis can be made. If the number is increasing myelomatosis is likely.

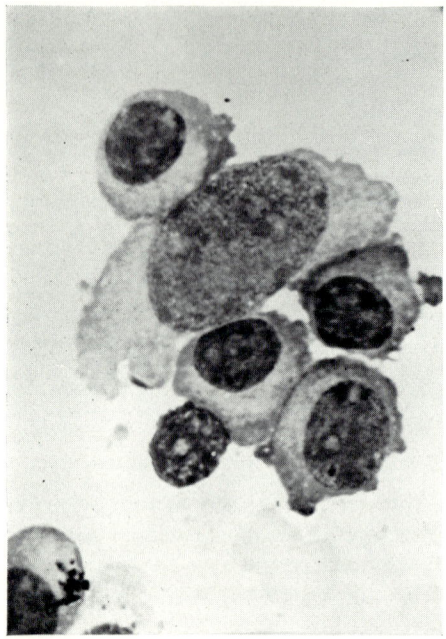 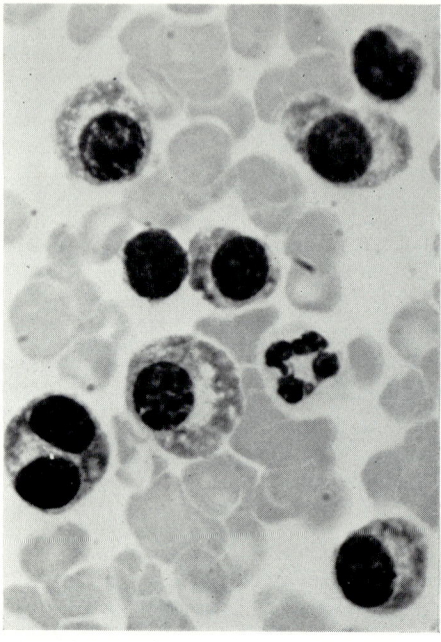

Fig. 61.—Myeloma marrow, showing variety of large 'rogue' and small myeloma cells. Female, aged 45 years. Hb, 33 per cent. Presented with bone lesions. (×1100.)

Fig. 62.—Myeloma marrow, showing myeloma cells, more like normal plasma cells. Female, aged 64 years. Hb, 83 per cent. Presented with abdominal pain. (×1100.)

CLASSIFICATION

Hobbs (1967) reported on 304 patients with paraproteinaemia whom he followed up for a minimum of 3 years or until a probable cause became apparent. The final classification was as follows:—

1. *Malignant*
   - Myelomatosis — 196
   - Lymphosarcoma — 5
   - Reticulosarcoma — 1
   - Waldenström's macroglobulinaemia — 19
   - Chronic lymphatic leukaemia — 2
2. *Benign*
   - Mainly static for 6 years — 68
   - Transient — 2
3. *Uncertain* — 11

He indicated that a follow-up for 10 years might be required before a certain diagnosis was made, and up to 20 years where solitary lesions or a trace of Bence Jones proteinuria were the presenting features.

As the main incidence of paraproteinaemia seemed to be in persons who were younger than those with myelomatosis, Waldenström (1960) suggested that a pre-myelomatous stage existed, which could persist for several years. It now seems generally recognized that this view has to be modified, because exclusion of those dying from unrelated disease still leaves an appreciable number in whom the cause remains obscure.

Although plasma cells form paraprotein, there are rare occasions when it cannot be detected in patients with myelomatosis. Usually, however, the amount of paraprotein in the serum is approximately proportional to the extent of the plasma-cell proliferation.

URINARY EXCRETION

Urinary excretion of paraprotein occurs when a sufficient amount of low molecular weight paraprotein has been formed. This is of the light-chain variety and can be detected by the Bence Jones reaction, or more accurately by immunoelectrophoresis of the urine. About half the patients with myelomatosis give a positive result, but although usually indicative of that disease it is not invariably so. A trace may be obtained whenever plasmacytosis occurs, provided the molecular size of the M-component is appropriate. A large quantity in the urine of patients with myelomatosis indicates gross abnormality of the plasma-cell system, and the prognosis is therefore poor.

AGE INCIDENCE

Hallen (1963) found paraproteins in 3 per cent of 294 largely healthy subjects over 70 years of age. Axelsson, Bachmann, and Hallen (1966) in Sweden studied the incidence in a larger sample. Serum was obtained from 6995 persons over the age of 25 (3400 males and 3595 females of whom 1041 males and 1002 females were over 60 years of age). The incidence of paraproteinaemia was as follows: men, 40–49 years, 0·1 per cent; 50–59, 1·0 per cent; 60–69, 2·0 per cent; 70–79, 2·4 per cent; 80–89, 9·2 per cent; and women, 30–39 years, 0·5 per cent; 40–49, 0·1 per cent; 60–69, 1·2 per cent; 70–79, 1·4 per cent; and 80–89, 1·6 per cent. IgG was the most common type (61 per cent), while IgA occurred in 27 per cent, and IgM in 8 per cent. Myelomatosis was suspected in 3 patients, 3 had had a neoplasm, and 1 suffered from lymphatic leukaemia. In the remaining 57 cases there was no apparent cause for the paraproteinaemia although an increase of marrow-plasma cells to a level above 3 per cent was observed in 23 per cent. None had Bence Jones proteinuria, and the E.S.R. in most patients was within the accepted normal range. Fine, Derycke, and Boffa (1965) discovered 16 cases with M-components among 500 subjects over the age of 68.

DIAGNOSTIC IMPLICATIONS

Despite advances in electro- and immunoelectrophoresis initial diagnosis still depends to a large extent on clinical assessment. The presence of skeletal pain, for example, in a person with small quantities of paraprotein in the serum and minimal proliferation of plasma cells in the marrow brings myelomatosis into the picture, whereas absence of skeletal pain and osteolytic lesions makes such a diagnosis less likely although gammopathy and plasma-cell proliferation may be more marked.

DISEASES

Hallen (1966) discussed the following clinical classification:—
1. Monoclonal gammopathy.
2. Waldenström's macroglobulinaemia.
3. Myelomatosis.
4. Lymphatic leukaemia.
5. Immune reaction diseases.
6. Neoplasms.

Monoclonal Gammopathy

An abnormal clone is thought to be present, which gives rise to the dysglobulinaemia. The existence of the disorder as an entity is based on the observation that M-components can remain unchanged—both in composition and quantity—for many years without the patient developing any disease that can be directly implicated. Hallen (1966) analysed 108 cases which fulfilled these criteria. Anaemia was present in 17 per cent, a lowered albumin in 12 per cent, and plasma cells above 3 per cent in almost a half. The gamma-globulins were lowered in 46 per cent and the M-components more than 1·0 g. per 100 ml. in a third. No fixed level, either of paraprotein or of plasma-cell proliferation, distinguished the disorder from early myelomatosis; the difference was apparent only when progress was assessed. The erythrocyte sedimentation rate was sometimes raised, and about 4 per cent excreted light-chain proteins in their urine. Of particular interest was the finding that only in a minority of patients did the presence of a macroglobulin indicate Waldenström's macroglobulinaemia.

The mean age of these patients was about 70 years. Many were in their eighties. None had relevant diseases, and discovery was by chance on routine testing of a large number of sera.

It could be argued that long-term follow-up over many years would perhaps show the development of myelomatosis or some other related disease in many of these persons, but it appears at present that elderly people do sometimes develop a paraprotein in their serum that does not influence their survival.

Waldenström's Macroglobulinaemia

This is a rare disorder which is almost confined to elderly males although 2 of the 4 cases described by Kok, Whitmore, and Ainsworth (1963) were women and the oldest 81. Lymphadenopathy, splenomegaly, hepatomegaly, anaemia, and a raised E.S.R. occur, in association with macroglobulinaemia. Marrow smears contain about 20 or 30 per cent mature lymphocytes with few plasma cells. Bence Jones protein is found in the urine of 10–15 per cent.

The abnormal protein coats the red cells causing tissue anoxia and a clotting abnormality, which could account for the bleeding diathesis that may be present. A mild degree of haemolysis can also be a feature, which probably explains the anaemia with increased marrow haemosiderin.

The histological picture of the enlarged lymph-nodes resembles that of a chronic inflammatory reaction.

Although anaemia may be present for several years, once the clinical disease develops survival is short and measured in months. Death may occur at any stage, even before nodal or visceral infiltration can be detected. Osteolytic bone lesions are not seen.

The condition has to be differentiated from lymphatic leukaemia, reticulosarcoma, and 'heavy-chain' disease.

HYPERVISCOSITY SYNDROME

The *hyperviscosity syndrome* was described by Fahey (1965) as a distinct entity. It is usually associated with macroglobulinaemia and excess of circulating IgM, but may also be found in IgA or IgG myelomatosis. Patients present with spontaneous haemorrhages and symptoms resulting from sludging in vessels supplying the eye and peripheral nerves.

HEAVY-CHAIN DISEASE

A group of patients have been described, usually middle-aged men, who present with painful enlarged lymph-nodes and weight-loss. Oedema and inflammation of the soft palate is a peculiar feature. Approximately half the cases deteriorate rapidly and die within a few months. The remainder may show temporary regression with survival for a few years.

The serum M-component in these patients gives a narrow band between the beta- and gamma-globulin peaks, and this has been shown to be the Fc fragment of the heavy chain of IgG. This protein also appears in the urine at a concentration of 50 mg. to 15 g. per 24 hours. It can be distinguished from light-chain Bence Jones protein by its failure to precipitate and redissolve when the urine is heated to boiling point.

As the disease progresses increasing quantities of the abnormal protein are produced, with a corresponding reduction of normal IgG. This results in an enhanced susceptibility to infection.

The diseased lymph-nodes show a proliferation of reticulum with an admixture of lymphoid and immature cells. Occasionally binucleated cells resembling those of Reed-Sternberg are seen.

MYELOMATOSIS

Since the discovery of the Bence Jones reaction in 1846 this disease has become well recognized. It interests the clinician, the pathologist, and the research worker alike, and much of the present knowledge on the size and structure of globulin molecules and the nature of paraproteins is a direct result.

Definition.—It is a skeletal disease with malignant proliferation of plasma-cell precursors and is usually associated with paraproteinaemia.

Incidence.—Martin (1961) stated that in most series the maximum incidence was between 50 and 60 years of age except in Sweden where the maximum was 20 years later. The reason for this is not known. It is possible that there is a sampling error, because since the development of geriatrics in this country the disease is often discovered in the late seventies and eighties. A preponderance of males was considered to be characteristic, but this view is no longer tenable as females appear to be affected as often as males.

The Cancer Registration returns in South Wales for the 5 years 1961–5 showed that the disease had been diagnosed in 69 males and 77 females, the highest incidence being in patients between 55 and 65 years of age. Above 65 years there were

18 males and 37 females, while beyond 55 years the corresponding numbers were 37 and 67. When standardized per million population, the rate in males was as follows: 55–65 years, 53; 65–75 years, 34; above 75 years, 39; while in females the relative rates were 45, 56, and 38. Analysis showed considerable difference when comparison in known incidence was made between urban and rural districts, between different counties, and also between different towns. Although the explanation is obscure the chances are that the criteria of diagnosis are not uniform, and that the true incidence is higher than that recorded.

In the M.R.C. Trial (Hobbs, 1969) the peak was between 60 and 70 years with the mean at 62 years of age.

The mode of presentation varies and three types are described:—
1. Multiple myelomatosis.
2. Solitary myeloma.
3. Extramedullary plasmacytoma.

MULTIPLE MYELOMATOSIS

The abnormal plasma-cell proliferation is prominent in scattered foci within the marrow. Diffuse infiltration is less marked.

Skeletal pain is usually present, particularly if the vertebrae, ribs, and long bones are affected. It may not be a feature if only the skull or pelvis is involved. Tenderness on percussion can usually be elicited. The disease can be present for many years before symptoms appear, with the result that widespread osteolytic lesions are visible radiologically when the patient is first seen. Sometimes the diagnosis is made during investigation of a patient with a high erythrocyte sedimentation rate.

Case 2.—This lady consulted her doctor at the age of 66 years with a prolapsed haemorrhoid of 6 days' duration. She then mentioned that she had been 'off colour' and had lost weight. Further investigation was undertaken because the Hb was 66 per cent and the peripheral blood contained nucleated red blood-cells. The serum protein showed a pre-gamma peak (beta- and gamma-globulins, 5·9 g. per 100 ml.). Chest X-ray showed osteolytic rib lesions, and the marrow confirmed the presence of myelomatosis. The blood paraprotein concentration initially 50 mg. rose within 2 weeks to 200 mg. per 100 ml.

This patient illustrates the non-specific and almost incidental way in which the disease may present, and also the value of laboratory screening.

Pathological *fractures* of ribs, femora, and vertebrae may result. Paraplegia due to compression fracture of the spine may be the presenting feature. General symptoms, such as anorexia and loss of weight, are often prominent.

Hypercalcaemia when pronounced can cause mental disturbances, nausea, and vomiting. Hyperviscosity of the serum, as is seen occasionally in patients with IgG myeloma, can lead to similar symptoms together with retinopathy, neuropathy, recurrent bleeding, cardiac failure, and lassitude. Blindness may develop.

Features of cardiac failure or renal failure may dominate the clinical picture, and gout can be precipitated by the associated hyperuricaemia.

Anaemia is usually present, but in about 30 per cent initial blood-counts are normal (Innes and Newall, 1961). There is nothing specific in the blood-film. A normocytic normochromic anaemia is the commonest picture, but a hypochromic, macrocytic, hypoplastic, refractory, or a leuco-erythroblastic type may be seen, and platelets may be reduced. Plasma cells are rarely present, although terminally they may be abundant. Examples of 'plasma-cell leukaemia' are very rare.

PROTEIN DISORDERS

Case 3.—This lady attended in 1964 at the age of 84 years because of abdominal pain. The liver was found to be enlarged. The haemoglobin was 50 per cent and white-cell count 10,000 per c.mm. with numerous atypical mononuclears that were difficult to classify. The serum protein showed a sharp peak in the gamma-globulin (2·24 g. per 100 ml.). The marrow showed large numbers of cells resembling those seen in the peripheral blood. The Bence Jones test on the urine was negative.

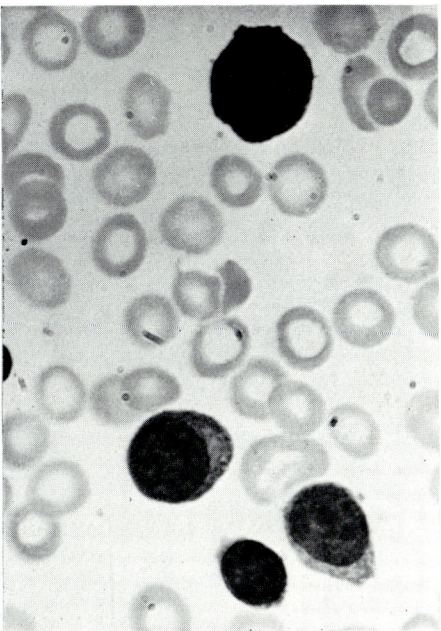

Fig. 63.—*Case* 3. Marrow smear showing myeloma cells. (×1100.)

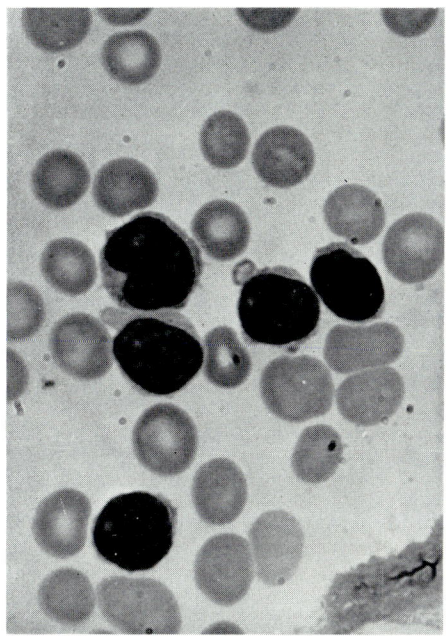

Fig. 64.—*Case* 3. Peripheral blood showing similar cells to the myeloma cells present in marrow. (×1100.)

Repeated examination of the blood showed cells of plasmablast type and the count rose to 20,000 per c.mm. with a platelet count of 85,000 per c.mm. Purpura developed.

A second marrow aspirate showed a picture of myelomatosis, the cells being of primitive leucoblastic type. The patient died within 4 months (*Figs.* 63, 64).

There were features of myelomatosis with plasma-cell leukaemia, which in its clinical course and cytological features resembled acute leukaemia.

Recurrent *infections*, particularly of the lungs and urinary tract, are noteworthy in the advanced stage, but may be early manifestations. Although the E.S.R. is usually raised, normal levels can be obtained. Hallen (1966) stated that the increase depended on many factors, particularly decreased albumin, increased fibrinogen and gamma-globulin, and especially the presence of M-components. There was a positive correlation between the E.S.R. and the concentration of the M-components when patients with lowered albumin and raised alpha-2-globulin were excluded.

Bence Jones proteinuria, as detected by routine urine testing, is present in approximately 50 per cent of cases, sometimes intermittently. A positive test is a good indication that the patient has myelomatosis, provided other features are also present, but it can occasionally occur in patients with other diseases such as macroglobulinaemia, lymphatic leukaemia, or malignant tumours, particularly when there are bone metastases. Albuminuria, other than Bence Jones proteinuria, is commonly found.

Osteolytic lesions are characteristic and may cause progressive destruction of the skeleton. The order of frequency seems to be spine, pelvis, skull, ribs, and long bones. They cause pain, fractures, or local swellings.

Changes in *serum protein* patterns have received considerable attention. The *total protein* level is usually raised and a level as high as 15 g. per 100 ml. has been reported. In the patients we have seen the commonest level is between 8 and 10 g. Occasionally a normal or a low level is obtained.

Electrophoretic analysis nearly always shows evidence of excessive synthesis of beta-globulin, of gamma-globulin, or of both. In 5 per cent of patients no electrophoretic abnormality is discovered (Martin, 1961).

The concentration of *paraproteins* in the serum is often about 2·0 g. per 100 ml. or less.

Hobbs (1969) recorded the data from 212 patients included in the M.R.C. Trial of cyclophosphamide and melphalan. The abnormal protein types were:—

	Per cent
IgG	53 (62 per cent being Bence Jones positive)
IgA	25 (70 per cent being Bence Jones positive)
Bence Jones only	19
IgD	1
Biclonal	2

Although there was no significant difference in the age of presentation of those in the IgG and IgA groups, certain trends appeared to be present. IgG myelomatosis was associated with a greater reduction of normal immunoglobulins and the IgA variety with a higher incidence of hypercalcaemia.

Normal *globulins* are displaced so that the concentration of gamma fractions may be only 0·3 g. per 100 ml. The alpha fraction is somewhat increased.

Serum *albumin* is usually deficient and levels below 2·5 g. per 100 ml. are common, but normal values do not exclude the disease.

Marrow smears contain excess plasma cells which may be mainly of the mature type, but almost invariably abnormal forms are present. Their number varies from around 8 per cent to 60 or 70 per cent, and it is only when a great excess of abnormal cells are seen that a definite diagnosis can be made by this means alone. Taken in conjunction with other clinical and pathological findings this mode of investigation is most valuable. Rare instances of megaloblastic erythropoiesis have been recorded, usually due to folic-acid deficiency. An increase of lymphocytes and of reticulum cells is sometimes noted.

Diagnosis: This depends mainly on the presence of bone pain, skeletal osteolytic lesions, and plasmacytosis in the marrow. When Bence Jones proteinuria is also a feature the diagnosis is usually clear. The findings of a specific M-protein in the serum establishes the diagnosis.

Often, however, the clinical picture is not straightforward. There may be no pain or osteolytic lesions, and the presenting feature may be loss of weight, anorexia, lassitude, or thrombosis. Bleeding from mucous membranes is fairly common and may be severe enough to warrant admission. Anaemia may be severe. Amyloid involvement of the heart or kidney can cause congestive cardiac failure or uraemia.

Infection, particularly of the lungs and urogenital tract, sometimes hides the underlying disease. The patient may be in hospital because of an unrelated illness, such as cerebral infarction, and it is only when the erythrocyte sedimentation rate is found to be considerably raised that the presence of another disease is suspected.

Carcinoma of the breast, prostate, and lung can be associated with paraproteinaemia, and when there is skeletal pain or secondaries the possibility of myelomatosis may not be considered. The marrow smears show plasmacytosis in both conditions. As a general rule, these changes are rare in carcinoma and common in myelomatosis, so that the chances are that the patient has myelomatosis, despite the presence of another disease.

Rheumatoid arthritis may also be associated with generalized bone pain, a high E.S.R., and paraproteinaemia, but here again the association is so rare that myelomatosis is likely.

A positive Bence Jones reaction in the urine is strong confirmatory evidence of myelomatosis, but can occasionally be obtained in patients with malignant disease and monoclonal gammopathy.

Similar comments apply to the presence of M-components in the serum. Although common in myelomatosis they are not in themselves indicative of that disease.

Discrete osetolytic lesions are present radiologically in about 80–90 per cent of these patients.

Prognosis.—When the full clinical picture has developed the average survival is usually less than a year, although there are exceptions. One of our patients lived for 3 years. Among the 119 cases described by Innes and Newall (1961) the 3-year survival rate was 5 per cent and none survived for 5 years. Bronchopneumonia, severe anaemia, uraemia, and cardiac failure are the common terminal events. According to Hallen (1966) a rise in the serum concentration of the paraprotein is of serious import. The presence of Bence Jones protein in the urine in excess of 1 mg. per 100 ml. also indicates a bad prognosis.

Isolated cases of longer duration have been described. Kesterton and McSwain (1952) reported a patient who survived 9 years, and there are others who have lived longer, but many presented with a local plasmacytoma. Hobbs (1969) claimed that an initial slow response to therapy might suggest a better prognosis. He estimated that the average doubling times for the production of the abnormal protein in myelomatosis was 10·1 months for IgG, 6·3 months for IgA, and 3·4 months for the Bence Jones type. He concluded from this that a single mutant cell would take approximately 32, 21, and 11 years respectively for clinical evidence of myelomatosis to develop.

Diagnosis is sometimes made during the premyelomatous phase, by the finding of M-components in the serum and abnormal plasma cells in the marrow. When such a patient progresses to myelomatosis and the date when the abnormalities were discovered is taken as the onset of the disease, duration can be considerable, because 10 years or more may elapse before the overt disease develops. The length of this 'prodromal' period probably varies, and in any case is of limited value prognostically, because it is only rarely observed.

Diffuse Myelomatosis

This implies diffuse infiltration of the marrow with plasma cells, many of which appear abnormal. No aggregation into discrete foci is visible. It is doubtful whether the clinical and pathological features are sufficiently definite and constant to justify its classification as a separate type, although it does form a fairly distinct subgroup of multiple myelomatosis.

Patients present with progressive anaemia which does not respond to treatment. Aplastic or leuco-erythroblastic anaemia may be diagnosed.

There are no symptoms referable to the skeletal system and radiological examination is negative. The E.S.R. is raised and the electrophoretic serum pattern similar to that seen in multiple myelomatosis.

Once severe anaemia develops survival is less than a year, but there is a prolonged asymptomatic phase. Investigation of a patient with a raised erythrocytic sedimentation rate may reveal excess plasma cells in the marrow smears, so that diagnosis is sometimes possible in the early stage. These patients may not become anaemic for many years.

Radiological evidence of generalized osteoporosis is common, but this is of no diagnostic value in the elderly.

Solitary Myeloma

In this variety the plasma-cell proliferation remains localized for a long period, but eventually progresses to the generalized type, indistinguishable from multiple myelomatosis. Death often supervenes from unrelated causes so that the final picture is not usually seen in the elderly.

Swelling, which is often painless and localized to a single bone—sternum, clavicle, skull, rib, humerus, or femur—is the most common finding. A pathological fracture may occur. Vertebral body collapse leads to spinal cord compression. In some patients, bone pain localized to the back is a troublesome complaint.

Radiological examination shows collapse of a vertebra, or the presence of a solitary cystic lesion in the involved bone. Tumours such as osteoclastoma, haemangioma, or secondary deposits are simulated.

Marrow aspiration of the lesion usually produces evidence of plasma-cell proliferation, but sometimes this is not a feature. The E.S.R. is often elevated and the electrophoretic serum pattern approaches that seen in multiple myeloma. A paraprotein is usually present, but the quantity is small unless dissemination is taking place.

Innes and Newall (1961) reported a 3-year survival rate of 32 per cent. The longest survivor in their series lived 10 years. Many died as a consequence of paraplegia and unrelated disease so that the true 3-year survival rate was probably higher.

Extramedullary Plasmacytoma

This is an uncommon variant. The patient presents with a plasma-cell tumour outside the skeleton, and diagnosis is made histologically. It may be found in the retropharyngeal region, in an enlarged lymph-node, in a muscle or subcutaneous mass, or in any viscus.

Sometimes the skeleton is involved although the symptoms can be minimal or absent. Typically, the tumour recurs after treatment, or appears in another site, until eventually there is widespread disease. Bone involvement is not characteristic, but usually occurs later. Several years may elapse before it becomes evident.

Extramedullary deposits are often found in patients with multiple myelomatosis. According to Hobbs and Corbett (1969) extra-osseous tumours can be detected during life in about 63 per cent of patients with IgD myelomatosis, and there is a tendency for this type to occur at a relatively young age, although 10 of the 30 cases they described were over 60.

Other Pathological Features

The serum *calcium* is sometimes raised when the disease is advanced, but the alkaline phosphatase is normal. The *uric acid* may also be elevated, presumably due to the increased breakdown of cells.

Amyloidosis is an important complication which influences the course of the disease. It is reputed to occur in about 25 per cent of cases. Presumably abnormal proteins leak out of the vessels into the surrounding tissue and are converted into amyloid. Sometimes an amyloid type of substance is seen which does not take up the usual amyloid stains. The distribution is not characteristic of either the primary or the secondary variety, although it approaches that of the primary. Widespread periarterial involvement is sometimes present, while in others it is localized to the myocardium. The kidney is affected in about a third of the cases.

Renal disease is often present and can cause death. It has been suggested that the kidneys are involved in approximately 60 per cent. The reason for this is not fully understood, but probably the excretion of abnormal proteins is a factor. Bence Jones protein may be toxic to the glomeruli and it can also precipitate as casts in the tubules. These changes, however, are also seen in patients who have had no Bence Jones proteinuria so, presumably, other proteins must be implicated.

There is often a foreign-body reaction around the casts. Protein droplets or crystals may be visible. Tubular dilatation proximal to the casts is common and, later, atrophy occurs. Sometimes there is diffuse plasma-cell infiltration.

Pyelonephritis is often present. The most common clinical manifestation is normotensive uraemia progressing to oliguric renal failure. In rare instances the tubules leak phosphate, amino-acids, and glucose. Urography has been considered dangerous, because of possible interaction between the substance used and the paraprotein, with consequent precipitation in the kidney, but Cwynarski and Saxton (1969) found the risk to be very small.

Post-mortem studies show that apart from skeletal disease there is widespread infiltration of other tissues in about 50 per cent of cases. The spleen, which may be moderately enlarged, is often infiltrated with plasma cells. Similar changes are seen in the liver, lymph-nodes, and, less frequently, other viscera.

Treatment

Myelomatosis is a fatal disease and there is no known effective treatment although sometimes the inevitable outcome can probably be delayed. Evaluation of therapy is difficult because the course of the disease is so variable.

A solitary myeloma may respond to X-ray therapy. When present in a limb, amputation may have to be considered despite the fact that the lesion is a manifestation of a generalized disease, but usually radical surgery is contra-indicated. An extramedullary plasmacytoma located in a lymph-node, the retropharyngeal region, or the intestines may also require X-ray therapy or surgery.

Multiple myelomatosis is a distressing condition and often the most important aspect of management is the alleviation of pain. Urethane is sometimes a useful drug for this purpose. Stilboestrol has also been given, though the reasoning behind this approach is puzzling.

Melphalan is perhaps the drug of choice. Approximately 5 mg. a day are given for 2 or 3 weeks and then discontinued for a week in order to assess its effect on the leucocytes and platelets. If there are no untoward effects the drug is resumed in a dosage of 2 mg. a day. Waldenström (1964) felt that a platelet count below 100,000 per c.mm. and a leucocyte count below 1500 per c.mm. were contra-indications. They should be counted two or three times a week at first and then at weekly or fortnightly intervals. Pain often disappears rapidly. Waldenström noted the following criteria: a decrease in the specific globulin fraction; an increase in serum albumin and in the normal gamma-globulin; improvement in the X-ray picture; and diminution in plasma cells on sternal puncture. In some patients melphalan therapy seemed successful except that no increase occurred either in antibodies or in the normal gamma-globulin. When judged by these criteria he felt that the drug was moderately effective and did offer some hope particularly when the disease was not advanced. He advocated that treatment be given, if possible, before skeletal lesions appeared. Mild anaemia was not a contra-indication. Speed, Galton, and Sivan (1964) administered 10 mg. orally for 5–7 days and then further courses of 50–70 mg. at approximately 6-weekly intervals. The total dose varied from 50 to 1348 mg. Apart from nausea and vomiting there were few side-effects. Mild renal damage was not aggravated. Some became anaemic and required blood transfusion, and a fall in neutrophil count was universal after the first course. There was relief of pain in 12 of 15 cases, and in half there was weight-gain and an increase in haemoglobin concentration, while in a quarter favourable biochemical changes were noted.

The addition of prednisolone to the régime is said to enhance the response.

It is generally accepted that melphalan therapy is contra-indicated when the presence of amyloidosis or 'myeloma' kidney is strongly suspected.

Cyclophosphamide: Malpas (1969) suggested an oral daily dosage of 2 mg. per kg., but indicated that it should be varied to avoid marrow suppression. Continued chemotherapy should be attempted, with a monthly check being kept on the white-cell and platelet counts.

Blood transfusion is often necessary. Infection of the lungs or urinary tract require therapy with the appropriate antibiotic. Pathological fractures should be treated. They usually heal as there is no abnormality of the osteoblasts. Hypercalcaemia requires rehydration and steroid therapy; hyperuricaemia responds to the appropriate drug—such as allopurinol—and retinal damage from hyperviscosity may need plasmaphoresis.

Lymphatic Leukaemia

M-components, usually of the macroglobulin type, have been found in lymphatic leukaemia. It is problematical whether such a disease should be regarded as Waldenström's macroglobulinaemia with lymphocytosis, or as leukaemia. The clinical course may be similar, but the weight of evidence suggests that the majority are true leukaemias. Hallen (1966) proved the existence of serum M-components in 8 of 59 patients with chronic lymphatic leukaemia. He estimated that this was about seven times greater than that expected in the general population matched for age and sex. Fifty-one of the patients were over the age of 60, 7 being over 80 years. Five had M-components. Only 1 of the 8 with M-components was a female. The quantity was small.

The presence of an abnormal protein is difficult to explain when there is no plasmacytosis. It is believed that lymphocytes produce immunoglobulins and therefore it is possible that occasionally they can synthesize an abnormal globulin. Indeed, it has been claimed that a macroglobulin has been extracted from leukaemic lymphocytes.

In rare instances M-components have been isolated from patients with acute and chronic myeloid leukaemia. Similar findings have been reported in patients with follicular lymphoma, lymphosarcoma, reticulum-cell sarcoma, myelosclerosis, and polycythaemia vera.

Waldenström (1960) explained that the overlapping of many of these diseases was due to the fact that they had a common stem cell—the 'reticulum' cell.

IMMUNE REACTION DISEASE

Occasionally M-components may be found. The triggering mechanism is not understood. Possibly the agent that stimulates the antibody mechanism can produce a wider effect, particularly when the patient is elderly or has a predisposing hereditary factor. Sometimes the abnormal globulin disappears, while in others it remains constant. Its presence does not seem to be of any prognostic significance.

A wide variety of diseases have been implicated, such as rheumatoid arthritis, polyarteritis, haemolytic anaemia, glomerulonephritis, liver cirrhosis, and acute infections.

NEOPLASM

In a series of 99 patients with paraproteinaemia, Lynch and Joske (1966) found that 9 had carcinoma without myeloma. Association with neoplasms in many sites has been described—lung, ovary, bladder, liver, skin, breast, stomach, colon, and prostate.

Case 4.—This lady attended in 1963, suffering from low back pain, and X-ray showed slight wedging of her dorsal vertebrae. She had had a right radical mastectomy 14 years previously. The serum protein showed a moderately sharp gamma-globulin peak at a concentration of 2·65 g. per 100 ml. The marrow showed an increased number of plasma cells. A first sample of urine was negative, and a second positive, for Bence Jones protein.

No evidence of recurrent neoplasm could be found, and because the features were not typical of myelomatosis she was given radiotherapy. However, at post-radiotherapy follow-up a lump was found in the left breast which proved to be a carcinoma with axillary metastases (*Figs.* 65–67).

The elderly are prone to develop neoplastic disease so that probably the association is often fortuitous. A person with monoclonal gammopathy could have an incidental carcinoma. Even patients with classic myelomatosis presumably have the same incidence of neoplastic disease as the general population, so that it is not unusual at necropsy to find an unrelated carcinoma.

On the other hand, it is possible that an unknown antigenic component produced by malignant cells can stimulate the production of an abnormal protein. Some cases in the literature suggest that this has been so, because the concentration of the protein has diminished greatly, or even disappeared, when the carcinoma has been treated. This has been noted, for instance, in carcinoma of the prostate. At present the problem is unsolved.

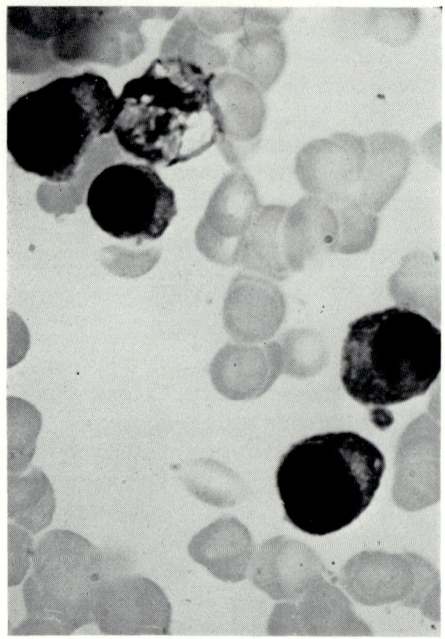

Fig. 65.—*Case* 4. Marrow smear showing excess of plasma cells. ($\times 1100$.)

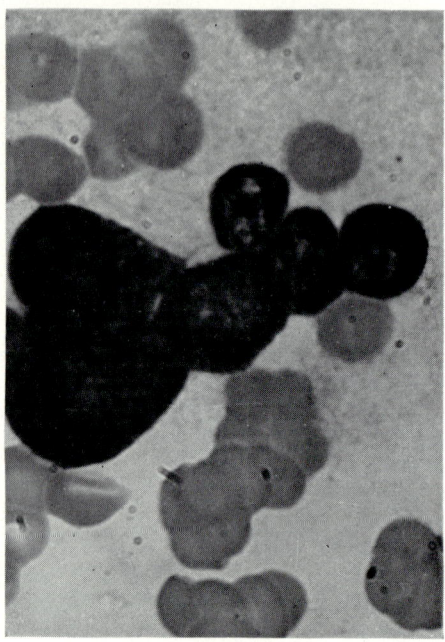

Fig. 66.—*Case* 4. Marrow smear showing group of carcinoma cells. ($\times 1100$.)

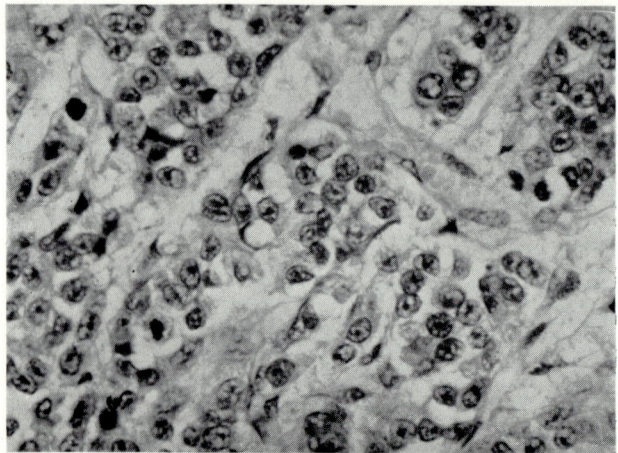

Fig. 67.—*Case* 4. Axillary lymph-node showing secondary breast carcinoma 14 years after mastectomy. ($\times 400$.)

The difficulty of arriving at a definite diagnosis is illustrated in the following case history (Powell and Thomas, 1967):—

Case 5.—A male, aged 97 years, was seen in 1962 with epistaxis, bronchitis, and mental confusion. His Hb was 70 per cent and E.S.R., 59 mm. in the first hour. A macrocytic anaemia was present

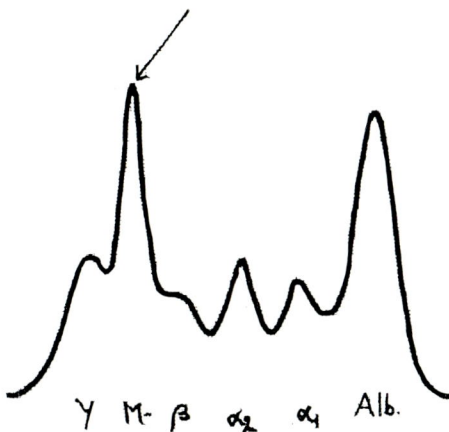

Fig. 68.—*Case* 5. Electrophoresis showing pre-gamma M-component 1·18 g. per 100 ml. Albumin, 1·78 g. per 100 ml. Alpha-1-globulin, 0·53 g. per 100 ml. Alpha-2-globulin, 0·68 g. per 100 ml. Beta-globulin, 0·59 g. per 100 ml. Gamma-globulin, 0·64 g. per 100 ml. Total protein, 5·4 g. per 100 ml. A/G ratio, 0·49 : 1.

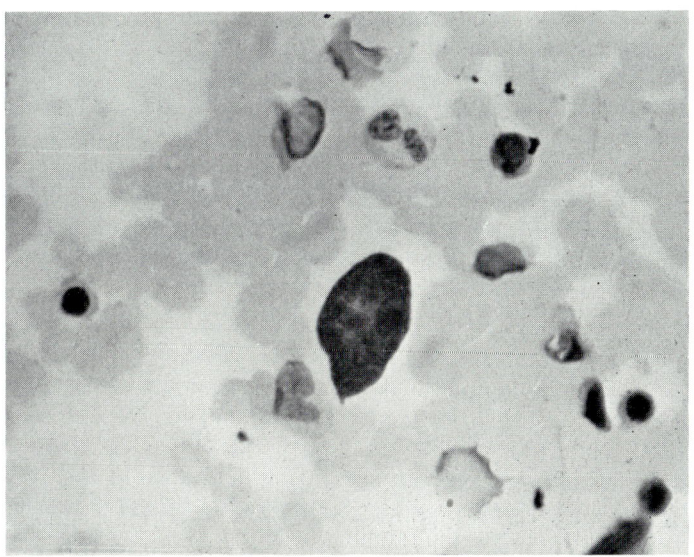

Fig. 69.—*Case* 5. Marrow showing 'rogue' plasma cell. ($\times$ 1100.)

and his serum vitamin-B_{12} was 250 pg. per ml. Blood-urea was 160 mg. per 100 ml., and R.A. latex test was positive. The serum protein measured 5·4 g. per 100 ml. (albumin, 1·78; alpha-1-globulin, 0·53; alpha-2-globulin, 0·68; beta-globulin, 0·59; pre-gamma peak, 1·18; gamma-globulin, 0·64). There was no Bence Jones proteinuria. An X-ray of the chest showed increased basal markings while those of the skull, pelvis, and spine were normal. Increased plasma cells were present in the sternal aspirate and some were large and atypical. He died 6 weeks after admission.

At necropsy there was amyloidosis with a bronchial adenoma which had metastasized to the liver (*Figs.* 68–72).

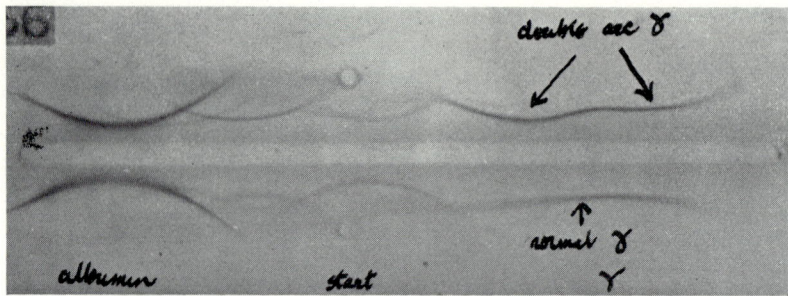

Fig. 70.—*Case* 5. Immuno-electrophoresis showing double gamma band. (*Dr. G. Franglen.*)

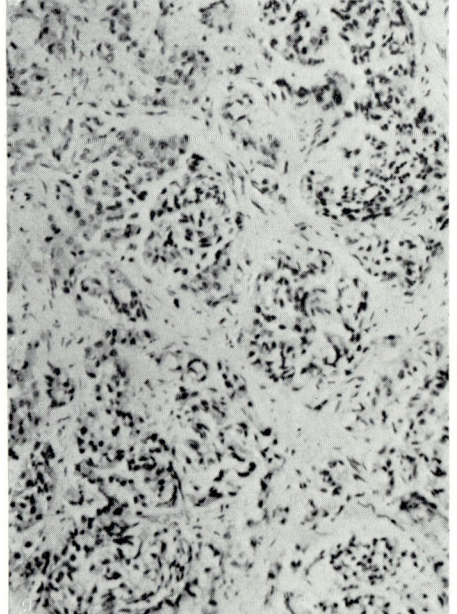

Fig. 71.—*Case* 5. Metastasis of bronchial adenoma to liver. (× 150.)

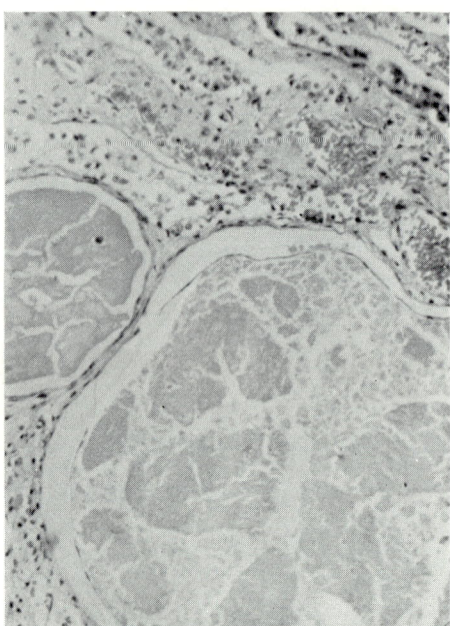

Fig. 72.—*Case* 5. 'Myeloma' casts in renal tubules. (× 150.)

The findings suggested several possibilities among which were the following: Monoclonal gammopathy with the other lesions being incidental; dysproteinaemia due to amyloidosis; premyelomatous phase of myelomatosis with associated amyloidosis; M-components produced as a result of the metastasizing adenoma; and even his advanced age could have been of some aetiological significance.

REFERENCES

Axelsson, U., Bachmann, R., and Hallen, J. (1966), *Acta med. scand.*, **179**, 235.
Cancer Registration (S. Wales), Welsh Hospital Board, Cardiff.
Cwynarski, M. T., and Saxton, H. M. (1969), *Br. med. J.*, **1**, 486.
Fahey, J. L. (1965), *J. Am. med. Ass.*, **194**, 255.
Fine, J. M., Derycke, C., and Boffa, G. A. (1965), Tenth Congress Soc. Europ. Haematol., Strasbourg (quoted by Hallen, J., *Acta med. scand.* (1966), Suppl. 462).
Hallen, J. (1963), *Acta med. scand.*, **173**, 737.
— — (1966), *Ibid.*, Suppl. 462.
Hobbs, J. R. (1967), *Br. med. J.*, **2**, 699.
— — (1969), *Br. J. Haemat.*, **16**, 599, 607.
— — and Corbett, A. A. (1969), *Br. med. J.*, **1**, 412.
Innes, J., and Newall, J. (1961), *Lancet*, **1**, 239.
Kesterton, J., and McSwain, B. (1952), *J. Bone Jt Surg.*, **34A**, 224.
Kok, D'A., Whitmore, D. N., and Ainsworth, R. W. (1963), *J. clin. Path.*, **16**, 351.
Lynch, W. J., and Joske, R. A. (1966), *Ibid.*, **19**, 461.
Malpas, J. S. (1969), *Br. med. J.*, **2**, 163.
Martin, N. H. (1961), *Lancet*, **1**, 237.
— — (1969), *J. clin. Path.*, **22**, 117.
Powell, D. E. B., and Thomas, J. H. (1967), *Br. J. geront. Pract.*, **4**, 127.
Speed, D. E., Galton, D. A. G., and Sivan, A. (1964), *Br. med. J.*, **2**, 1664.
Waldenström, J. (1960), *Proc. R. Soc. Med.*, **53**, 789.
— — (1964), *Br. med. J.*, **1**, 859.
W.H.O. Meeting on Nomenclature of Human Immunoglobulins (1964), *Bull. Wld Hlth Org.*, **447**, 30.

11

MYELOPROLIFERATIVE DISORDERS

MYELOFIBROSIS AND MYELOSCLEROSIS

MYELOFIBROSIS denotes the progressive replacement of haemopoietic marrow with fibrous tissue. The condition is termed 'myelosclerosis' when there is additional encroachment by cancellous bone. This disease occurs in patients who are usually over 50 years old, the most frequent distribution being between 60 and 70 years. The patient may present with the classic features of myelofibrosis, or as the terminal phase of another haematological disorder. The latter is considered later as part of the myeloproliferative syndrome.

LABORATORY FINDINGS

Peripheral Blood.—*Red blood-cells*: Myelofibrosis is one of the important causes of leuco-erythroblastic anaemia. The degree of anaemia may be minimal when the patient is first seen, but thereafter it is usually progressive. The erythrocytes are normochromic, except rarely when significant hypochromia is found. They also show anisocytosis, poikilocytosis, and polychromasia. Characteristic tear-drop and fragmented forms are seen. Careful examination will nearly always reveal the presence of nucleated red blood-cells, although the proportion present often varies widely in the same patient.

Reticulocytes may form 3–10 per cent of the red cells. Reticulocytosis of this degree can exist when red-cell production, as indicated by haemoglobin and radio-isotope studies, is not increased.

White blood-cells: The total leucocyte count is usually raised, although examples of leucopenia have been recorded. Immature forms—metamyelocytes, myelocytes, and blast forms—are seen. Basophilia and eosinophilia may be present.

Platelets: The platelet count is variable. Frequently thrombocytopenia is found, and regardless of the actual count bizarre giant platelets and megakaryocytic fragments may circulate.

Bone-marrow.—Aspiration of a satisfactory marrow smear is usually difficult, or impossible. The cortical bone is hard and the marrow cavity difficult to locate. Suction on the syringe yields scanty material, but examination can be informative if increased numbers of megakaryocytes are present.

Biopsy of bone-marrow is required for demonstrating the histological features of myelofibrosis. Various modified aspiration needles can be used for this purpose, for example, Westerman-Jensen, or large trephines such as Sacker-Nordin. The latter requires a large skin incision and may cause excessive bone damage where a bleeding tendency is present. The Gardner needle is more suitable and is used with a local anaesthetic. Surgical biopsy is seldom justified, or necessary in the elderly.

Bone-marrow sections show a marked increase in fibrous connective tissue encroaching on the marrow cavity. Reticulin and collagen stains are useful in highlighting the extent of this replacement. However, increased deposition of fibrous tissue is not diagnostic of myelofibrosis, as it occurs in many other diseases such as leukaemia, secondary carcinoma, bone disease, irradiation, and poisoning. Cancellous bone increases as the disease progresses. There is reduction in the amount of haemopoietic marrow, often with a relative increase in myelocytes, myeloblasts, and megakaryocytes.

Splenic Puncture.—This is seldom essential for diagnostic purposes in the elderly, but may yield useful information in difficult cases. Instead of the customary predominantly lymphocytic picture these cells are reduced to 20–50 per cent of normal with an admixture of normoblasts, myelocytes, metamyelocytes, and megakaryocytes.

Evidence of extramedullary haemopoiesis may also be found in other sites such as liver, retroperitoneal tissues, and lymph-nodes.

Folate and Vitamin-B_{12} Deficiency.—These haematinic factors may be deficient in myelofibrosis, probably due to increased utilization rather than defective absorption. Mixed pictures of both deficiencies with added iron deficiency may be seen. Such patients may become polycythaemic after treatment with folic acid or vitamin B_{12}.

Erythrokinetic Studies.—Radio-isotope studies can assist in diagnosis and also help in indicating the small group of patients in whom splenectomy may be beneficial.

Plasma-iron Clearance (P.I.C.).—This is a measure of the rate of clearance from the plasma of an injected dose of ^{59}Fe.

$$\frac{\text{Plasma Fe } (\mu\text{g. per 100 ml.}) \times (100 - \text{P.C.V.})}{T_{\frac{1}{2}} \times 100}.$$

($T_{\frac{1}{2}}$ = time taken in minutes for half the radioactivity to disappear from the plasma.)

The normal P.I.C. is approximately 0·7 mg. per 100 ml. per day. In myelofibrosis this is increased to over 3 mg. per 100 ml. per day.

Red-cell Iron Utilization.—Samples of blood are collected over 14–21 days, and the proportion of injected ^{59}Fe which has been incorporated into the erythrocytes is calculated. The results often show impaired iron utilization.

Red-cell Survival.—Survival is conveniently measured using ^{51}Cr. The majority of patients show diminished mean red-cell survival. In the patients studied by Szur and Smith (1961) the mean 50 per cent survival time ranged from 12 to 32 days (compared with the normal 25 ± 2 days). The relatively mild degree of impaired red-cell survival could be compensated for by a normally functioning marrow.

Surface Counting.—Surface radioactivity counts are made over the heart, liver, spleen, and sacrum. Patients with myelofibrosis often show raised initial counts over the liver and spleen, which are just above the normal range and not clearly related to red-cell survival or degree of splenomegaly. Evidence of extramedullary erythropoiesis may be obtained. In a majority of patients the spleen appears to be the seat of considerable red-cell destruction. When this is found, along with

BLOOD DISORDERS IN THE ELDERLY

Table XXVII.—Differential Diagnosis of Myelofibrosis

	Spleno-megaly	Hepato-megaly	Red Blood Corpuscles	Nucleated Red Blood Corpuscles	White Blood-cells	Leucocyte Alkaline Phosphatase	Platelets	Marrow	Average Survival
Myelofibrosis	++	±	Polychromasia Anisocytosis Poikilocytosis Tear drops	+	↑ with blasts	Normal	↓	Dry tap	1–10 yr.
Aplastic anaemia	–	–	Normal or Anisocytosis or Poikilocytosis	–	Normal or ↓	Normal	↓	Hypoplastic or maturation arrest	1 yr. <
Chronic myeloid leukaemia	++	+	Anisocytosis Poikilocytosis	+	↑ with myelocytes and blasts	↓	Normal, ↑, or ↓	(CML)	1–6 yr.
Chronic erythraemic myelosis	Late	Late	Anisocytosis Poikilocytosis	+	Normal, later ↑	Normal, later ↓ Probably normal	Normal	Erythroblastic	Near normal
Malignant myelosclerosis	–	–	Anisocytosis Poikilocytosis Polychromasia	+	↓ with blasts		↓	Dry	<18 mth.
Haemolytic anaemia	+	–	Anisocytosis Poikilocytosis Polychromasia Spherocytes	+	↑ slight	Normal	Normal	Normal or hypoplastic	? type
Leuco-erythro-blastic anaemia	–	–	Anisocytosis Poikilocytosis Polychromasia	+	↑ with blasts	Normal	Normal	Normal or primary condition	Duration of primary condition

marked impairment of red-cell survival, there may be sufficient indication for splenectomy.

Uric Acid.—Plasma uric-levels are often raised and associated with gout.

COURSE AND PROGNOSIS

The survival of patients suffering from myelofibrosis is peculiarly unpredictable. Many survive for 2–10 years—approximately 50 per cent survive more than 2 years. The prognosis is probably better than that of chronic myeloid leukaemia, but these elderly patients are often in a poor general state and prone to intercurrent infection. Progression of the disease is associated with increasing anaemia and a tendency to haemorrhage and thrombosis. The terminal phase may be that of an acute blast-cell transformation.

DIFFERENTIAL DIAGNOSIS (*see Table XXVII*)

The differential diagnosis is broadly that of leuco-erythroblastic anaemia, haemolytic anaemia, and the many conditions associated with splenomegaly.

Myeloid leukaemia may mimic the disease in its various phases, particularly when it is in an aleukaemic form. Marrow aspiration is usually diagnostic. The leucocyte alkaline phosphatase activity is normal or raised in myelofibrosis. However, frank leukaemia may develop.

Polycythaemia vera can terminate as myelofibrosis, so that transitional forms present difficulty. In such cases marrow sampling is the most important single diagnostic procedure.

The causes of leuco-erythroblastic anaemia are numerous, but careful examination of the peripheral blood-film for tear-drop cells is of some differentiating value. A primary haemolytic anaemia must be excluded, and other causes of leuco-erythroblastosis.

Chronic Erythraemic Myelosis.—The chronic form of Di Guglielmo's syndrome was only recognized subsequent to Di Guglielmo's (1928) description of acute erythraemic myelosis. Roath and Israels (1962) described 8 patients. All except 1 were over 55 years old. They presented with anaemia. The red cells showed anisocytosis and poikilocytosis. Occasional nucleated red blood-cells were seen. Bone-marrow aspiration smears were cellular and showed abnormal erythroblasts. Hepatomegaly and/or splenomegaly developed. No instance of 'malignant transformation' occurred. Provided the anaemia is treated the prognosis is probably little influenced by the disease process.

Malignant Myelosclerosis.—Lewis and Szur (1963) described 5 patients who showed features of an acute rapidly progressive illness such as is seen in the terminal phases of myelofibrosis, but in whom no chronic phase had been recognized. These patients were aged 43, 53, 55, 56, and 68 years. They presented with a rapidly developing anaemia and thrombocytopenia. They all showed a leucopenia and had nucleated red cells and leucoblasts in the peripheral blood. The spleen and lymph-nodes were not enlarged. Marrow aspiration yielded little or no cellular material. Bone biopsy showed a reduction of fat and haemopoietic tissue with a corresponding increase in collagen. Primitive reticulum cells and megakaryocytes were prominent. In all patients the condition pursued a relentless course and they were dead within 3–15 months.

THE MYELOPROLIFERATIVE SYNDROME

Polycythaemia vera, myeloid leukaemia, and myelofibrosis can be recognized as distinct entities. Patients are seen whose illnesses correspond to the classic description of these disorders. Nevertheless, it is clear that they can be interrelated in a continuous spectrum, and others, such as pernicious anaemia, can be interposed. The possible sequence of disease syndromes in such a spectrum is subject to wide variation. Thus a patient may present in a polycythaemic phase and progress through an anaemic to a myelofibrotic and terminally a leukaemic picture. The opportunity for witnessing progression of this nature is greater in the elderly who survive long enough to exhibit the interrelationship of various disease syndromes.

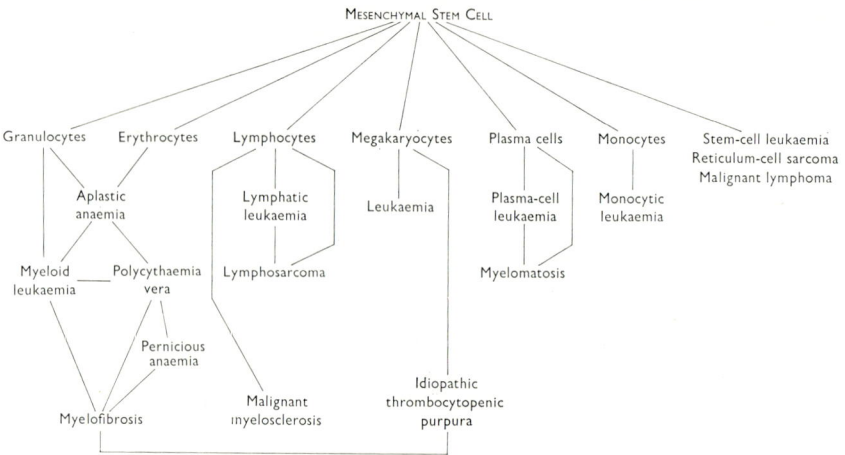

Fig. 73.—Interrelationship of diseases that may arise from abnormality of mesenchymal stem cell.

In clinical practice, however, the concept of 'the myeloproliferative syndrome' can all too readily serve as a refuge for the diagnostically destitute. The patient's interest is better served by as precise a diagnosis as possible.

The value of lumping together a variety of diseases into an interrelated scheme lies in its theoretical and prognostic implications, but it is then difficult to delineate a particular group. Indeed, the myeloproliferative syndrome can readily be expanded theoretically (and with some clinical justification) to include a major part of clinical haematology in the elderly (*Fig.* 73).

Megaloblastic erythropoiesis at some stage is common. Hoffbrand and others (1968) observed a group of 49 patients with myelosclerosis (age range 22–83 years, 32 of whom were over 60). Marked megaloblastic erythropoiesis occurred in 17 and mild changes in a further 16. The incidence was higher in the group with previous polycythaemia vera. Folate deficiency was the likely cause in 32 of these 33 patients.

Treatment

The problem devolves largely around the question of anaemia and spleen size. Iron deficiency is common in this age-group and should be corrected.

Megaloblastic anaemia may respond well to folic acid. Not only may the anaemia respond but so also may the thrombocytopenia. The latter sometimes occurs without any response in the haemoglobin.

Vitamin-B_{12} deficiency should be excluded or treated before giving folic acid.

Aplastic anaemia can occur, but is usually preceded by a hypoplastic stage, which may be a lone phenomenon or associated with combinations of haematinic deficiencies. Although blood formation is inadequate to cope with normal requirements and especially so when there is haemolysis or increased blood-loss—both of which are common in these patients—it is surprising how often a reasonably satisfactory haemoglobin level can be maintained for several months or even years when transfusions of packed red cells are given at intervals of 2 or 3 months. As the hypoplasia advances transfusions have to be given more often. Fresh blood is necessary if bleeding is due to gross thrombocytopenia.

Splenectomy: When this operation is considered three questions have to be answered:—

1. Is the patient suffering pain—that cannot be otherwise alleviated—because of the size of the spleen or the presence of perisplenitis?
2. Is the spleen participating in erythropoiesis to an appreciable degree?
3. Is red-cell destruction increased because of the splenomegaly?

Obviously the general health of the patient, the expected prognosis with and without operation, and the presence or absence of another disease or diseases are of paramount importance.

It is seldom necessary nowadays to operate because of pain. Treatment with modern analgesic drugs is usually effective. Extramedullary erythropoiesis occurs and is difficult to assess, but the state of the marrow can be judged in relation to the peripheral blood-picture. If there is a degree of hypoplasia, splenectomy is contraindicated unless it can be shown that the spleen is destroying red blood-cells. When it is enlarged and diseased the storage pool may be considerable and its destructive power a major factor in producing and maintaining anaemia. In these cases the spleen is greatly enlarged and the red cells abnormal either in shape, content, or covering. Their survival is decreased and the patient exhibits the characteristics of a haemolytic disease—but frank haemolysis need not be present. Increase in osmotic fragility and mechanical fragility, and a fall in the potassium: sodium ratio of red cells is known to occur within the spleen in certain conditions.

POLYCYTHAEMIA

Secondary Polycythaemia

Chronic tissue hypoxia can give rise to polycythaemia. Lung disease is a relatively more important cause than cardiac disease in the elderly. Chronic bronchitis, emphysema, and pneumoconiosis may be associated with a markedly raised red-cell count and increased blood viscosity. The mean corpuscular haemoglobin concentration is often reduced. The red-cell volume is increased, but the white-cell and platelet counts are not raised unless the primary condition has this effect. The arterial blood oxygen saturation is reduced to below 88 per cent, and cyanosis, both central and peripheral, may be profound. Splenomegaly is not a feature but the liver may be enlarged if congestive cardiac failure is present.

It is important that accompanying iron-deficiency is not missed. A degree of erythraemia hides this feature unless the blood-film is examined and the mean corpuscular haemoglobin concentration calculated. Serum-iron estimation and marrow aspiration may be indicated.

POLYCYTHAEMIA VERA

CLINICAL FEATURES

Definition.—Polycythaemia vera is characterized by an absolute increase in the total red-cell volume which is usually accompanied by increased leucocyte and platelet production, in the absence of a recognizable cause.

It is predominantly a disease of the middle aged and elderly. Males are affected more often than females and occasionally there is a familial incidence.

Age of Onset.—The age of onset of polycythaemia vera fits a normal distribution. Osgood (1965) found a median of 57 years with a standard deviation of 13 years. The incidence remained constant thereafter. Above the age of 55 years the incidence of new cases paralleled the number alive in the population. The survival times and age at death also followed a normal distribution. He concluded that polycythaemia vera was due to a single cause which was closely correlated with age. Furthermore, he pointed out that survival times in all malignancies studied fitted a log normal distribution, which suggested that polycythaemia vera was not a malignant process, at least in this respect. The age at which the patient first received ^{32}P was a major prognostic factor. Modan (1965a) carried out an epidemiological study in the Baltimore area. He found the mean age for newly diagnosed cases to be 60·3 years.

Symptoms.—Sometimes the diagnosis is made during routine examination or when a complication arises, but more frequently symptoms have been present for a year or more before the patient attends hospital. Headaches, which may have a migrainous or throbbing quality, are usually prominent, but vertigo, confusion, diplopia, loss of visual acuity, cranial nerve palsies, transient hemiparesis, drop attacks, fits, weakness, insomnia, and paraesthesiae may also be present. Lassitude and dyspnoea are common. Dyspepsia and abdominal pain due to perisplenitis or thrombosis of an intra-abdominal vessel can cause difficulty in diagnosis. Pruritus, particularly following a bath, is fairly frequent.

Clinical Examination.—The patient is plethoric and exposed surfaces are cyanosed. The cheeks, ears, and nose appear scarlet in a warm atmosphere and deep blue in the cold. The eyeballs are bloodshot and the retinal vessels congested. Papilloedema is seen only if thrombosis of the central vein has occurred.

The spleen is moderately enlarged in approximately 80 per cent of patients and the liver palpable in 50 per cent.

LABORATORY FINDINGS

Red-cell Mass.—The salient feature is an increase in the circulating red-cell volume, which must be distinguished from the finding of a raised red-cell count.

A variety of methods are available for estimating the total red-cell volume. Dye methods have generally been replaced by radio-isotopic techniques. Plasma volume can be measured using radio-iodinated albumin, and the red-cell volume calculated from the haematocrit. More commonly direct labelling of the patient's red cells with ^{51}Cr or ^{32}P is adopted. The greatest degree of accuracy is obtained when both plasma and red-cell volumes are determined, but we have found the ^{51}Cr method sufficiently accurate in routine work. The normal range, however, poses peculiar difficulties in the elderly. Several variables must be considered—such as sex, body-weight, and body composition. The results of red-cell volume estimations are accordingly expressed in several ways—as total volume; in relation to body-weight; in relation to body surface area; or as an expression of body composition. Probably the volume in relation to body-weight is the most generally useful. Normal ranges quoted are 32–36 ml. per kg. for males, and 34–38 ml. per kg. for females (Berlin, 1966). However, caution must be used in applying these figures to elderly patients. Piomelli, Nathan, Cummins, and Gardner (1962) compared the red-cell volumes of 91 octogenarian male veterans of the Spanish–American War with those of 19 healthy young men. The octogenarians showed a much greater variation in the relationship between red-cell volume and body-weight. The elderly group gave a mean red-cell volume of 25·7 ml. per kg. body-weight and a range of 16·2–36·0. The corresponding figures for the young men were 30·2 and 24·5–33·2 respectively. The octogenarians also showed poor correspondence between haematocrit levels and red-cell volume. The relationship between total body-water and body-weight was close in the young men, but less so in the elderly, although the mean of the red-cell volume/total body-water was the same in both groups (47·6 ml. per litre body-water in the elderly and 47·3 in the young), but the elderly gave a much wider range of values. Intracellular water formed a small fraction of the total body-water in the elderly—that is, the octogenarians were *relatively* fatter than the young men. Piomelli and others emphasized that their group of octogenarians was highly selective, so that their data are not necessarily applicable to those with a high incidence of morbidity. When the red-cell volume is related to total exchangable potassium it is found that the elderly may be more polycythaemic than a younger age-group (Nathan, 1966). The potassium total body-water ratio was raised in a group of elderly men who also showed a considerably increased extracellular compartment of total body-water. In other words, the lean tissues of the elderly were distributed differently. Diminished skeletal muscle mass had been replaced by a lean body mass in which the viscera had a relative preponderance over muscle. Nathan consequently suggested that red-cell volumes in the elderly should be related to the visceral mass, although there is no generally applicable formula available.

Peripheral Blood.—Red blood-count: Untreated cases of polycythaemia vera have red blood-cell counts usually in excess of 7 million per c.mm. The mean corpuscular volume is normal or reduced. Stained films often show exceptional crowding of erythrocytes which can be normochromic or hypochromic. There is frequently some degree of polychromasia or basophilic stippling, and an occasional normoblast is seen.

Haematocrit: The packed cell volume is raised above 60 per cent. Levels of over 80 per cent have been recorded.

Haemoglobin: The haemoglobin is raised, but this may bear little relationship to the presence or degree of polycythaemia. This is often the case in elderly patients who have a coincidental iron deficiency. In those already treated by venesection the haemoglobin value becomes even more unreliable.

White blood-cells: Approximately three-quarters have increased leucocyte counts, involving predominantly the granulocyte series, and stained films show a left nuclear shift with metamyelocytes and occasional myelocytes. The leucocyte alkaline phosphatase is usually increased. An absolute basophilia may be present and this has been invoked as an explanation for the occurrence of pruritus and peptic ulceration.

Platelets: Increased platelet counts are found in approximately 65 per cent of cases and their morphology may be abnormal, with large megakaryocytic fragments in the peripheral blood.

Blood viscosity: The earliest descriptions emphasized the thick viscid venous blood obtained from these patients, and attributed many of the clinical features and complications to this anomaly. Measurements of viscosity have shown an increase up to eightfold. The specific gravity of whole blood is also increased up to 1080 as compared with the normal 1055–1065. The E.S.R. is reduced to nearly zero.

Bone-marrow.—The bone-marrow is hypercellular, showing active proliferation of all stem lines. There is a corresponding reduction in marrow fat. Stainable iron is usually scanty. This contrasts with the findings in secondary polycythaemia where, as a rule, it is normal or increased.

Inconstant laboratory findings which are of little diagnostic significance include albuminuria, urobilinogenuria, hyperuricaemia, and hyperkalaemia in association with thrombocythaemia.

Vitamin B_{12} and Folic Acid.—Changes of doubtful significance in vitamin B_{12} and folic-acid metabolism occur. Kremenchuzky and Hoffbrand (1965) found that the mean serum vitamin B_{12} of 52 patients with polycythaemia vera was significantly higher than in their normal controls (578 and 472 pg. per ml. respectively). The serum folate was lowered in polycythaemic patients (mean level 5·4 compared with 9·6 ng. per ml. for controls). They also showed an increase in hypersegmented polymorphs. However, any folate deficiency that exists in polycythaemia is usually mild, and these authors do not appear to have taken any account of age in their comparisons.

DIAGNOSIS

Polycythaemia vera can be diagnosed only after the clinical and laboratory features have been considered together. Bodley Scott, Watkins, Fairley, and Scott (1967) made the diagnosis when the haemoglobin was greater than 17 g. per 100 ml. or the red-cell count over 6 million per c.mm., together with one other feature—a leucocyte count greater than 12,000 per c.mm., a platelet count greater than 300,000 per c.mm., or splenomegaly.

The presence of anoxia or chronic cardiovascular or pulmonary disease must be excluded.

When the clinical picture is suggestive of polycythaemia vera further investigation must be carried out. Obviously, a red-cell count, haematocrit, haemoglobin estimation, and white-cell and platelet counts should be routine procedures. A normal or only slightly reduced arterial oxygen saturation will also provide useful confirmatory evidence. The leucocytes show a raised alkaline phosphatase activity. An intravenous pyelogram is indicated if there is doubt as to whether the diagnosis is true polycythaemia. Brandt, Dacie, Steiner, and Szur (1963) investigated the renal tract of 91 patients in whom polycythaemia vera had been diagnosed. Eight (9 per cent) had renal lesions (neoplasms or cysts). All except 1 had associated splenomegaly and/or panmyelosis.

Dameshek (1966a) summarized the position by stating that the diagnosis of polycythaemia vera can be proved or disproved in 95 per cent of patients by a careful history; a physical examination, complete blood-counts, bone-marrow aspiration, and leucocyte alkaline phosphatase determination.

Red-cell volume estimations are only necessary in difficult cases, and even then the interpretation can be uncertain in the elderly.

Differential Diagnosis

'Stress' Polycythaemia.—The evaluation of polycythaemia is particularly difficult in obese, hypertensive males who have haematocrits of 50–60 per cent. As a rule the other features of polycythaemia vera are absent—namely, splenomegaly, leucocytosis, thrombocytosis, and increased leucocyte alkaline phosphate activity. It is in this group of patients that estimation of red-cell volume is of real value. Patients with 'stress' polycythaemia have a normal red-cell volume with a decreased plasma volume. The red-cell volume should be determined after abstinence from smoking. Unfortunately, as explained earlier, red-cell volume determinations may be misleading in the elderly and grossly obese, so that due attention must be given to the clinical findings and simpler laboratory tests.

Gaisböck's Disease.—Considerable confusion exists in the definition of Gaisböck's disease. Gardner (1966) claimed that Gaisböck's disease was identical with that of stress polycythaemia. Gaisböck described polycythaemia and hypertension in the absence of splenomegaly. The blood-volume was not estimated. Hall (1965) agreed that there was considerable overlap between Gaisböck's disease and stress polycythaemia, but suggested that there remained an entity which conformed to Gaisböck's description. These are patients with features of polycythaemia vera, including an increase in red-cell volume, but who have no panmyelosis or splenomegaly. Berlin (1966), however, stated that approximately 10 per cent of patients with polycythaemia vera have no splenomegaly or panmyelosis. Clearly such cases cannot be distinguished from the form of Gaisböck's disease delineated by Hall. The oldest patient in Hall's series of 20 men was 68 years, and 13 were aged between 30 and 50 years.

Benign Erythrocytosis.—Modan and Modan (1968) described 21 patients in whom a raised cell mass had been demonstrated. They showed neither splenomegaly, leucocytosis, nor thrombocytosis. There was a marked preponderance of males (17/21). Nineteen were aged over 40 years, and 15 over 50 years at the time of diagnosis. No myeloproliferative complications occurred in those who had not received radiation therapy, and the clinical course was relatively benign when compared with classic polycythaemia vera. The authors argued that these patients may be individuals who are at the upper end of the normal scale of red-cell mass. Nevertheless, they present with symptoms and complications that demand treatment. The difference between this entity and polycythaemia vera without splenomegaly and panmyelosis is probably purely semantic.

Erythropoietic Polycythaemia and Tumour-induced Polycythaemia.—These diseases with or without demonstrable erythropoietin must be considered in the differential diagnosis. Erythropoietin production has been demonstrated with cerebellar haemangioblastoma, renal tumours and cysts, and with phaemochromocytoma. Other tumours reported as giving rise to polycythaemia are adrenal cortical adenoma and carcinoma, ovarian carcinoma, hepatoma, and uterine fibroids. Some degree of polycythaemia is usually present in Cushing's disease. In most of these symptomatic polycythaemias splenomegaly and panmyelosis do not occur. Many of them reflect a real increase in total red-cell volume. Drugs have also been implicated. Androgen therapy for malignancy is one example.

COMPLICATIONS

These can be grouped into those that are due to the increased blood-volume and viscosity, and those arising in the other haematopoietic stem lines. The former are considered as part of the disease picture. The importance of iatrogenic complications must always be remembered.

Many of the complications are attributable to thrombosis and haemorrhage. Venous thrombosis, Raynaud's disease, thromboangiitis obliterans, gangrene, hemiparesis, ischaemic heart disease, and haemorrhage from various sites have been reported. Hepatomegaly, cirrhosis, hepatic vein, and portal vein thrombosis may occur.

Gout is found in approximately 5 per cent of patients, although the incidence of hyperuricaemia is higher.

There is an increased incidence of duodenal ulceration which could be related to the absolute increase of basophilic leucocytes releasing more histamine. This is also the probable explanation of the urticaria and itching that are often present after bathing.

Leukaemia and Myeloid Metaplasia.—In 10–15 per cent of patients the increase in leucocyte production becomes a predominant haematological feature and the leucocytes appear more primitive. It may then be difficult, or impossible, to distinguish between a process of myeloid metaplasia and leukaemia.

High neutrophil counts with a left nuclear shift, occasional myelocytes, myeloblasts, and nucleated red cells are seen. These are to be distinguished from leuco-erythroblastosis due to other causes. The film may even resemble that of chronic myeloid leukaemia. The increased alkaline phosphatase activity in polycythaemia provides a useful distinguishing test. The presence of the Philadelphia chromosome defect will also single out chronic myeloid leukaemia.

The reverse of this is seen when a patient is treated for chronic myeloid leukaemia only to develop an erythraemic picture. This may be indistinguishable from erythroleukaemia.

Extramedullary haematopoiesis is associated with the peripheral blood findings of myeloid metaplasia. It also contributes to the severity of the hepatosplenomegaly. Haematopoiesis can also take place in other sites, such as kidneys and lymph-nodes.

The frequency of acute leukaemia as a complication of polycythaemia vera is uncertain. The question is bedevilled by the possible role of radiotherapy. Modan and Lilienfeld (1964), reviewing 1222 patients seen at seven centres, found that 10 per cent developed leukaemia following ^{32}P and/or X-ray therapy, which compared with less than 1 per cent in the non-irradiated group. The risk appeared to be dose-dependent. Perkins, Israels, and Wilkinson (1964) did not find a single case of leukaemia in 127 non-irradiated patients. Halnan and Russell (1965), on the other hand, described 107 patients all of whom had been irradiated, but none had developed leukaemia. Szur and Lewis (1966) found 4 cases of leukaemia in 169 patients treated with ^{32}P—an incidence comparable to that found in the non-irradiated. The comparison of the variously reported series is difficult because of differing criteria of diagnosis for acute leukaemia (and even of polycythaemia vera). Further, irradiation may prolong survival and thereby allow more time for the development of complications. Dameshek (1966b) regarded the leukaemogenic effect of ^{32}P as a contra-indication to its use and stated that he had not observed a single case of acute leukaemia during a 10-year period in which he relied on phlebotomy and cytotoxic drugs.

Myelofibrosis.—The marrow of patients suffering from polycythaemia vera shows increasing fibroblastic activity as the disease progresses. The peripheral blood-picture is leuco-erythroblastic, with fragmentation and tear-drop erythrocytes. Attempted bone-marrow aspiration may result in a 'dry tap'. Bone-marrow biopsy shows fibrosis and foci of hypercellularity. Extramedullary erythropoiesis takes place.

The terminal haematological picture in polycythaemia vera depends on the duration of the disease, the complications that have occurred, and the type of treatment administered. It may be that of panmyelosis, leuco-erythroblastosis, pernicious anaemia, leukaemia, or aplastic anaemia.

TREATMENT

Survival time in untreated patients is difficult to gauge, but is sometimes about 18 months and consequently several forms of therapy have been introduced.

Venesection of 400 ml. to 800 ml. of blood every 6–8 weeks improves the patient, but on its own may be insufficient and there is a real danger of severe iron deficiency. A periodic check on the red-cell mass may help in assessment.

Radiophosphorus: After a preliminary venesection 2–8 g. of ^{32}P are given intravenously and the blood-picture studied 8 weeks later. A reduced platelet count is the first positive sign of a satisfactory response. A higher dose is necessary when the white-cell count is greatly raised. Adjustment of the blood-volume automatically follows. About 5–10 per cent of patients are refractory and follow-up is essential.

Side-effects are minimal, but the occasional development of acute leukaemia, acute erythraemic myelosis, and erythroleukaemia (Di Guglielmo's disease) have been noted in some series. Survival over 10 years is not unusual and death is almost invariably due to unrelated disease or vascular complications. Tubiana and others (1968) showed that although median survival after treatment was 14·5 years it was less in elderly patients and in those with short remissions after initial therapy. In 296 treated patients they followed up for over 5 years 145 had died, and of these 53 were known to have had a haematological complication: acute leukaemia in 29, chronic leukaemia in 4, myeloid metaplasia or myelofibrosis in 16, and aplastic anaemia in 4.

Nitrogen Mustard, 20–40 mg. weekly, may be given when treatment with radiophosphorus is not possible. Careful management of the dose and follow-up are necessary.

Chemotherapeutic agents (busulphan, thiotepa, nitrogen mustard, and pyrimethamine) after venesection: The danger of leukaemia is perhaps avoided, but agranulocytosis and aplastic anaemia sometimes occur. Side-effects such as nausea, vomiting, diarrhoea, and alopecia are fairly common. Thrombocytopenia may develop, particularly with pyrimethamine. The results are comparable with those obtained with radiophosphorus.

Anaemia developing in the course of the disease may be due to iron deficiency, leukaemia, myelofibrosis, vitamin-B_{12} and/or folate deficiency, or aplastic anaemia. Iron deficiency can mask deficiency of folate and therefore serum-folate estimation is always necessary. Where there is doubt a therapeutic trial with folate is justified.

Complications may need specific treatment. Gangrene of the extremity may require amputation; hemiplegia needs rehabilitative management; heart failure resulting from the increased work load requires urgent venesection; and haematemesis may be so severe that surgery is necessary. Gout can be troublesome.

Splenectomy is not indicated in uncomplicated polycythaemia vera, but sometimes in the course of the disease the advisability of such an operation arises. Considerable abdominal discomfort due to splenomegaly or perisplenitis can occasionally justify surgery, and haemolysis due to 'hypersplenism' is also a possible indication. The red-cell mass and the blood-volume both decrease after removal of a very large spleen, because its pooling effect can be considerable. However, surgery should not be undertaken lightly in these patients as they have a haemorrhagic and thrombotic tendency. Irradiation of the spleen may be preferable.

The deciding factors on which line of treatment to adopt in a specific case are complex. On the one hand, polycythaemia vera is often a slowly progressive disease which harms the patient by its hypervolaemia and hyperviscosity, while, on the other, it is associated with thrombocytosis and granulocytic proliferation. The first can be dealt with by repeated venesection, and the second by the use of myelosuppressive therapy. Moreover, the two forms of treatment can be combined. It is not surprising that opposing views are held. Those favouring venesection alone stress the side-effects of suppressive therapy, and others who use radiophosphorus or cytotoxic drugs believe that the increased erythrocytes, platelets, and granulocytes are in themselves harmful because of pruritus, peptic ulceration, hyperuricaemia, and thrombosis. The relative value of radiophosphorus and cytotoxic drug régimes has not yet been ascertained. If the incidence of leukaemia is increased then the use of cytotoxic drugs is perhaps preferable—but they also have their side-effects, including aplastic anaemia. Osgood (1964) summarized: 'Most persons would rather run some risk of dying of leukaemia at an advanced age than of dying younger without leukaemia. There is nothing we do in this world that does not carry some risk, and we must always weigh the benefits against the risk.'

Dameshek (1966b) stated that phlebotomy was the quickest way to relieve symptoms. In the feeble, 250 ml. should be removed initially and later 500 ml. He considered it inadvisable to wait longer than 4–5 days between phlebotomies. The development of iron deficiency was to be expected, but it was rarely permanent. He felt that by this means remission lasted longer than with phlebotomy alone. The haematocrit reading should be kept to a level below 55 per cent. He summarized: 'Phlebotomy, carefully performed and managed, should be capable of relieving symptoms and maintaining remission for many years in at least two-thirds of the patients. In the rest, the occasional addition of an oral alkylating agent may be desirable, and in rare cases ^{32}P may be used.'

Wasserman and Gilbert (1966) compared the result of using chlorambucil (6–8 mg. daily), cyclophosphamide (100–150 mg. daily), and busulfan (4–6 mg. daily). They accepted that phlebotomy could reduce quickly and effectively the increased blood-volume, but felt that it was also necessary to suppress the most actively proliferating cell line or lines at both intra- and extramedullary sites. Reduction of the W.B.C. was greater with busulfan than the others, and remissions tended to be longer. In order to minimize thrombocytopenia maintenance therapy with busulfan was not given, but prolonged remissions were maintained with chlorambucil and cyclophosphamide by using one-half the induction dose daily or full doses for 3- to 4-week periods, alternating with 3 to 4 weeks without treatment. Phlebotomy was rarely necessary once control was achieved with chemotherapy, thus avoiding chronic iron deficiency and abrupt haemodynamic changes.

Total body irradiation increases the risk of the development of leukaemia and the results are not as good as with ^{32}P (Osgood, 1965).

In the elderly—particularly the advanced elderly—overtreatment has to be guarded against. Symptoms can be relieved with phlebotomy, but frequent phlebotomies are difficult because of clotting. Moreover, such treatment causes iron deficiency which may be severe enough to precipitate mental confusion or heart failure. Leukaemia is not a contra-indication to treatment with radiophosphorus at this age, as the patient often dies from unrelated disease before leukaemia has time to develop. The myelosuppressive drugs now available are toxic to the marrow and have a tendency to cause nausea so that where possible they should be avoided.

In general, successful management depends on the relief of symptoms and the sensible balancing of risks.

REFERENCES

BERLIN, N. (1966), *Seminars in Hematology*, **3**, 209.
BODLEY SCOTT, R., WATKINS, P. J., FAIRLEY, G. H., and SCOTT, R. B. (1967), *Br. med. J.*, **2**, 664.
BRANDT, P. W. T., DACIE, J. V., STEINER, R. E., and SZUR, L. (1963), *Ibid.*, **2**, 468.
DAMESHEK, W. (1966a), *Seminars in Hematology*, **3**, 214.
— — (1966b), *Ibid.*, **3**, 226.
GARDNER, F. H. (1966), *Ibid.*, **3**, 175.
DI GUGLIELMO, G. (1928), *Haematologica*, **9**, 302.
HALL, C. A. (1965), *Archs intern. Med.*, **116**, 4.
HALNAN, K. E., and RUSSELL, M. H. (1965), *Lancet*, **2**, 760.
HOFFBRAND, A. V., CHANARIN, I., KREMENCHUZKY, S., SZUR, L., WATERS, A. H., and MOLLIN, D. L. (1968), *Q. Jl Med.*, **38**, 493.
KREMENCHUZKY, S., and HOFFBRAND, A. V. (1965), *Br. J. Haemat.*, **11**, 600.
LEWIS, S. M., and SZUR, L. (1963), *Br. med. J.*, **2**, 472.
MODAN, B. (1965a), *Blood*, **26**, 657.
— — (1965b), *J. chron. Dis.*, **18**, 605.
— — and MODAN, M. (1968), *Br. J. Haemat.*, **14**, 375.
— — and LILIENFIELD, A. M. (1964), *Lancet*, **2**, 439.
NATHAN, D. G. (1966), *Seminars in Hematology*, **3**, 216.
OSGOOD, E. E. (1964), *J. Lab. clin. Med.*, **64**, 560.
— — (1965), *Blood*, **26**, 243.
PERKINS, J., ISRAELS, M. C. G., and WILKINSON, J. F. (1964), *Q. Jl Med.*, **33**, 499.
PIOMELLI, S., NATHAN, D. G., CUMMINS, J. F., and GARDNER, F. H. (1962), *Blood*, **19**, 89.
ROATH, S., and ISRAELS, M. C. G. (1962), *Lancet*, **2**, 1140.
SZUR, L., and LEWIS, S. M. (1966), *Br. J. Radiol.*, **39**, 122.
— — and SMITH, M. D. (1961), *Br. J. Haemat.*, **7**, 147.
TUBIANA, M., FLAMANT, R., ATIE, E., and HAYAT, M. (1968), *Blood*, **32**, 536.
WASSERMAN, L. R., and GILBERT, H. S. (1966), *Seminars in Hematology*, **3**, 228.

12
BLEEDING AND COAGULATION DISORDERS
CLASSIFICATION OF BLEEDING DISORDERS

Platelet Abnormalities
  Thrombocytopenia
  Thrombocythaemia
  Thrombasthenia

Coagulation Defects
  Congenital deficiencies
    Haemophilia
    Christmas disease
  Acquired deficiencies
    Liver disease
    Drugs
  Hypofibrinogenaemia and fibrinolysis
  Circulating anticoagulants
  Disseminated intravascular coagulation

Capillary Defects
  Senile purpura
  Henoch-Schönlein purpura
  Symptomatic purpura
  Hereditary haemorrhagic telangiectasia
  Myxoedema coma

Combined Defects
  Von Willebrand's disease

Serum Abnormalities
  Hyperglobulinaemia
  Uraemia

PURPURA

Thrombocytopenic
  Symptomatic
    Systemic disease
    Infections
    Bone-marrow infiltrations
    Drugs
    Disseminated intravascular coagulation
    Thrombotic
  Idiopathic

Non-thrombocytopenic
  Senile
  Allergic. Henoch-Schönlein
  Infections
  Systemic disease
  Serum protein abnormalities
  Vitamin-C deficiency
Thrombasthenia
Thrombocythaemia
Combined Coagulation Defects—Von Willebrand's disease

Purpura is due to rupture of surface capillaries with subsequent spread of extravasated blood. The area involved can vary from pin-point petechiae to 2–3-cm. bruises, and they may be seen on skin, mucous membrane, and serosal surfaces.

Cutaneous purpura appears as red spots of varying size and shape, which are not raised above the skin surface. Blood-filled vesicles may, however, be found in the oral mucous membrane.

The chief clinical distinction that has to be made is between those where there is thrombocytopenia (less than 60,000 per c.mm.) and those where the count is normal.

Idiopathic Thrombocytopenic Purpura (I.T.P.)

Clinical Features

The family history may be entirely negative, or some relatives merely give a history of easy bruising or one suggestive of a minor bleeding disorder. Rarely, thrombocytopenia has been found as an autosomal dominant trait.

Approximately half present before the age of 15 years, but typical cases are seen in the middle-aged or elderly. There is a natural reluctance to dismiss the possibility of symptomatic thrombocytopenic purpura in the elderly, but several have been diagnosed as I.T.P. in their late seventies and follow-up for several years has failed to reveal a primary cause.

The disease is twice to four times as common in women as in men.

Although patients may first be seen with a chronic anaemia, it is far more likely for them to have purpura, excessive bruising, or epistaxis. Haematuria and postmenopausal bleeding may also occur. Melaena or haematemesis are seen infrequently. Intracranial haemorrhage is a rare complication, but an important cause of death.

Hess's test of capillary resistance consists of placing a sphygmomanometer cuff around the upper arm and inflating it for 10 minutes to 100 mm. Hg pressure, or to a pressure half-way between the systolic and diastolic blood-pressure if the former is less than 100 mm. Hg. The number of petechiae within a marked 3-cm. circle below the antecubital fossa are counted after congestion has faded. Normal adult subjects may have up to 10 petechiae; I.T.P. patients have over 100. In the elderly, however, the normal number varies and intermediate values are difficult to interpret because capillary fragility increases with age.

Splenomegaly is found in approximately a fifth.

The clinical course observed in the elderly often differs from that seen at younger ages, in that the acute self-limiting attacks of the young are uncommon, and the condition is more likely to pursue a chronic intermittent course.

Haematological Findings

The platelet count is very low when bleeding takes place. A level of approximately 60,000 per c.mm. appears to be critical, above which bleeding does not occur, but the converse does not apply as levels below this are not always associated with bleeding. Platelet morphology may be abnormal with giant or fragmented forms seen in the peripheral blood. Conflicting results have been reported for platelet antibodies, and this is not a helpful diagnostic procedure in I.T.P.

The bleeding time is prolonged to well in excess of 5 minutes in active phases.

Coagulation time is normal, but the clot fails to retract. The prothrombin consumption test is markedly reduced, but the other classic coagulation tests are normal.

The bone-marrow shows normal or increased numbers of megakaryocytes, although normal platelet budding is usually absent.

Pizzi, Carrara, Aldeghi, and Eridani (1966) found that in more than half the cases of chronic I.T.P. a plasma protein fraction (probably IgA) was strongly adherent to the surface of the megakaryocytes. This was not observed in secondary thrombocytopenia.

Diagnosis

The diagnosis may be made as the result of the investigation of a case of purpura or bleeding, or occasionally during the investigation of an anaemia. The first step is the demonstration of significant and persistent thrombocytopenia (below 60,000 per c.mm.) with the corresponding findings of increased bleeding time, decreased capillary resistance, and diminished clot retraction. The second stage involves the exclusion of a recognizable cause. Particular attention has to be paid to the drug history. Bone-marrow examination does not give diagnostic information, but is nevertheless essential in order to exclude a primary haematological disease such as leukaemia, myelofibrosis, or aplasia. The procedure is not associated with any increased bleeding hazard.

Latent systemic lupus erythematosus is a rare explanation in the elderly.

Treatment

Although spontaneous remissions are well recognized, particularly in younger patients with a short history, adrenocorticosteroid therapy and/or splenectomy has nearly always to be considered in the elderly.

In the acute phase prednisone in a dose of 40 mg. daily may tide the patient over the danger period, but if bleeding continues, or the disease enters a chronic relapsing stage, splenectomy may be necessary. It is not possible to predict which patient will benefit from the operation—probably only about half of the chronic elderly type will respond. The platelet count rises rapidly after splenectomy, although it may subsequently fall to its low preoperative level without necessarily inducing a recurrence of bleeding.

Blood Transfusion.—Lost blood should be replaced, but only temporary benefit is obtained from fresh platelet-rich blood, or even platelet transfusions.

Prognosis

Watson-Williams, Macpherson, and Davidson (1958) reviewed 93 cases of I.T.P., 21 of whom were over 50 years. Seven of these gave a short history (less than 100 days); in 5 splenectomy was performed within the first 100 days; and in 9 there was a long history. From their figures it is seen that those with a short history and better prognosis are by no means confined to the young. All 9 of their treated patients over 60 years were alive at the time of review, 6 months to 3 years later.

Intracranial haemorrhage is always a possible hazard, but despite this and the fact that response to treatment is unpredictable or even disappointing, life expectancy may be little affected.

Case 1.—This man presented in 1960 at the age of 76 years with melaena. All gastro-intestinal investigations were negative. Bone-marrow examination was also normal, and the only abnormality was a platelet count of 10,000 per c.mm. Steroid therapy was commenced. The platelets thereafter remained at levels varying from 5000 to 35,000. A papillary angiomatous lesion of the tongue was excised in 1963. The marrow examination was repeated in 1964, when nothing of significance was noted other than possibly fewer megakaryocytes than in 1960. He was readmitted in 1966 with another episode of melaena whilst still on steroids. When last seen in 1968 at the age of 84 years, he was symptom-free, although his platelet count was only 20,000 per c.mm.

Secondary Thrombocytopenia

Drugs

Thrombocytopenia may be a constant finding when certain drugs are given, as a result of their direct toxic action. Any of the drugs that cause aplastic anaemia can be implicated, although some have a predilection for suppressing platelet production. Alternatively, thrombocytopenia may be a sporadic manifestation of a patient's hypersensitivity to a particular drug.

The direct marrow toxins which can have a selective effect on platelets include gold, sulphonamides, organic arsenicals, cytotoxic drugs, colcemid, urethane, ristocetin, and chlorothiazide. The effect in these instances is largely dose-dependent.

The importance of hypersensitivity to drugs as a cause of thrombocytopenia was recognized following Ackroyd's observations (1949, 1955) that some patients after taking Sedormid (allylisopropyl-acetyl carbamide) for several months without ill-effect suddenly developed purpura. This feature was not dose-dependent. The platelets of sensitized patients could be agglutinated and lysed *in vitro* when they were exposed to similar concentrations of the drug. It appears that the drug combines with platelets to form an antigen which stimulates the production of antibody. Lysis requires the presence of complement. Subsequently, several other drugs have been shown to produce thrombocytopenia by a similar mechanism—for example, quinidine, quinine, sulphonamides, barbiturates, chlorpropamide, penicillin, chloramphenicol, tetracycline, para-aminosalicylic acid, paracetamol, tolbutamide, and desipramine.

Chlorothiazide cannot be assigned firmly to one or other type of thrombocytopenic-inducing mechanism. It may have a direct toxic action on megakaryocytes (Wintrobe, 1969), but is irregular in its effects. Nordqvist, Cramér, and Björntorp (1959) estimated that chlorothiazide gave rise to thrombocytopenia in approximately 1 per cent. They emphasized the desirability of doing blood-counts on elderly patients receiving this drug.

Constitutional symptoms often accompany the bleeding phase in hypersensitive patients. These and the purpura respond rapidly to withdrawal of the drug. Severe episodes may require fresh blood transfusion and steroids.

When thrombocytopenia is caused by one of the direct-acting marrow toxins the prognosis is better if the megakaryocytes are selectively damaged, rather than as part of a pancytopenia.

Barbiturates are usually safe sedatives in these patients, but carbromal and dichloralphenazone (Welldorm) should be avoided. Analgesics, such as aspirin, and those containing amidopyrine or phenylbutazone, may precipitate an acute attack.

INFECTION

Thrombocytopenia occurs occasionally in any infection, especially in septicaemia. However, purpura frequently occurs in conditions such as bacterial endocarditis, even when the platelet count is not significantly reduced, due presumably to a direct toxic action on the walls of capillaries.

OTHER BLOOD DISORDERS

Leukaemia.—Some degree of thrombocytopenia is the rule in acute leukaemia. It is also common in chronic lymphatic leukaemia, and the terminal stages of chronic myeloid leukaemia. In treated cases the effect of drugs cannot be distinguished from that due to the disease. Thrombocytopenic bleeding is a prominent feature in many and is often the cause of death.

Other haematological conditions that may present as thrombocytopenia include 'idiopathic' primary aplastic anaemia, myelofibrosis, multiple myeloma, malignant lymphoma, and neoplastic infiltration of the bone-marrow. Untreated pernicious-anaemia patients often show severe thrombocytopenia. Auto-immune haemolytic anaemia, complicated by persistent thrombocytopenic purpura, is known as 'Evans's syndrome'.

Any condition where the spleen is enlarged may have the same effect, whether due to chronic venous congestion, Felty's syndrome, or portal hypertension.

Paraproteinaemia, especially cryoglobulinaemia, may be associated with it.

Miscellaneous Conditions.—Hyperthyroidism, liver cirrhosis, massive whole-blood transfusion, and transfusion of incompatible blood can also cause thrombocytopenia. Platelet antibodies can often be demonstrated following multiple blood transfusion.

Thrombocytopenia may also be associated with carcinoma. Brodie, Bliss, and Firkin (1970) described 2 men, aged 72 and 52 years, who had carcinoma of the lung and developed severe thrombocytopenia without evidence of bone-marrow metastases, or consumption coagulopathy. The bone-marrow showed normal or increased numbers of megakaryocytes, and in 1 patient the platelet survival time was less than 24 hours. These features suggested that the depression of platelets was an immune reaction.

THROMBOTIC THROMBOCYTOPENIC PURPURA
(*Micro-angiopathic haemolytic anaemia*)

This condition is characterized by thrombocytopenic purpura, haemolytic anaemia, fever, and neurological signs. Renal involvement also is often present. Although predominantly a disease of children and young adults the elderly are by no means exempt. In a review of 163 cases Amorosi and Ultman (1966) stated that the age distribution extended to 77 years. Another, aged 84, was later described in the literature (Jacobson and Vickery, 1968).

Haemorrhage may occur from any site, and major gastro-intestinal or genito-urinary bleeding is often seen. The neurological signs fluctuate with headache, aphasia, confusion, psychosis, epilepsy, pareses, dysarthria, blindness, or coma. Renal involvement shows as proteinuria, haematuria, and uraemia. Arthralgia may be present. Hepatosplenomegaly and lymphadenopathy occur in a minority.

Malignant phase hypertension may be present, and Linton and others (1969) on the basis of a study of 9 patients who had both conditions suggested that the two could be related.

The peripheral blood findings include thrombocytopenia, anaemia, and reticulocytosis. Fragmented and bur red cells are seen. Red-cell survival is reduced, and indirect-reacting bilirubin levels are raised. The Coombs's test is negative. Haemoglobinaemia is present. There is a leucocytosis which may show leukaemoid features. Platelet life-span is markedly reduced.

Marrow examination does not usually show any diagnostic feature, and megakaryocytes are not depleted.

The diagnosis may be confirmed histologically. The hall-mark of thrombotic thrombocytopenic purpura is the finding of multiple hyaline thrombi—rarely they are seen in marrow biopsies but more commonly in viscera such as liver or kidneys. At post-mortem they are found particularly in the brain, heart, and kidneys.

The pathogenesis is not known. It appears that fibrin deposition in small blood-vessels provokes intravascular haemolysis and red-cell fragmentation by mechanical distortion (Rubenberg, Regoeczi, Bull, Dacie, and Brain, 1968). The thrombocytopenia could also have a similar explanation. Conflicting results have been reported in the few cases where detailed assessment of the coagulation factors have been made.

The majority of these patients succumb within 3 months, and only rarely does the disease become chronic or remit completely.

Heparin and/or steroids may be beneficial. Occasionally splenectomy improves red-cell survival.

Blood transfusion and control of hypertension may be required. Renal failure may need haemodialysis.

HAEMORRHAGIC THROMBOCYTHAEMIA

It is doubtful whether haemorrhagic thrombocythaemia is a distinct entity. Among Hardisty and Wolff's 5 patients (1955) 1 had chronic myeloid leukaemia, myelofibrosis, haemolytic anaemia, and had had a splenectomy; the second also had had a splenectomy; and the third had chronic myeloid leukaemia. A number of the reported cases have followed the removal of an atrophic spleen. Others subsequently develop leukaemia, polycythaemia, or myelofibrosis. Perhaps a good case can be made for considering this condition as one manifestation of the myeloproliferative syndrome. However, there remain a small number of patients who present with thrombocythaemia, and even after follow-up for many years have no new development, as in 1 of Hardisty and Wolff's patients who had been observed for 28 years. Furthermore, it is usually seen in the adult or elderly, in whom the life-span may be unaffected.

Haemorrhagic thrombocythaemia is much rarer than idiopathic thrombocytopenic purpura. Patients are seen because of spontaneous bleeding from the nose or gut, or bruising. Purpura is seldom present. Thrombotic episodes may occur in any organ in approximately one-third of the cases. The spleen is often palpable.

The platelet count varies from 500,000 per c.mm. to several millions and abnormal forms are present in the peripheral blood. There is a neutrophilia, and often some degree of polycythaemia—although if this is of significant degree the condition is indistinguishable from polycythaemia vera. Approximately one-half have an increased bleeding time. Platelets may show a qualitative defect in the thromboplastin generation test. Bone-marrow examination is always indicated and shows megakaryocytic hyperplasia. It also serves to exclude other primary haematological disease.

Treatment is by means of busulphan and/or radioactive phosphorus. Splenectomy is contra-indicated.

Thrombasthenia

Injury to a small blood-vessel, sufficient to bring blood into contact with connective-tissue collagen, results in platelet adhesion and aggregation with the release of adenosine diphosphate (A.D.P.). This in turn causes further aggregation and release of A.D.P. The phospholipid component (platelet factor III) is also made available for blood coagulation and is activated, particularly in the region of the platelet aggregate. Furthermore, platelets are also largely responsible for the incorporation of fibrin and clot retraction, so that a functional platelet defect can give rise to a bleeding tendency even when the count is normal.

Thrombasthenia, or Glanzman's disease, is a disease of the young, but failure of secondary platelet aggregation due to a defective A.D.P. release mechanism may be found in the elderly as a result of scurvy, uraemia, thrombocythaemia, and albinism. On the other hand, platelets from patients with ischaemic heart disease, and peripheral arterial disease, seem to be abnormally sensitive to A.D.P. (Bolton, Hampton, and Mitchell, 1967).

The tests which indicate abnormal platelet function are the bleeding time, clot retraction, platelet-aggregation tests (A.D.P.), platelet-adhesion tests, and platelet factor III availability.

Non-thrombocytopenic Purpura

Purpura, in the presence of a normal platelet count, usually denotes a different disease association in the elderly than in the young. Anaphylactoid purpuras (Henoch-Schönlein) are very rare, but nutritional deficiencies, metabolic diseases, dysproteinaemia, and, most common of all, senile purpura are often seen.

Senile Purpura

There is little purpose in giving figures for the incidence of senile purpura because they depend largely on its definition. Old people bruise readily, and this cannot be differentiated accurately from non-traumatic purpura. The more frequently and thoroughly old people are examined the higher will be the incidence of this condition.

Senile purpura occurs chiefly on the extensor surface of the forearms and hands, without involving the fingers. Similar lesions may be found near the spectacle-frame area of the face. The lesions may be up to 5 cm. in diameter and have sharp irregular outlines. They appear static on routine inspection, but if they are delineated, a changing colour and pattern will be demonstrated, with occasional disappearance in 2 or 3 weeks.

Skin changes sometimes seen in patients receiving adrenal corticosteroids resemble senile purpura in two basic respects (Scarborough and Shuster, 1960): degeneration of collagen occurs, and the inflammatory reaction to extravasated blood is impaired. These authors induced 'corticosteroid purpura' in 5 women on steroids by injecting 0·1 ml. of their own blood intradermally. Unfortunately, 3 of these suffered from rheumatoid arthritis and their mean age was 63 years, so that they might well have produced purpura apart from their steroid therapy, or even in response to any intradermal injection.

Senile purpura appears to be a direct expression of ageing. The thin, inelastic skin of the elderly slides over the underlying subcutaneous tissue to an abnormal degree. This subjects it to shearing stresses which rupture small blood-vessels. The atrophic tissues fail to contain the extravasated blood, and the phagocytic response may also be impaired. Measurements of capillary fragility show a progressive increase with age (Bell, Lazarus, and Munro, 1940; Hart and Cohen, 1969).

Vitamin-C Deficiency

Haemorrhagic features are usually prominent in fully developed scurvy, but their frequency in subclinical deficiency of ascorbic acid is not known. The possibility of deficiency states is increased in the elderly, particularly in high-risk groups, such as men living on their own, the poor, and those suffering from systemic or gastro-intestinal disease. Chronic alcoholism and hepatic cirrhosis are possible causes.

Andrews and Brook (1966) found no difference between the mean leucocyte vitamin-C content of patients with senile purpura and those without, but they did find sublingual petechiae in a group of 24 patients in whom the mean vitamin-C levels were 10·23 μg. per 10^8 leucocytes compared with 17·67 in a group of 64 without petechiae.

In states of deficiency sufficiently severe to give rise to scurvy, haemorrhagic features may predominate in any part of the skin, mucous membrane, or deeper tissue. Rarely, visceral haemorrhage occurs. The patient is usually anaemic, and often there is coexisting vitamin-B_{12}, folic-acid, or iron deficiency.

The diagnosis is confirmed by measuring the ascorbic-acid content of the patient's leucocytes, the ascorbic-acid saturation test, and the response to treatment, although large doses in the region of 1000 mg. daily are necessary.

Infections

Purpura may occur during acute infections even when the platelet count is normal. This is to be distinguished from allergic purpura which may be post-infective. The purpura of acute infections is commonly found in septicaemia, particularly bacterial endocarditis. The mechanism may be embolic or the result of a toxic vasculitis. A sudden onset of purpura with a normal platelet count in the elderly should indicate the possibility of septicaemia.

Although organisms, such as the meningococcus, are notorious for their possible association with a fulminating purpura, this is by no means confined to a few bacteria. Any toxigenic pathogen may produce a similar picture, as, for example, *Staphylococcus pyogenes* in the following case:—

Case 2.—An ex-coal miner, aged 70 years, gave a history of chronic bronchitis and valvular disease of the heart for many years. He showed progressive deterioration and was confined to bed for 3 weeks at home prior to his death. At post-mortem the body showed extensive, bright red, purpuric lesions involving the face, trunk, and legs. There was a fresh subarachnoid haemorrhage. The heart showed rheumatic type thickening of the aortic and mitral valves with thick,

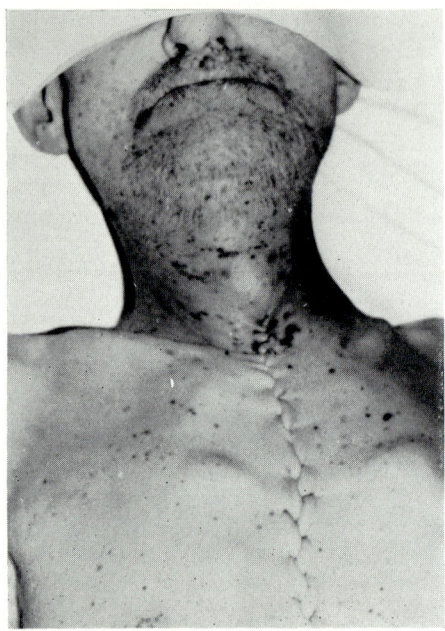

Fig. 74.—*Case* 2. Generalized purpura in staphylococcal septicaemia.

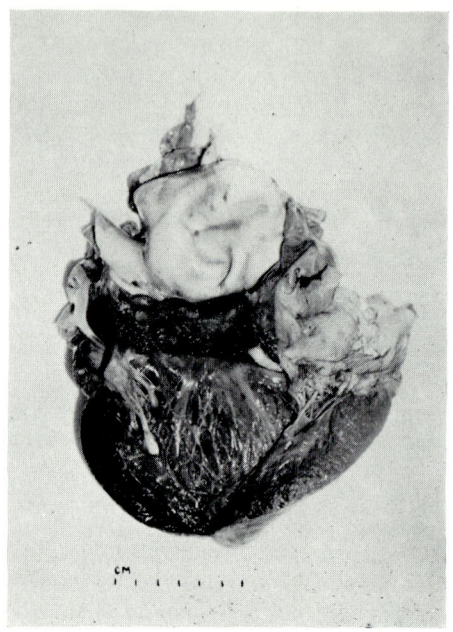

Fig. 75.—*Case* 2. Staphylococcal endocarditis affecting mainly the aortic valve, with a smaller area on the mitral valve.

fresh, friable vegetations covering the former. Histological sections of the kidneys, lungs, and brain showed foci of haemorrhage, which were striking in the case of the kidneys and could best be described as 'purpuric kidneys'. The blood and heart valve yielded a pure, profuse, growth of *Staphylococcus pyogenes* (*Figs.* 74–79).

DYSPROTEINAEMIA

Any of the conditions associated with abnormalities of the plasma proteins, especially of the gamma-globulin fraction, may cause purpura. This occurs in multiple myeloma, cryoglobulinaemia, macroglobulinaemia, and in association with any kind of hyperglobulinaemia. Waldenström (1948) described recurrent purpura with an increase of gamma-globulin, but it is doubtful whether this is a distinct entity because purpura may be associated with such a variety of differing protein abnormalities. Coagulation tests may be abnormal. Another factor is the possible infiltration of vessel walls—sometimes with amyloid.

Birch and others (1964) suggested that hyperglobulinaemic purpura could be due to auto-immunity, on the basis of a woman who presented at the age of 56 years with limb pains and 2 years later developed purpura. This was followed by features of Sjögren's syndrome, Raynaud's phenomenon, and hepatosplenomegaly. The serum beta- and gamma-globulins were raised. A thymic tumour was removed with resultant haematological improvement.

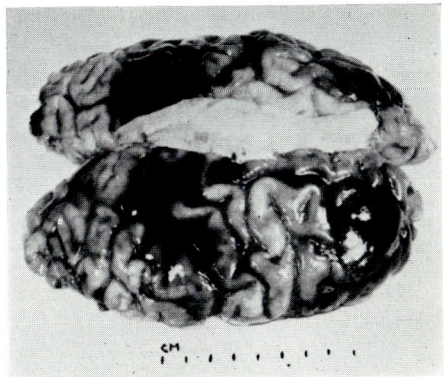

Fig. 76.—Case 2. Subarachnoid haemorrhage.

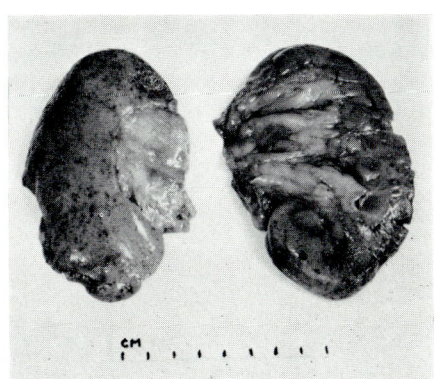

Fig. 77.—Case 2. Kidneys showing 'flea-bitten' appearance in staphylococcal septicaemia.

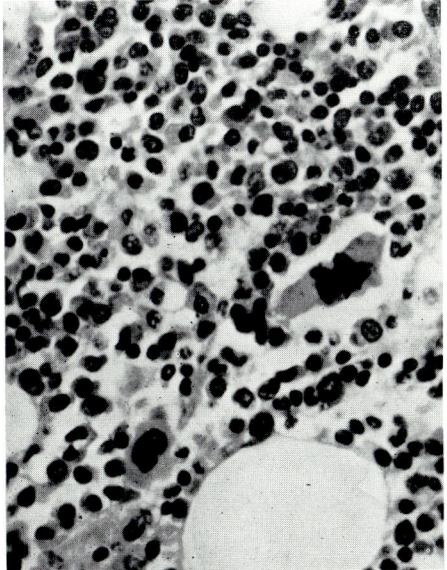

Fig. 78.—Case 2. Highly cellular reactive marrow. Megakaryocytes present. (Section of post-mortem marrow.) ($\times 150$.)

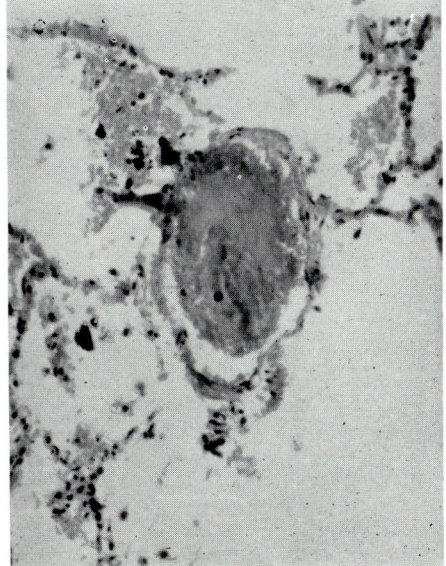

Fig. 79.—Case 2. Lung showing small-vessel thrombus and haemorrhage. ($\times 400$.)

MISCELLANEOUS CONDITIONS

Many of the factors implicated in thrombocytopenic purpura can also cause purpura without lowering the platelet count. This can be seen with drugs. Especially important in the elderly are diseases, such as chronic nephritis, uraemia, liver disease, carcinomatosis, and rheumatoid arthritis.

Myxoedema coma may be associated with severe haemorrhage, as in the 3 cases reported by Orr (1962) in women aged 72, 80, and 82 years. Multiple cutaneous and gastro-intestinal haemorrhages were present, and only 1 of them was thrombocytopenic. Hypothermia may be an important factor.

Uraemia can give rise to a variety of haemostatic defects, including thrombocytopenia, coagulation-factor deficiencies, platelet defects, and mixed abnormalities. Castaldi, Rozenberg, and Stewart (1966) carried out a detailed study on 19 patients at the time of bleeding. They concluded that bleeding in uraemia was due to a qualitative platelet defect which could be reversed by dialysis.

CLASSIFICATION OF COAGULATION DISORDERS

Congenital Coagulation Disorders
  Mild or late onset forms of haemophilia
  Christmas disease
  Von Willebrand's disease

Acquired Coagulation Disorders
  'Hypoprothrombinaemias'
  Deficiencies of factors II, V, VII, and X
    Chronic liver disease
    Intestinal malabsorption
    Biliary fistula
  Circulating anticoagulants
    (Factor VIII inhibitors)
  Defibrination syndrome
    Trauma, burns
    Postoperative
    Neoplasia (especially prostatic)
    Miscellaneous diseases
  Anticoagulant therapy
  Thrombolytic therapy

CONGENITAL DISORDERS OF COAGULATION

Haemophilia and Christmas disease are not diseases of the elderly and therefore only passing reference is made to them. Wilkinson, Nour-Eldin, Israëls, and Barrett (1961) in their survey of 267 patients suffering from haemophilia (229) and Christmas disease (38) did not find a single case that was first diagnosed after the age of 40 years. In fact, most cases were diagnosed before the age of 5. However, two aspects require attention. First, because of the continuing improvement in treatment, increasing numbers will live a normal life-span and be seen in old age. Secondly, mildly affected patients may have escaped detection. An interesting example of this was described by Borchgrevink (1959) in a man aged 68 years who sustained a fatal myocardial infarct despite mild haemophilia (factor-VIII level, 16 per cent).

The coagulation defect in von Willebrand's disease is not as severe as that in haemophilia, so that life expectancy may be normal. There is a prolonged bleeding time and a variable, although usually mild, depression of factor-VIII synthesis.

Blackburn (1961) reviewed 158 patients who had suffered from lifelong features of primary capillary haemorrhage. The presenting age ranged from early childhood to 65 years. Haemorrhagic episodes tended to decrease in frequency and severity with age in men, but not in women. They often tolerate surgery well. The severity of their symptoms is proportional to the degree of lowering of the factor-VIII level.

A further aspect of the congenital coagulation defects is that investigation of older, symptomless members of an affected child's family may be helpful in establishing the diagnosis. Mild cases and carriers may be found as a result of assaying the levels of factors VIII and IX.

The tests normally used in screening patients include: coagulation time (normal, Lee and White, 5–10 minutes); kaolin-cephalin time (normal, 35–50 seconds); and the thromboplastin-generation screening test (minimum times of 7–10 seconds). If these are abnormal it is necessary to carry out the thromboplastin generation test and assays of factors VIII and IX.

ACQUIRED DISORDERS OF COAGULATION

Spontaneous Factor-VIII Inhibitors

Non-haemophilic patients may develop inhibitors of the antihaemophilic globulin (factor VIII), usually in association with other diseases, such as rheumatoid arthritis, asthma, colitis, carcinoma, and drug reactions. Penicillin allergy has acquired a peculiar notoriety in this respect.

Green (1968) described 6 men, 4 of whom were over 50 years. The associated conditions were: penicillin allergy, rheumatoid arthritis, ulcerative colitis, hypersensitivity angiitis, and severe emphysema treated with steroids. Only 1 had no coexistent disease.

The inhibitor in cases of penicillin allergy is an IgG globulin which does not appear to be specifically related to penicillin antibody. Horowitz and Fujimoto (1962) reported the occurrence of penicillin allergy in a man, aged 83 years, who developed an inhibitor of factor VIII 90 days later. He was given prednisone and the inhibitor disappeared within 3 months. However, the clinical course of these patients is frequently relentless with failure to respond to any treatment. Steroid therapy should be tried initially, followed if necessary by immunosuppressive drugs. The cases associated with penicillin allergy have been treated with D-penicillamine and high concentrations of penicillin—the rationale of this being that strong solutions of penicillin may remove antibody globulin from the plasma. Clearly this is a hazardous procedure, and not entirely rational, as the inhibitor is not specifically related to the penicillin antibody.

Although the bleeding tendency due to inhibitors is often alarming, it does not necessarily afford protection against thrombotic cardiovascular disease. Green and Rizza (1967) reported a case of fatal myocardial infarction in a 57-year-old man who had a potent inhibitor of factor VIII. He had been taking prednisone for rheumatoid spondylitis.

Circulating anticoagulants may also develop to factors other than factor VIII.

The essential tests in cases of suspected circulating anticoagulants include: coagulation time; kaolin-cephalin time; thromboplastin generation test; and factor-VIII assay, with observation of the effect of plasma dilution.

THE DEFIBRINATION SYNDROME

Circulating blood contains an activating system which converts plasminogen to plasmin, which, in turn, splits fibrinogen:

Activating system + plasminogen → plasmin + fibrin
↓
split products

Fibrinogen and fibrin are both equally susceptible to digestion by plasmin *in vitro*, but in the circulation antiplasmin neutralizes released plasmin thereby protecting fibrinogen. Deposits of fibrin on blood-vessel walls include plasminogen which is capable of being activated with resultant lysis of fibrin. Thrombolytic drugs act similarly. In health, equilibrium exists between fibrin deposition and its removal, but many factors may influence the blood's spontaneous fibrinolytic activity. Age is one of them, although conflicting results have been reported by different workers. Buckell and Elliott (1959) found higher levels in younger men, but Hume (1961) reported that activity increased with age. Swan (1963) demonstrated a definite increase with age and indicated, on the basis of diluted plasma clot lysis times, that inhibitors could decrease with age. This may explain the discrepancies, because workers such as Buckell and Elliott used the euglobulin lysis time test. Fearnley and his co-workers (1963) found that a low fibrinolytic activity was especially common in atherosclerotic postmenopausal women.

Haemorrhage due to pathological fibrinolysis may be found in several conditions, the most important of which in the elderly are: carcinoma of the prostate, especially after surgery; hepatic cirrhosis; leukaemia; and conditions associated with shock or haemorrhage.

The prostate contains a high concentration of plasminogen activator, which can give rise to pathological fibrinolysis if a carcinoma of the gland has metastasized. Haemorrhage may be excessive, not only at the site of operation, but also in distant organs, with epistaxis or melaena. Profuse purpura may develop. As bleeding can be aggravated by the urokinase present in urine, fibrinogen infusion or epsilon-aminocaproic acid (EACA) therapy may be successful. Oestrogen treatment sometimes improves the generalized fibrinolytic state.

Other tumours can also disturb the fibrinolytic mechanism. Davidson, McNicol, Frank, Anderson, and Douglas (1969) described a 71-year-old housewife who presented with a secondary tumour deposit in the arm from a primary giant-cell carcinoma of the lung. The arm tumour was incised, after which it bled for 3 weeks until EACA was given. The patient's plasma showed a prolonged euglobulin lysis time, and the tumour fluid was rich in plasminogen activator.

An acute form can present within hours following shock or acute haemolysis. Another type is a subacute variety becoming apparent within days or weeks, usually associated with disseminated carcinoma. A chronic variant taking months to develop is related to anaemia, haemorrhage, or thrombosis (Merskey, 1968).

Diagnosis

The history and clinical picture should alert the clinician to the possibility of a state of pathological fibrinolysis, although the diagnosis entails the use of laboratory tests. These tests must be practicable under emergency conditions, and the results rapidly available. Screening tests should first be used:—

1. *Whole-blood clotting time*, with observation of the fate of any clot formed In severe cases the blood fails to clot, or if it does, the clot is poor and rapidly lysed
2. *Thrombin time and serial thrombin time*: The normal test: control is less than 1·3. This will be prolonged.
3. *Fibrinogen titre*: Normally, fibrin clots are seen in plasma dilutions up to $\frac{1}{128}$. The titre is 0–9 in severe fibrinogen deficiency. When tested with EACA fibrin will be seen at higher dilutions if fibrinolysis is present.
4. *Platelet count* or examination of blood-film.

If these tests suggest defibrination or fibrinolysis treatment should be given. Further confirmatory tests may be done if the facilities are available—for example, estimation of fibrinogen, euglobulin lysis time and plasminogen assay, and coagulation factors may be estimated by means of a thromboplastin-generation screening test. But under the conditions which so often obtain in the elderly these tests are seldom undertaken, or even necessary. They must be interpreted with the knowledge that defibrination, fibrinolysis, and disseminated intravascular coagulation present in a similar manner and frequently coexist.

TREATMENT

The underlying disease must be treated. Great care has to be taken if fibrinolytic inhibitors or fibrinogen are to be used.

Concentrated Fibrinogen.—This is obtainable from the Regional Blood Transfusion Centres. A rapid infusion of 5 g. in 400 ml. of distilled water can be given.

Dried Plasma.—Triple-strength plasma is a substitute for fibrinogen. Six bottles of freeze-dried plasma are reconstituted to 800 ml. This must be transfused with great caution in the elderly because of its osmotic effect.

Epsilon-aminocaproic Acid (EACA).—If active fibrinolysis has been demonstrated, and free blood-loss is taking place, 4–6 g. (40–60 ml. of a 10 per cent solution) of EACA is given over 30 minutes. Thereafter 0·1 g. per kg. body-weight can be given 4-hourly, or an oral dose of 3 g. every 8 hours.

If blood is loculated within a viscus or body cavity, EACA should not be given as it may cause fibrous organization.

It is possible to give anticoagulants simultaneously with EACA.

Trasylol.—This is a polypeptide which inhibits plasmin and plasminogen activator. It has been used in hyperfibrinolytic haemorrhage, and may be given in emergencies when precise distinction between excessive clotting or fibrinolysis cannot be made. It is given intravenously, 50,000–100,000 kallikrein international units, followed by the same dose hourly.

Inhibitors of fibrinolysis and replacement therapy may increase the danger of fibrin deposition and thereby perpetuate a vicious circle of intravascular coagulation with consumption of coagulation factors and further fibrinolysis. In such a situation heparin, followed by oral anticoagulants, may be beneficial.

Blood Transfusion.—This may be required, but should be used only to replace lost blood rather than in an attempt to correct the basic defect. Its effect is transient if active fibrinolysis is still proceeding.

Anticoagulants may be effective in subacute or chronic disease if maximal doses can be tolerated.

ANTICOAGULANT AND THROMBOLYTIC THERAPY

The place of anticoagulant therapy in ischaemic heart disease is still disputed, and the role of thrombolytic agents in thrombo-embolic disease even more so. In the elderly we have the paradoxical situation that the patients who are at greatest risk from thrombo-embolic disease may also show the highest incidence of toxic effects from the appropriate drugs.

Sevitt (1959) found thrombosis of the deep veins of the legs in 80 per cent of elderly patients dying following a fractured neck of femur, and in almost half the immediate cause of death was pulmonary embolism. Sevitt and Gallagher (1959) undertook a controlled trial of anticoagulant therapy—150 patients were given phenindione and compared with 150 controls. No embolism occurred in the treated patients, compared with an incidence of 18 per cent in the controls—which was fatal in 10 per cent. Necropsy studies confirmed this beneficial effect, and the authors concluded that if phenindione was given early, for sufficient time, and under laboratory control, it was both beneficial and safe for this type of patient. The danger of thrombosis has probably diminished since then owing to the practice of earlier mobilization, but where bed-rest is unavoidable venous thrombosis remains a hazard. As a result anticoagulants are frequently prescribed both for prevention and treatment, especially in high-risk patients who give a previous history of thrombo-embolic disease, or in whom there are early signs of such complications.

Anticoagulant therapy must be subject to particularly strict laboratory control because in the elderly tolerance is often impaired by chronic renal or hepatic disease. Good control may be impossible for several reasons: the difficulty of follow-up after the patient has been discharged; the onset of complications, such as bleeding from the gastro-intestinal tract or kidneys; the development of skin rashes; and the fact that blood dyscrasias occur more often than in younger persons.

ANTICOAGULATION

The coumarins and indanediones have no anticoagulant action *in vitro*, but act after they have been absorbed and metabolized by the liver, probably by reducing the synthesis of prothrombin, factors VII, IX, and X.

Phenindione (Dindevan) is in common use. A test dose of 25 mg. should be given, but the initial dose required is usually in the region of 200–300 mg. The maintenance daily dose is usually between 25 and 150 mg.

Three tests are in common use for the control of anticoagulant therapy: Quick's one-stage prothrombin time; the prothrombin-proconvertin test (P and P)—therapeutic range is 10–25 per cent; and the thrombotest—therapeutic range, 7–15 per cent. The latter two are the more sensitive but Quick's test has the advantage of simplicity. If this is used the ratio of test : normal time should be kept between 2·0 and 2·5. Elderly patients not on anticoagulants frequently give slightly elevated prothrombin times of 1·3–1·5.

In addition to the danger of intercurrent disease having a potentiating effect, drugs which bind with plasma albumin may also have a similar action—for example, salicylates, chlorpropamide, phenylbutazone, and chlorfibrate. The antidote for overdosage is vitamin K_1 (10–20 mg.), which acts almost as quickly orally as intramuscularly.

Heparin.—This is a mucopolysaccharide containing sulphate having a molecular weight of approximately 16,000. It is produced by mast cells and obtained commercially from animal tissues, such as beef lung. Its anticoagulant action is complex, affecting most stages. Thrombin is inhibited; the conversion of prothrombin to thrombin is impaired; and thromboplastin generation is impeded. High concentrations reduce platelet adhesiveness.

A dose of 10,000–15,000 units, injected intravenously, is repeated at 2 and 4 hours until stability is attained. After the initial emergency oral anticoagulants are given. Heparin dosage should be controlled by giving the dose that will keep the whole-blood coagulation time at two to three times the normal. Doses of 10,000 units 6-hourly may be given for 48 hours without laboratory control, but when treatment is prolonged the coagulation time or thrombin time should be used.

The antidote for serious bleeding is protamine sulphate, given intravenously as a 1 per cent solution (10 mg. per ml.). Approximately 1 mg. neutralizes 100 units of injected heparin, although an accurate dose is better calculated from a protamine titration. Protamine should be injected slowly to avoid hypotension and other side-effects.

Thrombolysis

Streptokinase.—Beta-haemolytic streptococci elaborate an enzyme which reacts with a proactivator or plasminogen, producing active plasmin which can break down most blood proteins, with the exception of fibrin.

Streptokinase is produced commercially from Lancefield group-C haemolytic streptococci. It has a molecular weight of approximately 50,000, but is not yet a pure substance. It can be antigenic, and produce pyrexial reactions. Dosage is difficult to control and severe haemorrhage may ensue. The usual method is to give a loading dose of streptokinase of 500,000 units in 30 minutes by intravenous infusion, followed by 900,000 units 6-hourly or 100,000 units hourly. This schedule may be combined with prednisolone 50 mg. by intramuscular injection given 1 hour before the infusion, and each 900,000-unit dose thereafter combined with 150 mg. hydrocortisone.

Verstraete, Vermylen, Amery, and Vermylen (1966) used a standard dosage scheme: initially, 1,250,000 units intravenously in 30 minutes; then 100,000 units hourly for 3 days. They claimed that laboratory control was not essential with this dosage, but this advice may not always be safe and generally the drug should not be used if laboratory control cannot be exercised. The tests used include: fibrinogen, fibrin plate assay, prothrombin time, euglobulin lysis time, plasma plasminogen, and thrombin clotting time.

If haemorrhage occurs the drug should be stopped and whole blood, preferably fresh, given. The antidote, EACA, may be dangerous and produce unlysable clots (McNicol and Douglas, 1969).

Arvin, a substance prepared from the venom of the Malayan pit viper, has been the subject of some encouraging reports (Ashford, Ross, and Southgate, 1968; Bell, Pitney, and Goodwin, 1968; Reid and Chan, 1968; Sharp, Warren, Paxton, and Allington, 1968). Although the venom is a coagulant when tested *in vitro* within the circulation it lowers the plasma fibrinogen, with the production of peptides having antithrombin properties.

The recommended schedule is an intravenous infusion of 1 unit per kg. body-weight in 100 ml. saline over 4–6 hours by means of a constant-infusion pump, followed by 1 unit per kg. body-weight in 20 ml. saline over 10 minutes, and thereafter 1–2 units per kg. body-weight every 12 hours.

The tests used for the control of therapy include plasma fibrinogen, which should be maintained around 50 mg. per 100 ml. A rough assessment is obtained by clotting dilutions of plasma with thrombin to halve the titre. Whole blood should show either no clot or a speck-clot.

The antidote to Arvin-induced haemorrhage is the specific antivenene and human fibrinogen.

Arvin is weakly antigenic, and Pitney, Bray, Holt, and Bolton (1969) described 2 patients who were resistant to a second course of treatment. This may be more likely following an initial intramuscular course than when the drug is given intravenously.

A comparison of the efficacy of heparin, streptokinase and Arvin was attempted by Kakkar, Flanc, Howe, O'Shea, and Flute (1969), although the total number of patients was only 30. They found a complete thrombolytic effect most frequently with streptokinase, but complications were least with Arvin.

Hirsh, Hale, McDonald, McCarthy, and Pitt (1968) treated 18 patients—7 over 60 years of age—who had had a major pulmonary embolus, with infusions of streptokinase. Clinical improvement was seen in 14, with angiographic confirmation in 12. Douglas (1969) advocated 'vigorous thrombolytic therapy' following massive pulmonary embolism, but he and McNicol (McNicol and Douglas, 1969) stressed the complications and limitations of this form of treatment.

REFERENCES

ACKROYD, J. F. (1949), *Clin. Sci.*, **7**, 249; **8**, 235, 269.
— — (1955), *Br. med. Bull.*, **11**, 28.
AMOROSI, E. L., and ULTMAN, J. E. (1966), *Medicine*, **45**, 139.
ANDREWS, J., and BROOK, M. (1966), *Lancet*, **1**, 1350.
ASHFORD, A., ROSS, J. W., and SOUTHGATE, P. (1968), *Ibid.*, **1**, 486.
BELL, G. H., LAZARUS, S., and MUNRO, H. N. (1940), *Ibid.*, **2**, 155.
BELL, W. R., PITNEY, W. R., and GOODWIN, J. F. (1968), *Ibid.*, **1**, 490.
BIRCH, C. A., COOKE, K. B., DREW, C. E., LONDON, D. R., MACKENZIE, D. H., and MILNE, M.D. (1964), *Ibid.*, **1**, 693.
BLACKBURN, E. K. (1961), *Br. J. Haemat.*, **7**, 239.
BOLTON, C. H., HAMPTON, J. R., and MITCHELL, J. R. A. (1967), *Lancet*, **2**, 1101.
BORCHGREVINK, CH. F. (1959), *Ibid.*, **1**, 1229.
BRODIE, G. N., BLISS, D., and FIRKIN, B. G. (1970), *Br. med. J.*, **1**, 540.
BUCKELL, M., and ELLIOT, F. A. (1959), *Lancet*, **1**, 660.
CASTALDI, P. A., ROZENBERG, M. C., and STEWART, J. H. (1966), *Ibid.*, **2**, 66.
DAVIDSON, J. F., MCNICOL, G. P., FRANK, G. L., ANDERSON, T. J., and DOUGLAS, A. S. (1969), *Br. med. J.*, **1**, 88.
DOUGLAS, A. S. (1969), *J. R. Coll. Phys., Lond.*, **3**, 171.
FEARNLEY, G. R., CHAKRABARTI, R., and AVIS, P. R. O. (1963), *Br. med. J.*, **1**, 921.
GREEN, D. (1968), *Br. J. Haemat.*, **15**, 57.
— — and RIZZA, C. R. (1967), *Lancet*, **2**, 434.
HARDISTY, R. M., and WOLFF, H. H. (1955), *Br. J. Haemat.*, **1**, 390.
HART, A., and COHEN, H. (1969), *Br. med. J.*, **2**, 89.
HIRSH, J., HALE, G. S., MCDONALD, I. G., MCCARTHY, R. A., and PITT, A. (1968), *Ibid.*, **4**, 729.

HOROWITZ, H. I., and FUJIMOTO, M. M. (1962), *Am. J. Med.*, **33**, 501.
HUME, R. (1961), *J. clin. Path.*, **14**, 167.
JACOBSON, B. M., and VICKERY, A. L., jun. (1968), *New Engl. J. Med.*, **278**, 36.
KAKKAR, V. V., FLANC, C., HOWE, C. T., O'SHEA, M., and FLUTE, P. T. (1969), *Br. med. J.*, **1**, 806.
LINTON, A. L., GAVRAS, H., GLEADLE, R. I., HUTCHISON, H. E., LAWSON, D. H., LEVER, A. F., MACADAM, R. F., MCNICOL, G. P., and ROBERTSON, J. I. S. (1969), *Lancet*, **1**, 1277.
MCNICOL, G. P., and DOUGLAS, A. S. (1969), *Br. med. J.*, **1**, 180.
MERSKEY, C. (1968), *Br. J. Haemat.*, **15**, 527.
NORDQVIST, P., CRAMÉR, G., and BJÖRNTORP, P. (1959), *Lancet*, **1**, 271.
ORR, F. R. (1962), *Ibid.*, **2**, 1012.
PITNEY, W. R., BRAY, C., HOLT, P. J. L., and BOLTON, G. (1969), *Ibid.*, **1**, 79.
PIZZI, F., CARRARA, P. M., ALDEGHI, A., and ERIDANI, S. (1966), *Blood*, **27**, 521.
REID, H. A., and CHAN, K. E. (1968), *Lancet*, **1**, 485.
RUBENBERG, M. L., REGOECZI, E., BULL, B. S., DACIE, J. V., and BRAIN, M. C. (1968), *Br. J. Haemat.*, **14**, 627.
SCARBOROUGH, H., and SHUSTER, S. (1960), *Lancet*, **1**, 93.
SEVITT, S. (1959), in *Modern Trends in Accident Medicine and Surgery* (ed. CLARKE, R., BADGER, F. G., and SEVITT, S.). London: Butterworths.
— — and GALLAGHER, N. G. (1959), *Lancet*, **2**, 981.
SHARP, A. A., WARREN, B. A., PAXTON, A. M., and ALLINGTON, M. J. (1968), *Ibid.*, **1**, 493.
SWAN, H. T. (1963), *Br. J. Haemat.*, **9**, 311.
— — WOOD, K. F., and DANIEL, O. (1957), *Br. med. J.*, **1**, 495.
VERSTRAETE, M., VERMYLEN, J., AMERY, A., and VERMYLEN, C. (1966), *Ibid.*, **1**, 454.
WALDENSTRÖM, J. (1948), *Schweiz. med. Wschr.*, **78**, 927.
WATSON-WILLIAMS, E. J., MACPHERSON, A. I. S., and DAVIDSON, L. S. P. (1958), *Lancet*, **2**, 221.
WILKINSON, J. F., NOUR-ELDIN, F., ISRAËLS, M. C. G., and BARRETT, K. E. (1961), *Ibid.*, **2**, 947.
WINTROBE, M. M. (1969), *J. R. Coll. Phys., Lond.*, **3**, 99.

13

HAEMOLYTIC ANAEMIAS

CLASSIFICATION

Congenital
  Spherocytic
  Non-spherocytic
  Elliptocytic

Acquired
  Primary
    Auto-immune
      Warm
      Cold
  Secondary
    Systemic disease
    Drugs
    Burns and trauma
  Cold-agglutinin syndrome
  Paroxysmal nocturnal haemoglobinuria
  Paroxysmal cold haemoglobinuria
  Micro-angiopathic haemolytic anaemia

HAEMOLYTIC anaemia exists when the regenerative capacity of the haemopoietic tissue fails to keep pace with the rate of red-cell breakdown.

The average red-cell life in health is 110–125 days. This is usually estimated by means of tagging the patient's cells with radio-isotopes such as ^{51}Cr or di-isopropyl-fluorophosphate labelled with ^{32}P. These techniques give a 50 per cent survival ($T_{\frac{1}{2}}$) of approximately 25 days, and this is the index most commonly taken when assessing the presence and severity of haemolysis.

Red-cell breakdown in health is probably confined to the reticulo-endothelial system. The haemoglobin is released and the globin bound to a circulating 2-muco-protein, haptoglobin. Other proteins, such as the beta-globulins and haemopexin, can also combine with haem.

If intravascular haemolysis occurs, albumin and haematin form methaemalbumin. When the amount of liberated haemoglobin exceeds the binding capacity of the serum proteins excess haemoglobin is excreted in the urine. Therefore, in health, haptoglobin binding is a means of preventing urinary loss of haemoglobin.

The haemoglobin molecule is catabolized to verdohaemoglobin (which still contains iron), and then split releasing iron and globin to form biliverdin, which, in turn, is rapidly reduced to bilirubin (*Fig.* 80).

HAEMOLYTIC ANAEMIAS

Circulating albumin binds with bilirubin and transports it to the liver, where the latter is converted from a fat-soluble pigment to one that is water soluble by conjugation with glucuronic acid—a reaction which is mediated by the enzyme glucuronyl transferase. This water-soluble conjugate gives an immediate red colour with diazotized sulphanilic acid (direct van den Bergh). The unconjugated

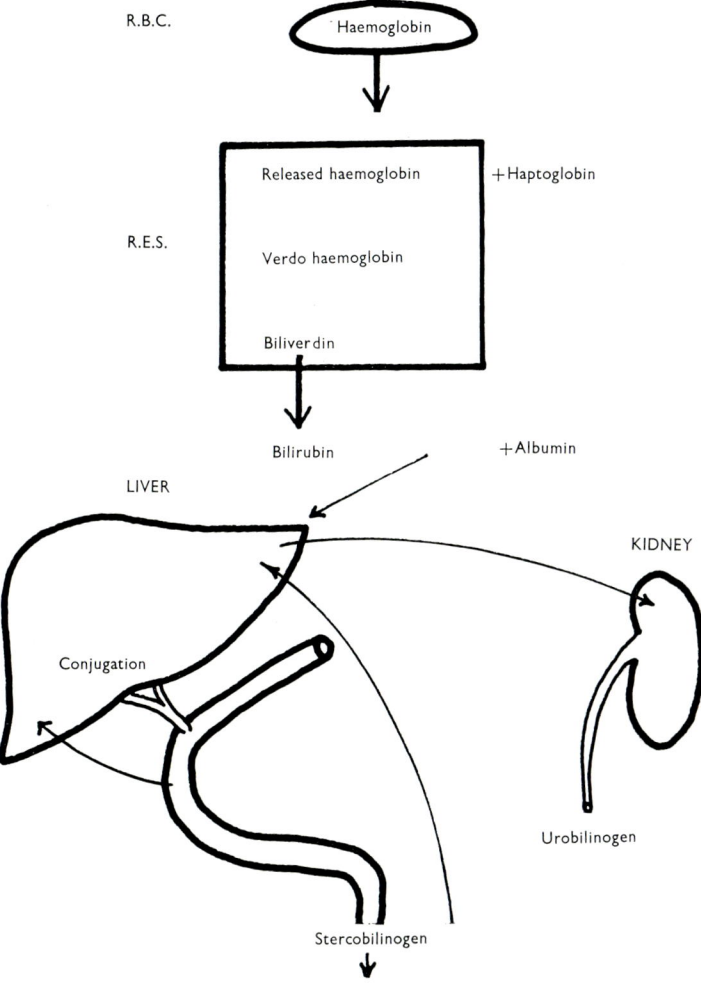

Fig. 80.—Haemoglobin catabolism.

fraction reacts only after the addition of alcohol (indirect van den Bergh). This test accordingly indicates whether excess bilirubin has passed through the liver cell, and in haemolytic states there is characteristically an increase in the indirect reacting fraction. Furthermore, because this fraction is only fat soluble it is not excreted in the urine (acholuric jaundice).

Bilirubin is excreted into the intestine where it is partly reabsorbed, and the remainder reduced by bacterial action to stercobilinogen, which, in turn, is again partly reabsorbed and excreted in the urine as urobilinogen.

Therefore a correlation is to be expected between the rate of haemoglobin catabolism and the amount of bile pigments excreted in faeces and urine. However, although increased excretion can usually be demonstrated and may be of some diagnostic help, the correlation is not close.

LABORATORY FINDINGS

Haemoglobin.—A rapidly falling haemoglobin, in the absence of demonstrable blood-loss, is strong presumptive evidence of increased haemolysis.

The peripheral blood-film shows anisopoikilocytosis with irregular fragmented red cells and microspherocytes. Polychromasia is seen in association with reticulocytosis and, in an acute phase, circulating nucleated red blood-cells appear. Occasionally a crisis occurs which is more aplastic than haemolytic, and in such cases polychromasia is not noticeable and the reticulocyte count is not increased.

The red cells may contain Howell-Jolly or Pappenheimer bodies. Heinz bodies are seen in some varieties.

Leucocytes.—A leucocytosis with neutrophilia is found during active haemolysis, but if the crisis is of the aplastic type a marked neutropenia may occur. This is also a feature of 'hypersplenism'.

A. Evidence of Red-cell Destruction

1. *Serum bilirubin.*—A slight to moderate elevation of serum bilirubin is often found (usually 2–5 mg. per 100 ml.) predominantly of unconjugated type.

2. *Urinary and Faecal Urobilinogen.*—These are increased if liver function is normal. The normal excretory rates are up to 4 mg. per 24 hours for urine and 40–300 mg. for faeces.

3. *Serum Iron and T.I.B.C.*—These are increased, but the elevation in iron is disproportionate so that the saturation is raised.

4. *Evidence of Intravascular Haemolysis.*—The plasma haemoglobin level is increased; haptoglobins are completely consumed; and excess haemosiderin appears in the urine. Methaemalbumin is found in the plasma. A variety of enzymes, such as serum aldolase, glutamic-oxalo-acetic transaminase, and lactic dehydrogenase, may be released.

The measurements most readily carried out for the detection of intravascular haemolysis are those for haemosiderinuria; Schumm's spectroscopic test for methaemalbumin; plasma haemoglobin (normal <1 mg. per 100 ml.); and electrophoresis for haptoglobins (normal 30–190 mg. per 100 ml. plasma).

B. Signs of Red-cell Regeneration

1. *Reticulocytes.*—The reticulocyte count is one of the best and most readily available indices of the activity of the marrow response, but a raised reticulocyte count does not necessarily indicate haemolysis. Equally high levels may be seen after haemorrhage or as a feature of treatment with specific haematinics. The normal reticulocyte count is below 2 per cent of the circulating erythrocytes.

2. *Peripheral Blood-picture.*—In addition to reticulocytosis the blood-film shows regenerative features in the form of marked polychromasia and punctate basophilia. During recovery from a severe haemolytic crisis nucleated red blood-cells may be numerous. Neutrophilia and thrombocythaemia may also be suggested by the film appearances.

3. *Bone-marrow.*—Active erythroid proliferation is seen with an increase in the sideroblast count and stainable iron content.

4. *Radio-isotope Studies.*—These show that the body iron turnover rate is increased.

DIAGNOSIS OF THE TYPE OF HAEMOLYTIC ANAEMIA

The main distinction that has to be made is between the type where the defect resides in the patient's erythrocytes and that where the plasma is at fault. These correspond broadly to the congenital and acquired groups, with the exception of paroxysmal nocturnal haemoglobinuria.

Congenital haemolytic anaemia may be spherocytic or less commonly non-spherocytic, the differentiation being based on the examination of the peripheral blood-film. The red-cell fragility is increased. Normally 50 per cent haemolysis takes place at 0·40–0·45 per cent NaCl at 20° C. Spherocytes show increased fragility, but this on its own is not diagnostic of congenital spherocytic anaemia because they may also be found in acquired secondary haemolytic states.

Further help may be obtained by testing the osmotic fragility after incubating defibrinated blood at 37° C. for 24 hours. The red cells from cases of spherocytic anaemia, and a subgroup of non-spherocytic haemolytic anaemia, show a greater enhancement of post-incubation fragility than normal.

Cases of hereditary spherocytosis also show an increased rate of autohaemolysis (when blood is incubated at 37° C.), but this is a feature shared with other types of haemolytic anaemia. If glucose is added, autohaemolysis is reduced in spherocytic cases as in normal blood.

Patients suffering from the acquired group of haemolytic anaemias are distinguished chiefly as a result of serological tests designed to indicate the presence of an auto-immune mechanism.

Antibody may be fixed to the patient's red cells, or be found free in the serum, and may be optimally active at 37° C. (warm) or at 0–30° C. (cold). Warm antibody is usually of the IgG type and often shows Rh blood-group specificity, whereas cold antibody is usually IgM and capable of binding complement.

The Direct Antiglobulin Test (Coombs)

This entails the suspension of patient's washed red cells in a saline dilution of serum containing antiglobulin. A 'broad-spectrum' activity against IgG and complement antibodies may be present. Following absorption with purified IgG an anti non-gamma serum remains which can be tested in a similar manner.

A positive direct antiglobulin test suggests the presence of auto-antibodies but does not necessarily indicate auto-immune haemolytic anaemia. Approximately 8 per cent of hospital patients give a weak positive non-gamma antiglobulin test, but a positive anti-gamma (IgG) test is very rarely found in health. Many drugs can give rise to a positive Coombs's test, and so can blood containing a high proportion of reticulocytes. If blood is allowed to stand at temperatures near 4° C. cold antibody and complement may be absorbed and give a positive reading.

Therefore, a positive result in the direct antiglobulin test must be interpreted with caution. Further information is obtained by carrying out a quantitative test and attempting to elute the antibodies prior to evaluating their specificity.

Testing for Antibodies in Serum (Indirect Test)

Cold-haemagglutinin disease is invariably associated with a demonstrable serum antibody. The cold agglutinin titre and its thermal amplitude should be determined. The IgM nature of this antibody can be confirmed by abolishing its agglutinating property with 2-mercapto-ethanol. The indirect antiglobulin test (indirect Coombs), where the patient's serum is tested against antiglobulin coated red cells, provides a measure of circulating free antibody.

Warm (IgG) antibodies are not so regularly demonstrable in auto-immune states, and are usually only found in active haemolytic phases. Enzyme-treated red cells are sensitive to these antibodies and the indirect antiglobulin test may be positive.

The possible blood-group specificity of serum antibodies should be established.

Ham's acidified-serum test for paroxysmal nocturnal haemoglobinuria should be done in atypical cases, and the Donath-Landsteiner test when paroxysmal cold haemoglobinuria is suspected.

Drug-induced haemolytic anaemia should be considered if Heinz bodies are demonstrable, or if sulphaemoglobin or methaemoglobin are present.

Enzyme-deficiency haemolytic anaemias are not a practical problem in the elderly.

HEREDITARY SPHEROCYTIC ANAEMIA

Although the majority of these patients present in childhood or early adult life classic cases may occur in the elderly.

Case 1.—This patient was first seen in 1962 at the age of 69 years. She had been 'anaemic' since the age of 23 and had been jaundiced three times in the past 20 years. A diagnosis of 'pernicious anaemia' was made in 1953, since when she had been receiving liver and vitamin-B_{12} injections.

In 1962 the haemoglobin varied between 59 and 72 per cent. The red cells were spherocytic and their fragility increased (68 per cent haemolysis at 0·5 per cent NaCl); reticulocytes, 3–15 per cent; bilirubin, 3·0 mg. per 100 ml. (indirect 2·5). The bone-marrow showed active normoblastic erythropoiesis.

The diagnosis and likely beneficial effect of splenectomy were explained to the patient in 1962, but she declined the operation.

Subsequently she remained in indifferent general health with chronic anaemia. Finally, in October, 1968, at the age of 75 years, she agreed to surgical treatment. An 800-g. spleen was removed (*Figs.* 81, 82), following which she recovered rapidly and has since maintained a normal haemoglobin. She now claims that she enjoys a greater sense of health and well-being than she has known for many years.

Clinical Features

The trait of spherocytosis may be dominant, although rarely sporadic cases are seen. Males and females are affected equally.

The characteristic clinical feature is that of recurrent crises of anaemia and jaundice. During these episodes the patient may be febrile and vomit. However, such clear-cut crises are not always discernible and it is much more difficult to recognize the real nature of a chronic, mild, intermittent anaemia.

HAEMOLYTIC ANAEMIAS

Some patients are first seen because of gall-stones. Other complications are chronic leg ulcers, chronic eczema, skin pigmentation, and skeletal developmental abnormalities.

Examination shows splenomegaly in most cases. Less frequently the liver and lymph-nodes may be enlarged.

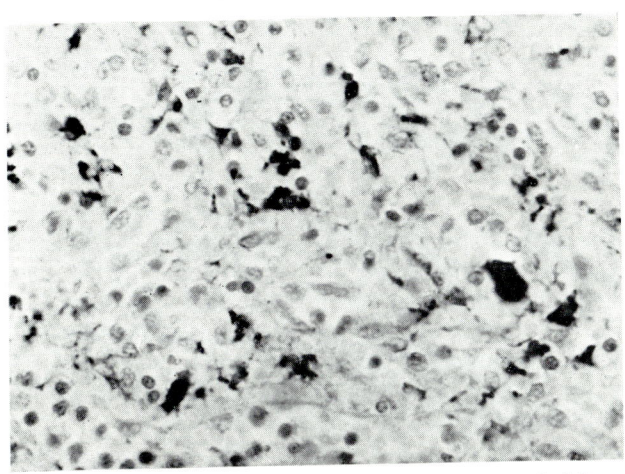

Fig. 81.—*Case* 1. Spleen containing haemosiderin in congenital haemolytic anaemia (Perls's stain). ($\times 400$.)

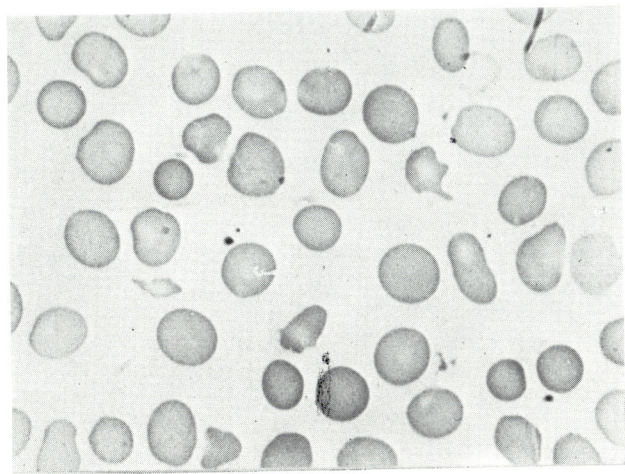

Fig. 82.—*Case* 1. Congenital spherocytic anaemia in a 75-year-old lady. ($\times 1100$.)

The typical laboratory findings are: spherocytic anaemia; reticulocytosis; increased red-cell fragility; raised indirect-reading serum bilirubin.

The urine may contain increased urobilinogen but no bile-pigments or salts (acholuric jaundice).

The bone-marrow shows erythropoietic hyperplasia. This is usually normoblastic, but features of folate deficiency have been reported.

Some, at least, of the anaemic crises are more aplastic than haemolytic. This is suggested by the occurrence of reticulocytopenia, leucopenia, thrombocytopenia, and hypocellular marrow smears. The serum bilirubin and urinary urobilinogen levels may also fall. Aplastic crises can be precipitated by an intercurrent infection.

The basic nature of congenital spherocytosis remains unknown. The concentration of aldolase within the red cell decreases with cell age. Chapman (1969) found reduced levels both in splenectomized and non-splenectomized cases of hereditary spherocytosis.

Treatment

Splenectomy is the only effective treatment. Although spherocytosis remains, the anaemia and other symptoms are nearly always greatly benefited if not completely cured.

CONGENITAL NON-SPHEROCYTIC HAEMOLYTIC ANAEMIA

An increasing proportion of non-spherocytic cases have been attributed to red-cell enzyme deficiencies, particularly pyruvate kinase and glucose-6-phosphate dehydrogenase, but such cases have not been reported in the elderly. However, as more of these are recognized it is likely that patients suffering from mild defects or carrier states will be found. Non-spherocytic cases rarely improve after splenectomy, although some with pyruvate kinase deficiency have done so.

ACQUIRED HAEMOLYTIC ANAEMIA

Primary, 'idiopathic', acquired haemolytic anaemia can be encountered at any age. It is diagnosed largely as a result of excluding any known cause of haemolysis—whether systemic disease, toxin, or intrinsic red-cell defect; and demonstrating the presence of auto- or iso-antibodies.

The antibody may be of warm or cold type. The warm variety is usually associated with more severe and intractable anaemia than the cold. Examples of severe anaemia are often associated with little free auto-antibody as demonstrated by the indirect Coombs's test. The clinical state and prognosis are most severe when the auto-antibody is a direct-acting saline antibody—especially if it is also haemolytic. The mortality-rate in this type may be up to 50 per cent.

In cold-agglutinin disease the clinical picture is much more chronic, and the severity is related to the thermal amplitude of the antibody—thus if the antibody is active at temperatures approaching that of the body, symptoms will be correspondingly constant.

Auto-immune haemolytic anaemia may be complicated by aplastic crises in the same way as congenital spherocytic anaemia, for example, Burston, Husain, Hutt, and Tanner (1959) described 2 men, aged 76 and 68 years, who showed bone-marrow aplasia and failure of red-cell production during the course of a Coombs-positive haemolytic anaemia.

Treatment

Blood transfusion is a hazardous procedure in these patients and must be attempted only in extreme situations. Recipient and donor should preferably be genotyped.

Steroid Therapy.—This provides the sheet anchor of treatment. The dose must initially be regulated to obtain a favourable haematological response. Oral prednisolone 40–100 mg. daily should be effective within 3 days, although sometimes the response is delayed for a week or so. The dose is subsequently reduced. Approximately three-quarters of the patients show an initial favourable response. Some do not relapse when steroids are gradually withdrawn, although others need maintenance therapy indefinitely.

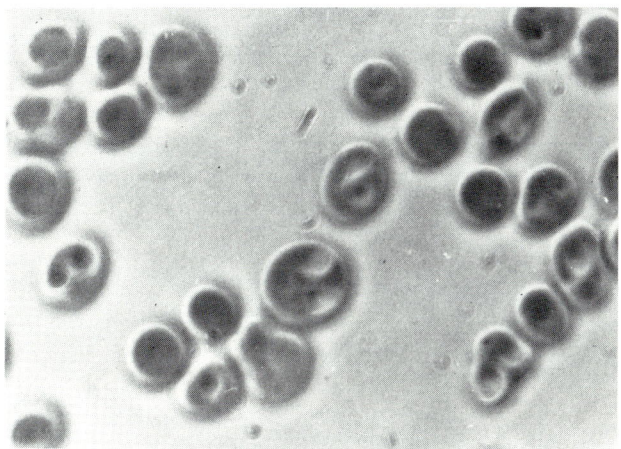

Fig. 83.—*Case* 2. Phase contrast photograph of red cells showing defective areas. (×1100.)

Cold-antibody cases respond poorly, if at all, to steroids.

Splenectomy is of limited value in these cases, although it may be entertained if there has been no adequate response to steroids. It should not be performed unless there is excessive destruction in the splenic circulation as demonstrated by means of radio-isotopes. Other features which may be associated with a favourable response are splenomegaly, incomplete antibodies in small amounts, and the presence of warm antibodies.

Cytotoxic Drugs.—These are usually reserved for refractory cases where steroids have been ineffective and splenectomy not indicated.

Any of this group may be given a trial but the ones favoured for warm-antibody cases are 6-mercaptopurine or azothioprine, whilst those with cold antibody may be given chlorambucil or cyclophosphamide.

Case 2.—This man, aged 67 years, was admitted giving a 2-month history of weight-loss and anorexia. He was orthopnoeic and showed bilateral ankle oedema. The urine had been dark brown for 3–4 weeks. Both liver and spleen were moderately enlarged, and axillary lymph-nodes were palpable.

The principal laboratory findings were: Hb, 47 per cent; P.C.V., 20 per cent; W.B.C., 7300 per c.mm. (neutrophils, 77 per cent); E.S.R., 31 mm. in the first hour. The blood-film showed marked polychromasia with fragmented cells, microspherocytes, and numerous normoblasts. The reticulocyte count varied from 27 to 50 per cent. Many of the red cells showed irregular punched-out areas, especially in wet preparations. (*Fig.* 83.)

Sternal marrow smears were highly cellular with brisk normoblastic erythropoiesis and erythrophagocytosis. Red-cell fragility was slightly increased; serum bilirubin, 5·0 mg. per 100 ml. (indirect 4·0); serum iron, 90 μg. per 100 ml., T.I.B.C., 400 μg. per 100 ml. (saturation, 23 per cent); folate, 2·0 ng. per ml.; and vitamin B_{12}, 180 pg. per ml.

Shumm's test, Donath Landsteiner test, and Ham's test were all negative.
Red-cell survival using ^{51}Cr, $T_{\frac{1}{2}}$ was 4 days.
Direct Coombs's test was positive at 4° and 37° C. using gamma and non-gamma sera. The patient's serum also agglutinated his own cells at 4° and 21° C., but not at 37° C. Cord blood-cells were not agglutinated and the antibody was identified as anti-I.
The Wassermann and V.D.R.L. tests were positive, but were probably non-specific because the FTA, RPCFT, and T.P.I. were negative.
An axillary node biopsy showed non-specific reactive changes.
An initial response was obtained to prednisone 30 mg. t.d.s., but he soon relapsed and showed no further response to mustine, vincristine, or procarbazone and died in congestive cardiac failure 6 weeks after admission.
Post-mortem showed pulmonary embolism and bronchopneumonia. There was advanced congestive failure. The spleen weighed 400 g. and showed features of severe blood destruction, but no primary cause was found.

Comment.—This man had a fulminating auto-immune haemolytic anaemia showing anti-I specificity, not responding to any treatment, and without a recognizable primary cause at autopsy.

SECONDARY ACQUIRED HAEMOLYTIC ANAEMIA

This group shares many of the clinical and laboratory features of the primary type, except that another disease is recognized as the cause of the haemolytic process.

PRIMARY HAEMOPOIETIC DISEASE OR MALIGNANT LYMPHOMA

Leukaemia.—Some degree of haemolytic anaemia is common in all types of leukaemia. In acute leukaemia the picture may be difficult to distinguish from the leukaemoid reaction that is sometimes associated with haemolytic anaemia, but the direct Coombs's test is seldom positive. Increased haemolysis is also often seen in the terminal stages of chronic myeloid leukaemia, although it is seldom possible to demonstrate an auto-immune mechanism.

Chronic lymphatic leukaemia is a frequent cause of auto-immune haemolytic anaemia, occurring in some 10–25 per cent of cases. It may become manifest at any stage of the disease. The spleen is greatly enlarged. There is often an accompanying thrombocytopenia. The direct Coombs's test is positive and the antibody is of the warm IgG type, rarely showing any specificity.

Reticulosarcoma and Lymphosarcoma.—Haemolytic anaemia, when it occurs, resembles that associated with chronic lymphatic leukaemia, except that the direct Coombs's test is often of cold type and shows anti-I specificity. If a warm antibody is present it may show anti-Rh specificity.

Hodgkin's Disease.—Haemolytic anaemia is a common complication, but tests for auto-antibodies are usually negative although warm and cold auto-antibodies have been found—in some series up to 25 per cent of patients.

Myelosclerosis.—Approximately 15 per cent of patients have a haemolytic anaemia, and a higher proportion have occult haemolysis. The direct Coombs's test is negative. If tests show evidence of increased red-cell destruction in the spleen, the patient may benefit from splenectomy.

Multiple myeloma is very rarely associated with haemolytic anaemia.

Waldenström's macroglobulinaemia has been seen with auto-immune anaemia.

Carcinoma.—Haemolytic anaemia is found in up to 5 per cent of patients although radio-isotope studies show a much higher incidence of diminished red-cell survival. The leuco-erythroblastosis that may accompany malignant disease is often a reflection of increased haemolysis.

Ovarian Dermoids.—A peculiar association has been reported with ovarian dermoid tumours or teratomata. These are direct Coombs's positive. Removal of the tumour produces a dramatic response in the anaemia and disappearance of the Coombs's reaction.

Renal failure with elevated blood-urea levels tends to be overlooked as a possible cause of refractory anaemia with diminished red-cell survival. Similarly, general toxaemia—'haemopathic haemolytic anaemia'—may be encountered in very ill elderly patients with no recognized pathogenic mechanism.

Arteritis.—Cold agglutinins may be associated with dysglobulinaemia in conditions such as polyarteritis nodosa and Wegener's granulomatosis. Flanagan, McCracken, Jones, and Cross (1965) reported the case of a 74-year-old man who had a necrotizing, giant-cell arteritis and died from severe haemolytic anaemia associated with cold agglutinins and positive direct Coombs's test.

Collagen Diseases.—Systemic lupus erythematosus is rarely encountered in the older patient, but variants are sometimes seen. Coexistent anaemia is largely due to haemorrhage, infection, or renal failure. The presence of a positive direct Coombs's test does not necessarily signify a haemolytic anaemia. However, a severe auto-immune type may develop in any of the collagen diseases and be associated with pancytopenia and thrombocytopenic purpura. The antibody responsible is warm, and often both anti-gamma G and non-gamma. Complement is fixed, and the serum complement low.

Warm-type auto-immune haemolytic anaemia has been recorded in the presence of ulcerative colitis.

Case 3.—Female, aged 58 years. In 1967 a partial thyroidectomy had been performed for a goitre following which she developed a rash on face, limbs, and trunk. There was also malaise. The L.E. latex test was positive on several occasions, although L.E. cells could not be demonstrated. A skin biopsy gave features consistent with systemic lupus erythematosus. Hb then was 88 per cent (12·9 g. per 100 ml.); W.B.C., 3500 per c.mm. (neutrophils 13 per cent). Prednisone was given.

In 1969 at the age of 60 years she had weakness and dyspepsia. Hb was 39 per cent (5·8 g. per 100 ml.); W.B.C., 2600 and platelets, 15,000 per c.mm. After repeated blood transfusion the haemoglobin again fell rapidly. The direct Coombs's test was negative, but the saline fragility showed a definite increase. Red-cell survival studies were not undertaken because of the necessity for frequent blood transfusion. A.N.F. antibodies were present on her last admission.

This patient who is suffering from S.L.E. in her sixties has developed a haemolytic anaemia. Neither condition appears to be readily controlled by steroid therapy.

Felty's Syndrome.—This comprises arthritis, splenomegaly, anaemia, and leucopenia in adults. It appears to be a variant of rheumatoid arthritis. As a rule haemolysis is not significantly increased in rheumatoid arthritis. Dyshaemopoiesis and chronic haemorrhage (due to salicylates) are more important causes of the refractory anaemia which these patients often show. The anaemia of Felty's syndrome is usually normocytic with features of an acquired auto-immune haemolytic anaemia. Its severity is not necessarily related to that of the arthritis. Systemic symptoms of malaise and fever are, however, prominent. Marked neutropenia may give rise to intercurrent infection. A few of these patients, particularly those with severe neutropenia, may benefit from splenectomy.

Hepatic cirrhosis frequently gives rise to increased haemolysis, but this is seldom severe. The direct Coombs's test is usually negative, but may be positive. The peripheral blood shows, in addition to anisocytosis and polychromasia, increased numbers of spherocytes and target cells.

Zieve's syndrome comprises jaundice, hyperlipaemia, hypercholesterolaemia, and haemolytic anaemia. These features develop transiently in chronic alcoholics.

Drugs and Chemicals.—Drugs may cause haemolysis as a result of a direct toxic effect on the red cells. This is a regular and predictable phenomenon with drugs such as phenylhydrazine, phenacetin, nitrobenzene, sulphones, arsine, and lead.

The second haemolytic mechanism is where the drug rarely has this effect, and does so only in people who are exceptionally susceptible, possibly due to an enzyme defect or to absorption of the drug on to the red-cell surface. A wide variety of antipyretics, antimalarials, nitrofurans, and sulphonamides produce haemolysis in patients whose red cells are deficient in glucose-6-phosphate dehydrogenase.

The peripheral blood-picture in these patients shows the usual characteristics of haemolysis, including spherocytosis. Additional features suggestive of a drug reaction are methaemoglobinaemia, sulphaemoglobinaemia, and Heinz bodies within the red blood-cells. The direct Coombs's test is usually negative when haemolysis is caused by direct toxic action or where there is an underlying enzyme defect.

Quinine, salicylates, and phenacetin are among the drugs to which some people are hypersensitive. Penicillin sometimes gives rise to an auto-immune haemolytic anaemia. White, Brown, Hepner, and Worlledge (1968) reviewed 12 published cases and described 2 of their own, a woman aged 64 and a man aged 66, in whom a strongly positive direct Coombs's test was obtained due to IgG antibody. Penicillin combines with proteins to form a hapten-protein complex on the red-cell membrane. Sensitization is more likely to occur when high doses are given. IgM in vitro-agglutinating antibodies have been found in up to 90 per cent of patients after penicillin therapy, but is harmless unless IgG antibody is present. These authors stressed the danger of attributing progressive anaemia in subacute bacterial endocarditis to the disease when it could be the result of penicillin therapy.

Methyldopa may cause anaemia. However, many more patients show laboratory evidence of sensitization to the drug than actually develop haemolytic anaemia. Carstairs, Breckenridge, Dollery, and Worlledge (1966) found that approximately 20 per cent of treated patients had a positive direct Coombs's reaction of IgG type. The incidence of sensitization paralleled the dose of the drug and duration of treatment. None of these patients had overt haemolytic anaemia. Worlledge, Carstairs, and Dacie (1966) studied 30 patients with haemolytic anaemia while on methyldopa therapy, and found that the anaemia developed insidiously between 3 and 37 months of commencing treatment. There was a rapid response, either to cessation of the drug or to steroids. They estimated that the incidence of anaemia was 0·15–0·3 per cent.

Therefore, a positive direct Coombs's test is not an indication to stop the drug. Regular haemoglobin measurement should be a sufficient check. The case of a man, aged 71, reported by Clark (1967) may be more ominous in that his patient developed auto-immune haemolysis and agranulocytosis when on methyldopa. The mixed antiglobulin reaction for auto-antibodies on the patient's white cells was strongly positive.

Scott, Myles, and Bacon (1968) reported that mefenamic acid could give rise to a Coombs's positive (IgG) auto-immune haemolytic anaemia and described 3 such patients over the age of 50.

Infection.—Dacie (1962) found that 12 per cent of 175 patients with auto-immune haemolytic anaemia had had a preceding infection. A clear causal relationship could not be seen in the warm-antibody type, but cold antibody was associated with primary atypical pneumonia.

Infection may often produce anaemia as a result of disseminated intravascular coagulation. Any infection can do this, and particular attention has been given to the role of Gram-negative endotoxins in the generalized Schwartzman phenomenon, but Gram-positive organisms may be equally dangerous in this respect. In a study of 49 cases of staphylococcal septicaemia, 17 of whom were over 50, Powell (1961) found that small-vessel thrombosis and fibrinoid necrosis were notable findings. The renal component, with tubular necrosis, made a significant contribution to the fatal outcome. Any infection can give rise to haemolysis. This may be acute and dramatic as in clostridial and streptococcal infections, or barely perceptible as in chronic granulomatous conditions.

Malaria and leishmaniasis provide a large number of cases in endemic areas.

Trauma.—Massive injury, burns, and the use of prostheses in cardiovascular surgery can cause severe haemolytic anaemia.

PAROXYSMAL COLD HAEMOGLOBINURIA

In this condition acute haemolysis follows exposure to cold. The degree of cold need not be extreme and symptoms appear at variable intervals, up to 8 hours afterwards. Haemolysis is associated with rigors, fever, limb pains, headache, and possibly vomiting. The first specimens of urine passed are dark in colour. Slight jaundice and splenomegaly may develop. Urticarial features have also been reported. Recovery is usually rapid and complete.

The laboratory findings are those of an acute haemolytic anaemia with leucopenia. Erythrophagocytosis is often seen. Later in the attack a leucocytosis with left nuclear shift develops.

The haemolytic mechanism involves a cold phase, during which antibody and some components of complement are fixed to the red-cell surface, and this is followed by the warm reaction in which C_2 and C_3 fractions are fixed to produce haemolysis. The Donath-Landsteiner test is based upon this reaction. A rough qualitative assessment may be obtained by observing haemolysis when the patient's blood is allowed to clot at 0° C. as compared with a 37° C. sample. The more accurate indirect method involves testing the patient's serum against group-O, P-positive red cells, at 0° and 37° C. A mixture of the patient's serum with normal serum is also tested because complement may be deficient after haemolysis. An indirect antiglobulin technique can also be used.

The Donath-Landsteiner antibody is a 7S IgG, and has to be distinguished from cold agglutinin. It has a specific anti-P effect.

The direct Coombs's test may be positive during an attack, but subsequently becomes negative.

The Wassermann reaction is often positive in these patients, but this does not always indicate syphilis, although cold agglutinins have a particular tendency to be associated with that disease.

The urine in the early stages of an attack contains oxyhaemoglobin and methaemoglobin. A positive test for albumin is also obtained.

Cold Agglutinin Haemoglobinuria and Raynaud's Syndrome is predominantly found in persons over 50 years. These patients show susceptibility to cold with attacks of haemoglobinuria and Raynaud's phenomenon. The spleen may be slightly enlarged. The cold agglutinin titre can be as high as 1/512,000, and the direct Coombs's test positive.

Cold Agglutinins with Primary Atypical Anaemia.—These are commonly associated. *Mycoplasma pneumoniae* is the organism responsible, although less commonly influenza has given rise to the same condition. Many of these patients are elderly. Lawson and others (1968) reported the additional complication of acute renal failure in 2 women aged 64 and 54. They both recovered following dialysis.

PAROXYSMAL NOCTURNAL HAEMOGLOBINURIA

This is mainly a disease of early adult life but examples may be found in the elderly. It appears to be an acquired defect of erythrocytes.

The presentation is usually that of a chronic refractory anaemia with episodes of exacerbation, in association with weakness, jaundice, abdominal pain, fever, and splenomegaly. Haemoglobinuria may be noted in urine passed at night, but not in that voided during the day.

A persistent pancytopenia gives rise to considerable diagnostic difficulty if the underlying nature of the disease is not suspected. There is a macrocytic anaemia with reticulocytosis, and an occasional normoblast is often seen. Plasma haemoglobin is raised, and methaemalbumin found. Leucocyte alkaline phosphatase activity is reduced.

Significant quantities of iron are lost in the urine as haemosiderin, and this can be sufficient to cause iron-deficiency anaemia.

Diagnosis is aided by the exclusion of other diseases such as pernicious anaemia, congenital spherocytosis or acquired haemolytic anaemia, and aleukaemic leukaemia. The most important diagnostic test is Ham's acidified serum test, in which the patient's red cells are incubated at 37° C. in the presence of serum (the patient's or normal) acidified to pH 6·5–7·0. The percentage haemolysis is measured. In paroxysmal nocturnal haemoglobinuria 10–50 per cent lysis is found in the acidified sample.

The clinical course of the disease is protracted and compatible with a normal life-span. It may tend to become milder in its intensity. Venous thrombosis is a common complication. Increased susceptibility to infection and haemorrhage also occurs.

Hitherto three examples of its termination in acute leukaemia have been recorded (Damashek, 1969) and the disease may form part of the spectrum of the myeloproliferative disorders.

Transfusion of saline-washed red cells is indicated for severe anaemia, and any superimposed iron deficiency should be corrected.

MICRO-ANGIOPATHIC HAEMOLYTIC ANAEMIA

Irregularly distorted ('bur') red cells have long been recognized as a feature of renal failure, but these cells may be seen in many other conditions. A haematological and histological study of 18 patients who had overt haemolytic anaemia during acute or chronic renal failure was reported by Brain, Dacie, and Hourihane

(1962). Four further patients with disseminated carcinoma were added. They emphasized the aetiological role of pathological changes in small blood-vessels. Fragmentation of red cells could then result from mechanical damage. The same team of workers (Rubenberg, Regaeczi, Bull, Dacie, and Brain, 1968; Bull, Rubenberg, Dacie, and Brain, 1968) produced red-cell fragmentation *in vitro* by strands of less than 1 μ diameter, such as would occur *in vivo* by deposition of fibrin strands. They likened the pathological picture to that found in the generalized Schwartzman phenomenon and the state of disseminated intravascular coagulation.

Whatever the mechanism may be, the fact remains that patients with various diseases such as disseminated carcinoma, leukaemia, and oligaemic shock (with or without uraemia) may develop haemolytic anaemia with fragmented cells and often severe thrombocytopenia. This is considered further under thrombotic thrombocytopenic purpura (*Chapter* 12).

Hypersplenism.—The concept of hypersplenism has been the subject of argument for many years. However, there is no doubt that patients are seen with splenomegaly; anaemia, which is often haemolytic; leucopenia; and thrombocytopenia. Furthermore their blood-picture responds to splenectomy. The direct Coombs's test is usually negative, although positively reacting cases have been reported.

Hypersplenism with Hypogammaglobulinaemia.—These patients suffer from repeated infections and often have an underlying malignant lymphoma.

General Comments

The clinical features and diagnostic criteria have been reviewed briefly, but it must be stressed that many elderly patients show haemolytic features in their terminal illnesses which cannot be classified. Moreover, fulminating sepsis, severe hepatic insufficiency, renal failure, or disseminated carcinoma may so dominate the clinical picture that the associated haemolysis is irrelevant or overlooked.

References

Brain, M. C., Dacie, J. V., Hourihane, D. O'B. (1962), *Br. J. Haemat.*, **8**, 358.
Bull, B. S., Rubenberg, M. L., Dacie, J. V., and Brain, M. C. (1968), *Ibid.*, **14**, 643.
Burston, J., Husain, O. A. N., Hutt, M. S. R., and Tanner, E. I. (1959), *Br. med. J.*, **1**, 83.
Carstairs, K. C., Breckenridge, A., Dollery, C. T., and Worledge, S. M. (1966), *Lancet*, **2**, 133.
Chapman, R. G. (1969), *Br. J. Haemat.*, **16**, 145.
Clark, K. G. A. (1967), *Br. med. J.*, **3**, 94.
Dacie, J. V. (1960, 1962, 1967, 1968), *The Haemolytic Anaemias*, Parts 1-4, 2nd ed. London: Churchill.
Damashek, W. (1969), *Blood*, **33**, 263.
Flanagan, P., McCracken, A. W., Jones, F. R., and Cross, R. M. (1965), *J. clin. Path.*, **18**, 588.
Lawson, D. H., Lindsay, R. M., Sawers, J. D., Luke, R. G., Davidson, J. F., Wardrop, C. J., and Linton, A. L. (1968), *Lancet*, **2**, 704.
Powell, D. E. B. (1961), *J. Path. Bact.*, **81**, 141.
Rubenberg, M. L., Regoeczi, E., Bull, B. S., Dacie, J. V., and Brain, M. C. (1968), *Br. J. Haemat.*, **14**, 627.
Scott, G. L., Myles, A. B., and Bacon, P. A. (1968), *Br. med. J.*, **3**, 534.
White, J. M., Brown, D. L., Hepner, G. W., and Worledge, S. M. (1968), *Ibid.*, **3**, 26.
Worledge, S. M., Carstairs, K. C., and Dacie, J. V. (1966), *Lancet*, **2**, 135.

14

MARROW FAILURE

CLASSIFICATION OF MARROW APLASIA

Predominant Presentation
  Pancytopenia
  Red-cell aplasia
  Agranulocytosis
  Thrombocytopenia

Aetiological Types
  Drugs
    a. Direct marrow toxins, e.g., benzene and derivatives, cytotoxic drugs, arsenic
    b. Unpredictable, e.g., chloramphenicol, phenylbutazone, gold compounds, anticonvulsants, organic arsenicals, insecticides
  Ionizing Radiations—direct marrow toxin
  Infections
  Systemic Disease
    Carcinoma
    Liver disease
    Endocrine—Addison's disease; Simmonds's disease; Hypothyroidism
    Renal disease and Uraemia
    Chronic disorders

Bone-marrow Disorders
  Neoplasia
    a. Primary.—Leukaemia; Lymphoma; Myeloma
    b. Secondary.—Carcinoma; Sarcoma
  Fibrosis and Sclerosis
  Leuco-erythroblastic

Sideroblastic
Hypersplenism
Thymoma
Paroxysmal Nocturnal Haemoglobinuria

Idiopathic (50 per cent)

Marrow failure as a cause of anaemia was first recognized by Ehrlich in 1888, and until the early 1930's it was a well-defined entity manifested by progressive anaemia, leucopenia, and thrombocytopenia occurring as an acute illness in adolescents or young adults. The diagnosis could always be made by finding an aplastic bone-marrow.

Since then the concept has been widened to include instances where there is an aplastic blood-picture and a hypercellular marrow, or a hypocellular marrow with a regenerative blood-picture, provided the disorder is not clearly secondary to general disease and that haematinic therapy is unsuccessful. The present approach allows erythropoiesis to be viewed dynamically, and recognizes not only that the appearance of a smear or section is not necessarily representative of the marrow as a whole, but also that haemopoietic requirements have to be considered. A marrow sufficiently active to deal with normal needs can still be inadequate under stress. A state of 'relative' hypoplasia can exist. This may be seen, for instance, when a patient with a neoplasm or renal disease is anaemic, and has haemolysis of a degree that would be insufficient to cause anaemia were the marrow functioning normally.

Mild relative hypoplasia seems to be fairly common in the elderly and is usually secondary to low-grade infection or occult disease. There are also instances when the marrow response to haematinic therapy in the deficiency anaemias is so slow and inadequate, despite the absence of an apparent cause, that hypoplasia cannot be excluded. These patients usually stabilize their haemoglobin fairly satisfactorily in the region of 60–65 per cent, but are incapable of maintaining a higher level unless transfused. The marrow smear usually shows a regenerative pattern, though occasionally there is some diminution of erythroid precursors. It is possible that hitherto unknown haematinic factors are deficient, or that incorporation of all the necessary metabolites within the developing erythron is impaired.

There is no rigid division between 'refractory' anaemia and 'aregenerative' or 'aplastic' anaemia, and the terms are often synonymous; but 'refractory' anaemia implies a lack of response to seemingly correct treatment. Even when the roles of vitamin B_{12}, folic acid, pyridoxine, and intercurrent disease are considered, they are still commoner at this age than at any other.

Havard (1962) reported on 24 cases of refractory anaemia. None had myelosclerosis or evidence of a dominating systemic disease. He concluded on the basis of radio-isotope studies that four patterns of anaemia could be recognized, namely:—

1. Normocytic, or macrocytic anaemia, and normal leucocyte and platelet counts, with normoblastic hyperplasia of the marrow. There was evidence of impaired synthesis of haemoglobin, which he considered to be probably due to a myeloproliferative disorder.

2. Pure red-cell anaemia, or pancytopenia, with hypoplastic bone-marrow. Red-cell survival was reduced and the Coombs's test positive. He postulated that the anaemia was the result of auto-immune damage to the bone-marrow.

3. Pure red-cell anaemia, or pancytopenia, with a cellular bone-marrow. Red-cell life was reduced and the Coombs's test negative. He believed that this was a heterogeneous group in so far as haemolysis was concerned, but that in each case the underlying reason for the anaemia was an inadequate marrow response due to a lack of reserve. It is interesting that in five instances examination of sternal marrow smears gave a false impression of hypocellularity.

4. Pancytopenia with an acellular bone-marrow. Red-cell life was normal and the Coombs's test negative. Injected ^{59}Fe disappeared slowly from the plasma. He felt that anaemia in this group was due to primary marrow aplasia. Eight patients were included, ranging in age from 21 to 82 years, 4 being over 65.

Havard and Scott (1963) later reported on an extended series of 101 patients. Although they were not able to classify this series similarly because radio-isotope studies were not carried out, they grouped them on the basis of the marrow findings into:—

Group I: with reduced bone-marrow cellularity: (*a*) generalized hypoplasia (49 cases); (*b*) erythroblastic aplasia (6 cases).

Group II: without reduced bone-marrow cellularity: (*a*) with erythroblast preponderance (35 cases); (*b*) with myeloid preponderance (11 cases).

Patients with features of myelosclerosis and acute or chronic neutropenia were excluded.

Aplastic Anaemia

General and Age Incidence

The general incidence is low. Among 2700 patients over the age of 65 admitted to hospital during an 18-month period, 174 had a haemoglobin level below 10 g. per 100 ml., 5 of whom had aplastic anaemia (Evans, Pathy, Sanerkin, and Deeble, 1968); but despite its relative rarity, the number over the age of 60 years possibly equals the total of those seen below that age, for example, 11 of the 20 cases reported on by Rankin (1961) were in this age category.

In Havard and Scott's series (1963) the mean age in the group with generalized bone-marrow hypoplasia was 45 years (range 35–82), and the sexes were equally affected. The second group, with a cellular bone-marrow and erythroblastic preponderance, showed a marked concentration in the fifth and sixth decades, the mean age being 58 years (range 24–88). Eight out of 45 of Israels and Wilkinson's series (1961) were over 60 years.

Aetiology

The two main clinical groups of aplastic anaemia are those where a definite or likely cause is recognized, and the remainder which are idiopathic. The group with a known or presumed cause can be further subdivided—for example, into those where the marrow is directly involved in some organic disease, or those where a systemic condition or poison affects haemopoiesis.

Bone-marrow Disease.—Myelofibrosis, myelosclerosis, myelomatosis, leukaemia, malignant lymphoma, secondary carcinoma, or sarcoma are all important causes of aplastic anaemia in the elderly. Their recognition is difficult if aspiration of the marrow fails to reveal the primary condition.

Drugs and Poisons.—Comparatively few elderly, anaemic patients are seen who have not previously taken a variety of prescribed or privately purchased drugs. Mohler and Leavell (1958) reviewing 302 cases from the literature, including 50 of their own, considered that drugs were probably responsible for 21 per cent. Rankin (1961) stated that in 15 of the 20 cases he studied, there was a convincing history that a drug capable of affecting the bone-marrow had been taken. The more carefully the drug intake of these patients is ascertained, the more difficult it becomes to exclude this factor as a possible cause.

It would be impossible to give a comprehensive list of all the drugs that have been incriminated. Drugs can act as direct poisons and regularly suppress haemopoiesis in a dose-dependent fashion. These may be recognized with reasonable accuracy, but it is more difficult to establish a cause-and-effect relationship with drugs that do so in an unpredictable manner.

Wintrobe (1969) listed the drugs associated with cases of aplastic anaemia reported to the American Medical Association Registry for 1965 and 1967 as follows:—

Total Reports in Registry	1067
Chloramphenicol	376
Sulphonamides (antibacterial)	137
Acetylsalicylic acid	97
Insecticides	56
Phenylbutazone	43
Solvents	33
Diphenyl hydantoin sodium	28
Mephenytoin	26
Sulphonamide (non-antibacterial tolbutamide, etc.)	26
Gold compounds	13

Other less commonly incriminated substances include quinacrine, potassium perchlorate, tetracycline, penicillin, hair dyes, dinitrophenol, carbon tetrachloride, amphotericin B, thiosemicarbazone, meprobamate, phenothiazines, and heavy metals.

Drugs which act as direct marrow toxins include busulphan, 6-mercaptopurine, nitrogen mustard, cyclophosphamide, melphalan, antifolic compounds, benzene and its derivatives, and inorganic arsenic.

Ionizing radiations act in a similar dose-dependent manner. The haemopoietic tissues are most sensitive, and the extent of reaction depends upon the intensity and duration of exposure. Routine radiotherapy may produce lymphocytosis and thrombocytopenia, but anaemia is rare and permanent blood changes seldom result. Late changes in the elderly are more likely to be seen following long-lasting internal radiation—for example after ingestion or injection of radio-isotopes, such as radium and mesothorium. Thorium dioxide (Thorotrast) was used between 1930 and 1947, since when several reports confirmed its neoplastic effects (MacMahon, Murphy, and Bates, 1947; Horta, Abbat, da Motta, and Roriz, 1965). Langlands and Williamson (1967) followed up 37 survivors of 137 patients who had received intra-arterial Thorotrast in Edinburgh between 1930 and 1947. Eighteen men (mean age 52·4, range 37–71 years) and 17 women (mean age 56·6, range 33–78 years) were investigated. They found that although the Hb, W.B.C., and platelet counts were within the normal ranges, all except 1 showed peripheral blood abnormalities—such as anisocytosis, macrocytosis, bur cells, stipple cells, Howell-Jolly bodies, and giant platelets. These findings suggested a progressive loss of splenic function after a latent interval of 20 years or more. Therefore, a history of exposure to ionizing radiations, even many years previously, should be specifically sought in the elderly.

Renal Failure.—This has already been referred to in Chapter 2, but its importance is re-emphasized in this context. Not infrequently, patients suffering from a refractory anaemia are found to have an elevated blood-urea level. This need not amount to a state of clinical uraemia, but quite small rises to levels of 60–100 mg. per 100 ml. may be associated with failure to respond to haematinics. The anaemia shows features which are partly haemolytic and partly aplastic. Thus a moderate reticulocytosis usually distinguishes it from other forms of aplasia. Shaw and Scholes (1967) found that the reticulocyte counts rose (*a*) as the red-cell survival time fell; (*b*) as the blood-urea rose; and (*c*) as the haemoglobin level fell. Low reticulocyte counts were seen in those with high blood-urea levels following blood transfusion, in some with acute renal failure, and in a few who were severely ill. They concluded that the reticulocyte count gave an approximate indication of red-cell production at low urea levels, but was not reliable at high levels because of a delay in reticulocyte maturation.

The Anaemia of Malignancy.—Friedell (1965) defined this as 'an incompletely compensated haemolytic anaemia which is not associated with overt haemorrhage or nutritional deficiency'. However, the evidence for haemolysis (for example, red-cell survival, reticulocyte count, and red-cell osmotic fragility) may be slight or minimal, and such that a healthy patient would readily compensate. Patients with malignant disease therefore may show 'ineffective erythropoiesis', and this failure to produce red cells is probably of greater significance than the increase in haemolytic destruction. Friedell postulated that the primary cause of the red-cell deficit in the cancer patient was 'an increased rate of destruction of immature red blood-cells by a hyperplastic reticulo-endothelial system'. Some of the findings, such as a lowering of serum total iron-binding capacity, resemble that reported in cases of the 'anaemia of chronic disorders'. However, as pointed out in Chapter 2, we found that the incidence of attendant or coincident iron deficiency is so high in elderly hospital patients that the T.I.B.C. is often elevated.

Pure red-cell aplasia secondary to neoplasia is well recognized with thymoma, but appears to be very rare in carcinoma. Entwistle, Fentem, and Jacobs (1964) recorded an exceptional case in a man aged 68 years with bronchogenic carcinoma. The patient's serum contained a factor which inhibited erythropoiesis in rabbits, but disappeared following irradiation of the tumour.

The Pathogenesis of Aplasia.—This is not known. Furthermore, it may vary with the cause, or the patient. Thus chloramphenicol can cause acute haemopoietic depression during therapy, which is dose-related and seen with blood-levels above 35 μg. per 100 ml. (Scott, Fitzgerald, Belkin, and Laurence, 1965). More usually there is no anaemia, but evidence of impaired erythropoiesis is found—increased serum iron and transferrin saturation, delayed plasma-iron clearance, and reticulocytopenia. The bone-marrow remains cellular. This may be due to an interaction with messenger RNA. Yunis and Bloomberg (1964) suggested that there is an inherited enzymic deficiency preventing the normal metabolism of chloramphenicol in susceptible persons. A variety of *in vitro* biochemical abnormalities have been described in patients recovering from blood dyscrasias due to drugs, but no tests are yet available to enable their prior detection, such as exist with glucose-6-phosphate dehydrogenase and haemolytic anaemia.

CLINICAL FEATURES

Males seem to be affected more often than females. The mode of onset is usually chronic, but was acute in 3 of 8 cases occurring in patients 60 years of age or over reported on by Boon and Walton (1951). The early symptoms depend on which of the haemopoietic stem lines is mainly deranged. Lassitude, increasing exertional dyspnoea, pallor, and the other indications of progressive anaemia are common features. Deterioration may be rapid over 2 or 3 weeks, or persist for 6 months to a year before becoming pronounced. Evidence of thrombocytopenia usually develops sooner or later with bruising, petechial haemorrhages, or blood-loss—usually from the gums, nasopharynx, or gastro-intestinal tract. These can occur at any stage and may be the reason for admission. The danger of haemorrhage is greater when there is concomitant infection (Vincent and de Gruchy, 1967). Bronchitis, bronchopneumonia, tonsillitis, or infection elsewhere is often present and, if the granulocytes are severely depressed, pyrexia may be marked and mucosal ulceration develop. Terminally, there is extreme pallor, infection, buccal ulceration, and haemorrhagic features.

Auto-antibodies against all three types of cells can develop (Heilmeyer, 1957).

Case 1.—Ulcerative colitis was diagnosed in 1964 when this lady was 52, and sulphaphthalidine given. A second attack occurred 2 years later when salazopyrin was prescribed. This and prednisolone were given in 1968 prior to her readmission with exacerbation of colitis and extensive bruising and petechial haemorrhages. Her Hb was 68 per cent; P.C.V., 33 per cent; W.B.C., 1200 per c.mm. (neutrophils, 55 per cent), and platelets 15,000 per c.mm. No haematological abnormality, other than anaemia, had been noted previously. The marrow showed a promyelocytic maturation arrest with only a few megakaryocytes and no budding activity. Sideroblasts were present.

Salazopyrin was discontinued. The blood-picture improved over the next 2 years, but the platelets remained at near 10,000 per c.mm., with the W.B.C. at 3000–5000 per c.mm.

Total colectomy was performed in October, 1968, after readmission with a Hb of 38 per cent; W.B.C., 1600 per c.mm.; and platelets, 12,000 per c.mm. In 1969 the W.B.C. was 3000–5000 and the platelets, 10,000–50,000 per c.mm.

Considerable difficulty had been encountered in giving blood transfusions owing to severe pyrexial reactions not due to demonstrable serological incompatibility. The direct Coombs's, Ham's, Donath-Landsteiner and cold auto-antibody tests were all negative.

Although this patient's pancytopenic picture was originally attributed to salazopyrin the later course suggests an unrelated hypoplasia, or one due to the primary disease.

Examination of the patient may not assist greatly in the diagnosis although petechiae, spontaneous bruising, and bleeding gums indicate thrombocytopenia, and pallor of the mucous membrane beyond that expected from the known blood-loss arouses suspicion of marrow disease. The absence of hepatosplenomegaly and of enlarged lymph-nodes favours primary marrow aplasia.

Usually the only clinical feature is an insidious anaemia, and the diagnosis then depends on haematological investigation.

Enlargement of liver, spleen, or lymph-nodes may be secondary to myelofibrosis, leukaemia, or haemolytic anaemia, and polycythaemia can progress to aplasia even when myelosuppressive drugs are withheld. On the other hand, similar features are seen in primary aplastic anaemia. Of the 50 cases described by Mohler and Leavell (1958) splenomegaly was present in 34 per cent, hepatomegaly in 32 per cent, and enlarged lymph-nodes in 24 per cent.

INVESTIGATION

A. BLOOD-PICTURE.—The *red-cell count* is almost invariably below 3 million per c.mm.

The *haematocrit* is usually between 15 and 20 per cent and the M.C.H.C. normal or slightly reduced.

The *reticulocyte count* may be zero, and is usually below 1 per cent, but occasionally a normal or even a raised level is found.

The *haemoglobin level* is variable. Occasionally it is as low as 30 per cent, but usually a level of 60–70 per cent (6·8–8·6 g. per 100 ml.) is present when the patient is first seen, and the mildness of the anaemia may hide the seriousness of the disease.

The *white-cell count* is less than 2000 per c.mm. in the average case, and polymorphs amount to 10–30 per cent of the total. A lymphopenia may also exist.

The *platelets* are usually below 50,000 per c.mm. and sometimes as low as 10,000. This is a constant feature and essential for diagnosis (Lewis, 1969). A response in the anaemia is presaged by a rising platelet count.

The *erythrocyte sedimentation rate* is normal, unless the cause of the anaemia, or an unconnected disease, is characterized by an elevation.

The *blood-film* shows anisocytosis and poikilocytosis, possibly with hypochromia or macrocytosis.

When there is pancytopenia, with gross diminution of reticulocytes, the diagnosis is usually clear, though marrow examination is still necessary.

Serum-iron levels and the degree of transferrin saturation are usually raised, unless there has been a state of preceding severe iron deficiency.

The *bleeding time* is prolonged, and clot retraction impaired. These findings are related to the severity of the thrombocytopenia. Tests of coagulation are normal.

Erythrocyte protoporphyrin is increased.

Ferrokinetic studies:—

a. Plasma-iron turnover is measured by following the rate of disappearance of intravenously administered ^{59}Fe-labelled plasma from the circulation. This rate is determined by various factors such as the relative amounts of iron in the plasma and stores, the rate of iron transfer to the red cells, and the speed of equilibration with the labile iron pool. The normal time taken for half the radioactivity to be lost ($T_{\frac{1}{2}}$) is 60–140 minutes. This is prolonged in aplastic anaemia.

Plasma iron turnover may then be calculated:—

$$\frac{\text{Plasma Fe} \times \text{plasma volume} \times 0.693 \times 24 \text{ hours}}{T_{\frac{1}{2}} \text{ (hours)}}.$$

This gives a measurement in mg. per day. The normal range is between 20 and 42 mg. It is reduced in aplastic anaemia.

b. Red-cell utilization of iron is a more accurate measurement. In this test, blood is sampled at intervals up to 3 weeks following the ^{59}Fe injection.

Red-cell turnover rate = plasma iron turnover × max. blood activity.

Normally this is 0·47 mg. Fe per kg. per day and is greatly reduced in aplastic anaemia.

c. Surface counting of radioactivity: ^{59}Fe activity is measured over the heart, liver, spleen, and sacral marrow. Measurements are made frequently during the first hours after injection and then gradually spaced out on alternate days for 10 days. In aplastic anaemia the proportion of ^{59}Fe taken up by the blood and bone-marrow is reduced and delayed, whilst the liver and spleen counts are increased (*Figs.* 84, 85).

Although ferrokinetic studies are not essential for diagnosis, they can help in delineating the type of anaemia in difficult cases. Thus Singh, Shinton, and Williams (1970) studied 10 patients with primary acquired sideroblastic anaemia, 7 of whom were over 60 years, and showed by repeated testing that a progressive change occurred from an initially mild degree of impaired haemoglobin synthesis, to a phase of ineffective erythropoiesis, culminating in complete erythropoietic failure.

B. BONE-MARROW.—Examination of both smear and biopsy material are necessary before a definite diagnosis is made. Typically, there is progressive hypocellularity until eventually the marrow is composed almost entirely of fat globules, lymphocytes, plasma cells, and reticulum cells and fibres. The increase in fibrous tissue gives an appearance superficially resembling early myelofibrosis.

Erythropoietic activity is diminished, though usually it remains normoblastic with the normoblasts numbering less than 10 per cent of the nucleated cells. Many

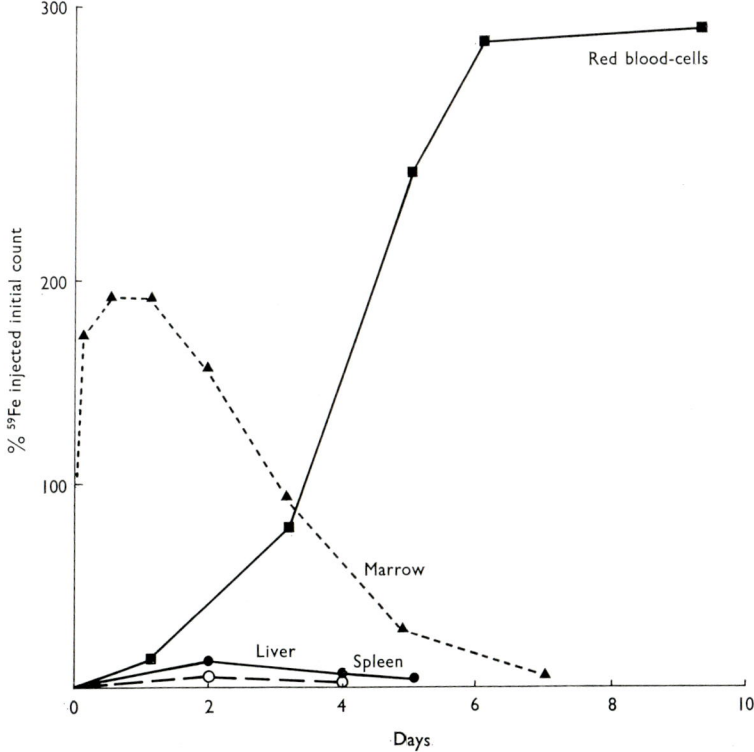

Fig. 84.—Ferrokinetic studies showing distribution of injected ^{59}Fe (normal).

may contain iron granules. In aplastic anaemia 70 per cent or more of the normoblasts may be sideroblasts, but a similar ratio can occur in patients with vitamin-B_{12} or folate-deficiency anaemia. When anaemia is due to infection, or malignancy, the proportion is less—perhaps 20–30 per cent. An occasional megaloblast or macro-normoblast is often seen.

Granulopoietic activity is greatly reduced and immature forms, insufficient to suggest leukaemia, can be present. Lymphocytes predominate.

Megakaryocytes are scanty or absent and their shape often abnormal. There is little, if any, evidence of platelet budding.

Pancytopenia is not always present. The appearance may vary from aplasia to hyperplasia in different sites, and haemopoietic depression may be confined to a single stem line.

Aspirated marrow may provide films that are not comparable with those obtained from biopsy material, and the degree of cellularity can change from hyperplasia to aplasia in succeeding specimens. Boon and Walton (1951) found a hypercellular marrow in 5 of their 25 cases. There is often no correlation between the findings in a single specimen and the course or severity of the disease. It is imperative that in atypical cases the relationship between the blood-picture and the marrow findings is assessed repeatedly.

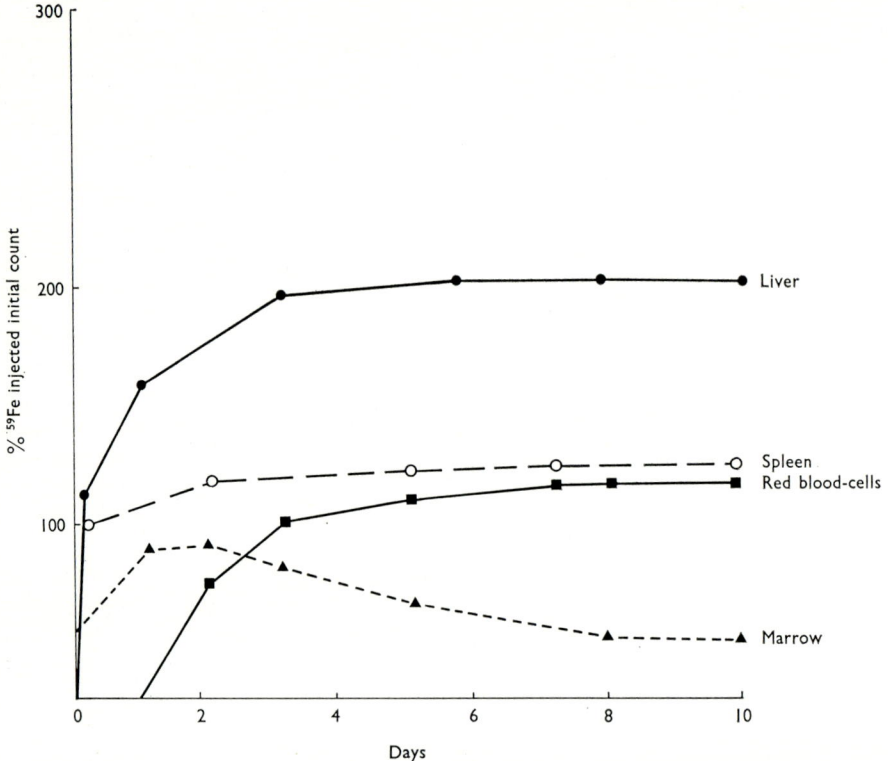

Fig. 85.—Ferrokinetic studies showing distribution of injected ^{59}Fe (aplastic anaemia).

The main difficulty lies in the differentiation from aleukaemic leukaemia and myelofibrosis, and sometimes it cannot be made until an adequate time interval has elapsed.

At autopsy there may be fibrosis of liver and pancreas due to accumulation of iron in the reticulo-endothelial cells, and the siderosis may be sufficiently pronounced to simulate haemochromatosis. This is due to multiple blood transfusions, continued absorption of medicinal iron given for the anaemia before hypoplasia was diagnosed, or the occasional presence of haemolysis or of hypersplenism. Haemorrhages into the skin, serous membranes, viscera, pharynx, and gastro-intestinal tract are usually present, together with sepsis and urinary infection.

TREATMENT

The drug history has to be reviewed and any drug that the patient is taking should be discontinued if there is the slightest possibility that it is implicated. Substitution with another drug should not be undertaken lightly.

The giving of iron, vitamin B_{12}, folate, vitamin C, and pyridoxine is always justified, after a specimen for serum measurements of the main haematinic factors has been taken, because they are often deficient at this age. On the other hand, there is no purpose in continuing therapy for longer than a few weeks when the anaemia is stationary or becoming more pronounced.

Prednisolone, in a dosage of 20–30 mg. daily, may be valuable because of the possibility of haemolysis or of auto-immune effects.

Eventually blood transfusion is necessary. This form of treatment should not be delayed when the haemoglobin is falling, or has reached a level of 50 per cent (7·3 g. per 100 ml.), as left ventricular failure, mental confusion, or some other manifestation of anaemia may develop rapidly. Packed cells should be given in an effort to maintain a reasonably high haemoglobin for as long as possible. An average level of 60–70 per cent is the best that can be achieved. Usually 450 ml. of packed red cells every 2–3 weeks is sufficient, but continuation of this form of therapy is difficult in the very old, because attendance is often erratic and complications such as thrombosis, infection, and psychological upsets are prone to develop. Splenectomy is sometimes indicated when there is haemolysis or hypersplenism.

Israels and Wilkinson (1961) emphasized the importance of conserving veins for repeated life-saving transfusions, and described modifications to the standard giving sets.

One of the major problems is the control of haemorrhage. Platelet transfusions will help in critical situations, but offer no long-term solution. Oestrogen–progestogen compounds may aid haemostasis.

Androgens sometimes simulate haemopoiesis—for example, a weekly injection of 500–600 mg. of testosterone propionate or oenanthate, for a period of several months. Early encouraging results using phytohaemagglutinin have not been fulfilled.

Dimercaprol (B.A.L.) may be useful in gold or arsenical poisoning.

Prognosis

The course of the disease depends upon the cause and the type of haematological reaction. Those that present acutely with a severe systemic illness usually pursue a relentless fatal course. Aplastic anaemia is always to be regarded seriously but is by no means uniformly fatal. The longer the patient survives, the better are the prospects for ultimate recovery (Lewis, 1969). Very low platelet counts and extreme neutropenia are serious omens.

If exposure to a known marrow toxin can be stopped the marrow may recover. For example, Wijnja, Snijder, and Nieweg (1966) described 5 patients who had pancytopenia with a history of chronic self-medication with acetylsalicylic acid (for up to 50 years in a 79-year-old woman, who had taken an estimated total of 20 kg.). The blood-picture returned to normal, or near normal, in all once the drug was discontinued. Unfortunately, other drugs, such as chloramphenicol, initiate an aplastic process which is uninfluenced by cessation of treatment—although obviously all such drugs should be withdrawn in these patients.

The influence of age on prognosis is debatable. Some series appear to show an improved prognosis in the elderly. In Havard and Scott's (1963) series the groups that had a cellular bone-marrow and included a higher proportion of the elderly fared better (3 per cent dead within 6 months and 38 per cent within 3 years) than the younger hypoplastic group (20 per cent dead within 6 months and 63 per cent within 3 years). However, the proportion alive after 5 years was similar in both groups, although this could have been partly accounted for by death from unrelated disease in the elderly. Israels and Wilkinson (1961) divided their series of 45 patients into three groups—those in remission; those surviving more than 3 months; and

Table XXVIII.—Haematological Characteristics of 14 Patients over the Age of 60 (Mohler and Leavell, 1958)

Sex	Age	Cause	Marrow	Blood	Duration	Comments
M.	65	Idiopathic	Hypocellular	Pancytopenia	1 yr. 5 mth.	Spontaneous remission
F.	62	Idiopathic	Hypocellular	Anaemia	9 yr.	Remission after splenectomy
M.	82	Idiopathic	Hypocellular	Anaemia	1 yr. 3 mth.	Remission with cortisone
M.	73	Idiopathic	Hypocellular	Pancytopenia	4 yr. 9 mth.	Remission with cortisone
M.	62	Benzol	Hypocellular	Pancytopenia	6 yr.	—
M.	78	Idiopathic	Hypocellular	Pancytopenia	8 mth.	Staphylococcal septicaemia
M.	79	Idiopathic	Hypocellular	Pancytopenia	5 mth.	Platelet rise with cortisone
M.	65	Idiopathic	Hypocellular	Anaemia, leucopenia	4 yr. 6 mth.	Acute myeloid leukaemia
F.	69	Idiopathic	Hypocellular	Pancytopenia	10 mth.	Haemorrhage, severe thrombocytopenia
M.	71	Idiopathic	Hypocellular	Pancytopenia	1 yr. 3 mth.	Refused transfusion
M.	68	Idiopathic	Normocellular	Anaemia, leucopenia	4 yr. 6 mth.	Erythroid hypoplasia
F.	71	Idiopathic	Hypocellular	Anaemia, thrombocytopenia	2 yr. 4 mth.	Septicaemia, haemochromatosis
M.	63	Idiopathic	Normocellular	Anaemia, leucopenia	4 yr. 10 mth.	Atrophy of testes
M.	66	Drug	Normocellular	Pancytopenia	2 yr. 3 mth.	Multiple drug medication before anaemia

those surviving less than 3 months. The last category included 20 patients, 9 of whom were over 40 years and 7 over 50 years. Lewis (1965) also found a graver prognosis in those over 40. Therefore, it seems that the prognosis is more serious in the elderly, except when they are segregated on the basis of their bone-marrow findings.

The general picture that is often obtained is illustrated in *Table XXVIII* (abstracted from Mohler and Leavell's series).

Other Haematological Complications.—Aplastic anaemia may precede myelofibrosis, myelosclerosis, or leukaemia. It may also be a stage in the progress of polycythaemia vera or pernicious anaemia. The prognosis is then that of the predominant condition.

Paroxysmal Nocturnal Haemoglobinuria (PNH).—Aplastic anaemia may terminate in PNH—just as PNH itself can pass into an aplastic phase. Lewis and Dacie (1967) described 6 such patients including a 64-year-old woman. Approximately 15 per cent of cases in a general population will develop a PNH-like defect in their red cells, which may even cause death.

RED-CELL APLASIA

Pure red-cell aplasia is rare, but 5 of the 16 patients with aplastic anaemia studied by Lange, McCarthy, and Gallagher (1961) had normal myeloid and platelet activity, with a lack of erythroid precursors in the marrow. Three of the patients were in their late sixties; 1 was considered to have acute erythroid hypoplasia, and 2 the chronic form. Reticulocytes were absent in 2 and 0·2 per cent in the others. Some of these cases have an associated thymic tumour. Entwistle and others in 1964 stated that there were 44 recorded instances of this association, and many have been described subsequently.

Red-cell aplasia can also occur with increased activity of the white-cell series, and in these patients early leukaemia has to be excluded. The patients can be kept reasonably symptom-free with repeated blood transfusions. Other forms of treatment are contra-indicated.

AGRANULOCYTOSIS

The cause can be ascribed to a drug or toxin in about half the cases. Wintrobe (1969) listed the drugs associated with leucopenia that had been reported to the American Medical Association Registry on Adverse Reactions, Council on Drugs, Chicago, April–May, 1965, and 1 June, 1967 (*Table XXIX*).

Any drug or toxin that can cause aplastic anaemia occasionally produces lone aplasia of the white-cell series. Even drugs that are primarily known for their possible haemolytic effect may also do so. For example, Clark (1967) described agranulocytosis with an auto-antibody in a man aged 71 years who was taking methyldopa—although chlorpropamide had also been taken.

Drugs may induce granulocytopenia by one of at least two mechanisms:—

a. An Immune Mechanism.—In these instances a small test dose of the drug in a previously sensitized individual has been shown to produce extreme granulocytopenia within a few hours. This, of course, should not be a routine method of ascertaining the patient's hypersensitivity. Increased peripheral destruction of the leucocytes takes place, and drug-dependent leucocyte agglutinins can be demonstrated. These antibodies are different from leucocyte iso-antibodies, such as are formed following multiple transfusion, pregnancies, collagen diseases, viral pneumonia, liver disease, and paroxysmal nocturnal haemoglobinuria.

The drugs that exhibit this immunological type of mechanism include amidopyrine, sulphonamides, chlorpropamide, meprobamate, antithyroid drugs, hydrazoline, and mercurial diuretics.

b. Direct Marrow Toxicity.—This is usually dose related, and such drugs can be shown to inhibit DNA synthesis in suspensions of marrow cells. Drugs that may act in this manner include chlorpromazine, phenothiazines, sulphonamides, hydantoins, and antithyroid drugs. Some drugs are capable of depressing granulopoiesis by either or both of these mechanisms.

CLINICAL FEATURES

The relationship to an offending drug will depend upon the type of mechanism responsible. In the hypersensitivity group the amount of drug taken may be small, and the onset of agranulocytosis sudden and unpredictable. In the dose-dependent

Table XXIX.—DRUGS ASSOCIATED WITH LEUCOPENIA

	No. Reported*	
	Total	Drug alone
Total Reports in Registry	1337	
Analgesics		
Amidopyrine	70	15
Dipyrone	64	22
Phenylbutazone	44	17
Acetylsalicylic acid	87	4
Antibacterial agents		
Sulphonamides	121	26
Chloramphenicol	75	18
Penicillin	97	7
Sulphonamide derivatives		
(non-antibacterial)	47	21
Anticonvulsants	66	15
Phenindione	23	10
Diphenylhydantoin sodium	43	5
Meprobamate	35	2
Phenothiazines	467	143
Chlorpromazine	227	83
Promazine	69	30
Mepazine	34	13
Imipramine	33	5
Prochlorperazine	30	4
Antithyroid drugs		
Thiouracil, propylthiouracil	34	23

* Panel on Haematology, Registry on Adverse Reactions, Council on Drugs, A.M.A., Chicago, April–May, 1965, and 1 June, 1967.

type the drug has usually been taken over a long period. Thus in the case of thiouracil and phenothiazine derivatives the drug may have been taken for several weeks during which leucopenia develops gradually.

There may be a prodromal period of 2 or 3 weeks when there is lassitude, fatigue, and anorexia, but usually the onset is sudden. The patient has a rigor, develops soreness of the mouth, and within 24–48 hours is seriously ill with a temperature of 103–105° F. (39–40·5° C.). Oral ulceration develops rapidly with cervical adenitis, and other superficial lymph-nodes enlarge. The spleen is rarely palpable. Pulmonary or renal infection is often present although this may have been the reason for therapy with the causative drug.

Unless arrested the disease is rapidly fatal. Infection increases and the patient dies within a few days. Paradoxically, some patients are found to have persistent, severe, drug-induced neutropenia with little or no constitutional upset.

Marrow Examination

This reveals a marked reduction of the granulocytic series, and terminally the aplasia is complete. In the classic case there is no disturbance of erythropoiesis and the megakaryocytes are normal.

Treatment

Treatment consists of discontinuing the causative drug, combating infection, and giving steroids in an effort to diminish any antibody effect that is present.

Diagnosis

Diagnosis is usually straightforward although differentiation from aleukaemic leukaemia can be difficult. Occasionally, the disease is less acute, and then benign neutropenia has to be considered.

Prognosis

The prognosis in agranulocytosis is poor, particularly when the patient has reached an advanced age. Confusion, drowsiness, skin ulceration, and the development of pneumonia or urinary infection are poor signs. The younger patient may recover if the cause can be removed and infection combated. The first sign of improvement is the appearance of myelocytes, and possibly myeloblasts, in the peripheral blood. Mature granulocytes appear later, and there may be transient leucocytosis or a leukaemoid reaction before a normal picture returns.

Other causes of neutropenia include acute and chronic infections, chronic disease and inanition, liver cirrhosis, Felty's syndrome, hypersplenism, systemic lupus erythematosus, and any primary or secondary neoplastic process involving the bone-marrow.

Case 2.—This man, aged 64, was seen in 1966. He had suffered from rheumatoid arthritis for 11 years. In the first 2 years he was given gold and salicylate therapy. At that time his Hb was 80 per cent (11·7 g. per 100 ml.), and W.B.C., 9600 per c.mm., with a normal differential. The gold injections were repeated in 1964 and generalized erythema developed 2 weeks later. Indomethacin was started in January, 1966. A routine blood-count in April, 1966, showed Hb, 83 per cent (12·1 g. per 100 ml.); W.B.C., 2100 per c.mm. (neutrophils, 5 per cent; lymphocytes, 63 per cent; monocytes, 2 per cent; eosinophils, 30 per cent); and platelets, 200,000 per c.mm. He had no symptoms referable to the neutropenia. The white cells increased during the ensuing months but then reverted to leucopenic levels, the last count being 1800 per c.mm., with neutrophils, 32 per cent. A marrow examination when the neutropenia was first diagnosed showed simple hypoplasia.

He had been given gold and indomethacin prior to the neutropenia, but this has persisted without associated symptoms. He subsequently developed all the features of Felty's syndrome.

Chronic Idiopathic Neutropenia

The polymorphs can be greatly reduced. Although there is no progressive aplasia of the granulocyte series mature polymorphs can be virtually absent in marrow smears from patients with chronic idiopathic neutropenia, probably due to maturation arrest. Recurrent or cyclical granulopenia is seen. These patients usually have a long history of recurrent mucosal ulceration with spontaneous recovery, each attack lasting 10 days or so, with an interval of about 2–6 weeks. There may be splenomegaly, adenopathy and arthralgia. Malaise, fever, and infection are often present. Marrow examination may reveal arrested production of neutrophils during the acute episodes.

Relative Marrow Failure

A healthy marrow can cope with any deficiency anaemia, provided the cause of the anaemia is removed. Erythropoiesis increases four to six times without an appreciable time lag. There is no definite evidence that this reserve power diminishes with ageing despite reduction of the red marrow.

Measurement of the rate of disappearance of ^{59}Fe from the serum and its timed reappearance in haemoglobin is probably a fairly accurate method of assessing marrow activity, but in most hospitals reliance has to be placed on noting the response to treatment and the degree of cellularity in a marrow smear. Both observations are of limited value. In the deficiency anaemias there is a variable delay because the stores are repleted before sufficient haematinic factor reaches the marrow, and without information on the extent of the depletion it is impossible to decide when a full marrow response is to be expected. Similarly, hypercellularity of the marrow may be localized and does not exclude hypoplasia. More information is obtained from bone-marrow biopsy material, but examination of succeeding specimens is necessary before a progressive response can be assessed. In ordinary clinical practice such repeated procedures may not be justified. Generally speaking some guidance is obtained from a single specimen, whether smear or biopsy, provided it is suitably timed. Correlating the increase of erythropoiesis with that expected from the degree of anaemia is useful when the disparity is pronounced, but is otherwise too inaccurate to be relied upon.

There are four main causes of marrow hypofunction, namely chronic infection, liver damage, renal disease, and cancer. The first indication of their presence may be an inadequate marrow response to anaemia and its treatment. Mild haemolysis, with reduction of red-cell survival to 70 or 80 days, is insufficient to cause anaemia when marrow function is unimpaired. The finding of a normal blood-picture does not necessarily indicate a healthy marrow, because it is only when there is 'stress' that its reserve power can be assessed.

References

Boon, T. H., and Walton, J. N. (1951), *Q. Jl Med.*, **20**, 75.
Clark, K. G. A. (1967), *Br. med. J.*, **4**, 94.
Ehrlich, P. (1888), *Charité Ann.*, **13**, 300.
Entwistle, C. C., Fentem, P. H., and Jacobs, A. (1964), *Br. med. J.*, **2**, 1504.
Evans, D. M. D., Pathy, M. S., Sanerkin, N. G., and Deeble, T. J. (1968), *Geront. clin.*, **10**, 228.
Friedell, G. H. (1965), *Lancet*, **1**, 356.
Havard, C. W. H. (1962), *Q. Jl Med.*, **31**, 21.
— — and Scott, R. B. (1963), *Lancet*, **1**, 461.
Heilmeyer, L. (1957), *Blood*, **12**, 194.
Horta, J. da S., Abbatt, J. D., da Motta, L. C., and Roriz, M. L. (1965), *Lancet*, **2**, 201.
Israels, M. C. G., and Wilkinson, J. F. (1961), *Ibid.*, **1**, 63.
Lange, R. D., McCarthy, J. N., and Gallagher, N. I. (1961), *Archs intern. Med.*, **108**, 850.
Langlands, A. O., and Williamson, E. R. D. (1967), *Br. med. J.*, **2**, 206.

Lewis, S. M. (1965), *Br. med. J.*, **1**, 1027.
— — (1969), *Jl R. Coll. Phys. Lond.*, **3**, 253.
— — and Dacie, J. V. (1967), *Br. J. Haemat.*, **13**, 236.
MacMahon, H. E., Murphy, A. S., and Bates, M. I. (1947), *Am. J. Path.*, **23**, 585.
Mohler, D. N., and Leavell, B. S. (1958), *Ann. intern. Med.*, **49**, 326.
Rankin, A. M. (1961), *Med. J. Aust.*, **2**, 95.
Scott, J. L., Fitzgerald, S. M., Belkin, G. A., and Laurence, J. S. (1965), *New Engl. J. Med.*, **272**, 1137.
Shaw, A. B., and Scholes, M. C. (1967), *Lancet*, **1**, 799.
Singh, A. K., Shinton, N. K., and Williams, J. D. F. (1970), *Br. J. Haemat.*, **18**, 67.
Vincent, P. C., and de Gruchy, G. C. (1967), *Ibid.*, **13**, 977.
Wijnja, L., Snijder, J. A. M., and Nieweg, H. O. (1966), *Lancet*, **2**, 768.
Wintrobe, M. M. (1969), *Jl R. Coll. Phys. Lond.*, **3**, 99.
Yunis, A. A., and Bloomberg, G. R. (1964), *Progress in Haematology*, **4**, 138.

INDEX

ACETYLSALICYLIC acid causing aplastic anaemia 265
— — blood-loss 7
Achlorhydria, histamine-fast, in iron-deficiency anaemia 131
— — pernicious anaemia 91
— tests for 91
Acholuric jaundice complicating haemolytic anaemia 243, 247
Addisonian anaemia (*see* Pernicious Anaemia)
Addison's disease 55
Adrenal gland disease 55
Adrenocorticosteroid therapy in idiopathic thrombocytopenic purpura .. 226
Age distribution of lymphoid tissue tumours .. (*Figs.* 32, 33) 143
Ageing, biological and pathological aspects of 1
— haemopoiesis and .. .. (*Fig.* 1) 5
— low serum vitamin B_{12} due to .. 108
— — — iron due to 65
— role of, in incidence of leukaemia (*Figs.* 41–43) 167
— — — Hodgkin's disease 150
Agitation in iron-deficiency anaemia .. 74
Agranulocytosis 267
Albumin, decrease of, with age .. 10, 11
— level, association of, with disease categories 11
— serum, in infection and in vascular disease 23
Alcohol intolerance in Hodgkin's disease 152
Alcoholism, chronic, folate deficiency associated with 118, 119
Aleukaemic leukaemia 183
— — diagnosis of, in macrocytic anaemias 107
Amyloidosis complicating myelomatosis 203, 204
— in Hodgkin's disease 151
Anaemia, aplastic (*see* Aplastic Anaemia)
— associated with bed-sores 23
— — carcinoma .. .. (*Fig.* 2) 23
— — cirrhosis of the liver 33
— — infection, chronic 21
— — surgery 25
— — trauma 28

Anaemia in atherosclerosis 49
— causes of 7
— clinical examination in 15
— complicating polycythaemia vera .. 222
— in Cushing's syndrome 55
— diffuse myelomatosis 202
— due to gastro-intestinal disease .. 41
— early detection of 137
— — — in special risk cases 138
— Felty's syndrome 44, 45
— folate deficiency with .. 111, 116
— haemolytic (*see* Haemolytic Anaemia)
— of Hodgkin's disease 151, 153, (*Fig.* 36) 158, 159
— hypothyroidism 54, 125
— investigation of 15
— and jaundice, recurrent crises of .. 246
— leuco-erythroblastic, in myelofibrosis 210
— in leukaemia, acute 173
— — chronic myeloid 176–177
— lupus erythematosus 51
— of lymphatic leukaemia 181
— malignancy 250, 260
— management of 139
— marrow failure as cause of 256
— megaloblastic (*see* Megaloblastic Anaemia)
— micro-angiopathic haemolytic .. 228
— morbidity and mortality in 4
— in multiple myelomatosis 198
— osteo-arthritis 49
— pernicious (*see* Pernicious Anaemia)
— prevalence of 2
— prevention of 133
— — primary 136
— recurrence of 139
— 'refractory' 257
— in renal disease 37
— rheumatoid arthritis 43
— secondary refractory, in chronic bronchitis 21
— sideroblastic .. .. (*Fig.* 31) 126
— — following isoniazid and P.A.S. therapy 21
— types of 13
Anaplastic sarcoma .. 147, 148, 156
Angiitis 53

272

INDEX

Angina pectoris associated with iron-deficiency anaemia 75
— — preceding pernicious anaemia 94, 96
Antibody(ies) components, decrease in, with age 13
— in pernicious anaemia 92
— serum, testing for 246
Anticoagulant(s), circulating, complicating traumatic bleeding 30
— — essential tests for 235
— — therapy 238
— — tests for control of 238
— — in thrombosis 31
Anticonvulsant therapy causing pseudolymphoma 162
— — relation of, to folate deficiency 114, 117
Antiglobulin test, direct, in haemolytic anaemia 245
— — indirect, in haemolytic anaemia .. 246
Antihaemophilic globulin inhibitors .. 235
Apathy in iron-deficiency anaemia .. 73
— pernicious anaemia 94, 106
Aplasia, pathogenesis of 260
Aplastic anaemia 258
— — aetiology of 258
— — clinical features of 260
— — investigation of 261
— — in myeloproliferative syndrome .. 215
— — prognosis in 265
— — red-cell aplasia in 267
— — terminating in paroxysmal nocturnal haemoglobinuria .. 267
— — treatment of 264
— crises in auto-immune haemolytic anaemia 248
— — congenital spherocytic anaemia .. 247
Apoferritin 59, 61
Arterial disease .. .. (*Figs.* 5–9) 49
Arteritis causing haemolytic anaemia .. 251
— giant-cell or temporal 50
Arvin for thrombolysis 239
Ascorbic acid, iron, vitamin B_{12}, folic acid, interrelation of 128
— — in scurvy 123
— — supplementary to iron therapy .. 80
Astrafer (iron-dextrin) 81
Atherosclerosis 49
Atrial fibrillation in iron-deficiency anaemia 76
Augmented histamine test for achlorhydria 91
Autoanalyser technique for serum iron estimation 77
Auto-immune disease and Hodgkin's disease 161
— disorders, pernicious anaemia and .. 103
— haemolytic anaemia 245, 248

Auto-immunity and hyperglobulinaemic purpura 232
Azotaemia in iron-deficiency anaemia .. 77

BASOPHILIC leukaemia 183
Bed-sores, anaemia in patients with .. 23
Behavioural problems in iron-deficiency anaemia 75
Bence Jones protein 190
— — — urine tests for 191
— — proteinuria in multiple myelomatosis 199, 201
Biochemical abnormality, presence of, in erythropoiesis 147
Bleeding disorders (*Figs.* 74–79) 224–234
— — classification of 224
— investigation into presence of 70, 72
— traumatic 30
Blind-loop syndrome causing low serum vitamin B_{12} 108
Blood disorders associated with general disease .. .. (*Figs.* 2–9) 18–57
— peripheral, in polycythaemia vera .. 217
— transfusion in aplastic anaemia .. 265
— — iron-deficiency anaemia 83
— — packed red cells, in myeloproliferative syndrome 215
— — in pernicious anaemia 104
— viscosity in polycythaemia vera .. 217
Blood-cell anomalies in obstructive jaundice .. .. (*Fig.* 3) 32
Blood-loss, anaemia due to, in renal disease 37
— causing anaemia 7, 30
— in gastro-intestinal disease causing anaemia 41
— tests for 15
Blood-picture(s) in acute leukaemia (*Figs.* 48, 49) 173
— in aplastic anaemia 261
— bizarre, complicating diagnosis of tuberculosis 20
— of folate deficiency 111
— peripheral, in red-cell regeneration .. 245
— in pernicious anaemia 89
Blood-urea, raised, in renal disease anaemia 37, 38
Bone involvement in reticulosarcoma .. 147
Bone-marrow cytology in rheumatoid arthritis 47
— Hodgkin's disease .. (*Fig.* 36) 158
Brill-Symmers disease (*see* Lymphoma, Follicular)
Bronchial adenoma, paraproteinaemia associated with .. (*Figs.* 68–72) 207
Bronchitis, chronic, causing polycythaemia 21

INDEX

Bruising, excessive, in elderly .. 30
— — idiopathic thrombocytopenic purpura 225
— spontaneous, in pernicious anaemia 98
Buffy coat in blood-picture of pernicious anaemia 89
Busulphan in myeloid leukaemia 186, 187

Capillary defects causing bleeding .. 224
— haemorrhage, primary 235
Carcinoma associated with paraproteinaemia .. .. .. (Figs. 65–67) 205
— — — thrombocytopenia 228
— blood changes associated with (Fig. 2) 23
— causing aplastic anaemia 260
— — haemolytic anaemia 250
— — iron-deficiency anaemia 72
— gastro-intestinal, recognition of presence of 140
— haemorrhage due to pathological fibrinolysis in 236
Cardiac failure, congestive, anaemia precipitating 139
— — — in iron-deficiency anaemia .. 76
— — — pernicious anaemia .. 96, 98, 106
— — — folate deficiency associated with 118
Cardiovascular system, symptoms of iron-deficiency anaemia in 75
Catalases 62
Cervical node enlargement in Hodgkin's disease 150, 152
Chemicals causing haemolytic anaemia 252
Chemotherapy in Hodgkin's disease .. 153
— polycythaemia vera 221, 222
Chlorambucil in Hodgkin's disease .. 154
Chloramphenicol causing impaired erythropoiesis 260
Chlorothiazide causing thrombocytopenia 227
Christmas disease 234
Chromosome, Philadelphia 178
Cirrhosis of liver 33
— — associated with anaemia 125
— — in haemochromatosis .. 35, 36
Clinic, central, in prevention of anaemia 134
Clotting-factor deficiencies complicating traumatic bleeding 30
Coagulation defects causing bleeding .. 224
— — in cirrhosis 35
— disorders, acquired 235
— — classification of 234
— — congenital 234
Cobalt salts supplementary to iron therapy 80
Cold agglutinins with primary atypical anaemia 254
— haemoglobinuria, paroxysmal .. 253

Cold-haemagglutinin disease, serum antibodies in, tests for 246
Collagen diseases, angiitis in .. 52, 53
— — causing haemolytic anaemia .. 251
Combined therapy in acute leukaemia .. 185
Congenital haemolytic anaemia, diagnosis from other macrocytic anaemias 107
Coombs's test in haemolytic anaemia .. 245
— — indirect, in haemolytic anaemia .. 246
Corpuscular haemoglobin concentration, mean (see M.C.H.C.)
'Corticosteroid purpura' 231
— therapy complicating tuberculosis .. 20
— — giant-cell arteritis 50
— — Hodgkin's disease 154
Cranial nerve involvement in iron-deficiency anaemia 75
Crohn's disease, folate deficiency associated with 118
Cushing's syndrome 55
Cyanocobalamin in pernicious anaemia 104
Cyclophosphamide in Hodgkin's disease 154
— multiple myelomatosis 204
Cytochromes 62
Cytotoxic drugs in acquired haemolytic anaemia 249

Defibrination syndrome 236
— — tests for 237
— — treatment of 237
Deficiency anaemias in aged 13
— — inadequate marrow response to haematinic therapy in 257
— — prevention of 133
— — relation between 128
— states giving rise to macrocytic or megaloblastic anaemia (Fig. 31) 123
Dementia in iron-deficiency anaemia 74, 75
Depression in iron-deficiency anaemia .. 74
— pernicious anaemia 94, 106
Dermatitis, exfoliative, folate deficiency in 120
Dermoids, ovarian, causing haemolytic anaemia 251
Desquamation, folate and iron lost in .. 120
Diabetes mellitus 55
— — associated with haemochromatosis 36
Diagnex Blue test for gastric acid secretion 90, 91
Dicopac test in pernicious anaemia .. 92
Disease, general, vitamin-B_{12} deficiency associated with 103
— iron deficiency associated with .. 67
— folate deficiency associated with .. 118
Diverticula of jejunum associated with vitamin-B_{12} deficiency 101

INDEX

Diverticula of jejunum with folate deficiency 114
Donath-Landsteiner test 253
Drug(s) associated with leucopenia .. 268
— causing agranulocytosis 267
— — aplastic anaemia 258
— — haemolytic anaemia 252
— — thrombocytopenia 227
— hypersensitivity causing thrombocytopenia 227
— used in treatment of Hodgkin's disease 153
— — — leukaemia 186
— — — myeloma 203
— — — polycythaemia vera 221
Drug-induced sideroblastic anaemia .. 127
Dyshaemopoietic anaemia with ringed sideroblasts in marrow 126
Dysphagia, iron-deficiency 72
— in pernicious anaemia 98
Dyspnoea in iron-deficiency anaemia 75, 77
Dysproteinaemia 232

Electrocardiographic changes due to anaemia .. .. .. (*Fig.* 20) 77
— — in pernicious anaemia 96
Electrophoretic analysis in detection of paraproteins 190, 192
— — multiple myelomatosis 200
Endocarditis, bacterial, blood changes associated with 19
Endocrine disease 54
Enzyme assays in iron deficiency .. 68
— systems, iron-dependent 62
Eosinophilic leukaemia 183
Epilepsy, folate deficiency associated with drug therapy for .. 114, 117
Epistaxis in idiopathic thrombocytopenic purpura 225
Epsilon-aminocaproic acid (EACA) in defibrination syndrome 237
Erythraemic myelosis, chronic 164, 183, 212
Erythrocyte protoporphyrin 70
— sedimentation rate (E.S.R.) 9
— — — in infection 19
— — — rheumatoid arthritis 43
Erythrocytosis, benign 219
Erythrokinetic studies in myelofibrosis .. 211
Erythroleukaemia 183
Erythropoiesis, decreased, in renal disease anaemia 39
— effect of ageing on 7
— ineffective, in malignant disease .. 260
— megaloblastic 214
Erythropoietic polycythaemia 219
Erythropoietin, diminution of, causing erythropoiesis 40
Evans's syndrome 228

Extramedullary plasmacytoma .. 202, 203
Extrinsic factor (*see* Vitamin B_{12})

Factor-VIII inhibitors, spontaneous .. 235
Felty's syndrome 44
— — causing haemolytic anaemia .. 251
Ferrioxamine test, differential 70
Ferritin 59, 61
Ferrivenin (saccharated iron oxide) .. 81
Ferrokinetic studies in aplastic anaemia (*Figs.* 84, 85) 262
Fibrinogen, concentrated, in defibrination syndrome 237
Fibrinolysis, pathological, haemorrhage due to 236
Fibrinolytic mechanisms, hyperactive, complicating traumatic bleeding .. 31
FIGLU test .. .. (*Fig.* 26) 112
Folate deficiency .. 86, (*Figs.* 25–30) 110–121
— — associated with other diseases (*Figs.* 27–30) 118
— — — vitamin C deficiency 114, 123
— — causes of 113
— — clinical features of 115
— — complicating pernicious anaemia treatment 106
— — laboratory and diagnostic features of .. .. .. (*Fig.* 26) 111
— — in myelofibrosis 211
— — symptoms and signs other than anaemia 116
— — treatment of 121
— — with anaemia 116
— hepatic 113
— malabsorption causing anaemia .. 8
— metabolism and rheumatoid arthritis 46
— red-cell 110, 112
— serum, level of, in folate deficiency .. 111
— — renal disease 40
— — low, occurring alone 115
— — — with normal liver folate .. 116
— — in pernicious anaemia 91
— — and red-cell, normal levels .. 110
— — values following trauma 28
Folate-clearance test 113
Folate-deficiency anaemia .. 13, 111
— — in relation to other deficiencies 129
Folic acid coenzymes, impaired production of 128
— — iron, vitamin B_{12}, and ascorbic acid, interrelationship of .. 128
— — preparations 121
Folic-acid absorption tests 113
— antagonists 110
— metabolism .. .. (*Fig.* 25) 110
— — in polycythaemia vera 218
Folinic acid 110

INDEX

Follicular lymphoma (*see* Lymphoma, Follicular)
Foodstuffs, iron content of 58
Fracture, pathological, in multiple myelomatosis 198, 204

GAISBÖCK'S disease 219
Gamma-globulin(s), increase in, with age .. 10, 12
— levels in disease categories 12
— serum, in infection and in vascular disease 23
Gammopathy, monoclonal 196
Gastrectomy, anaemia following .. 138
— pernicious anaemia following 98, 104
Gastric acid secretion in pernicious anaemia 90
— atrophy and iron deficiency .. 69, 72
— — in pernicious anaemia .. 93, 94
— carcinoma, bleeding due to, causing anaemia 41
— — and pernicious anaemia .. 94
— herniation leading to anaemia .. 138
— mucosa, changes in, in iron deficiency 69
— neoplasm, recognition of presence of 140
Gastrin, synthetic, in test for achlorhydria 91
Gastro-enterostomy and vagotomy, anaemia following 27
Gastroferrin 35
Gastro-intestinal blood-loss, causes of .. 7
— — investigation of 71, 72
— disease 41
— disturbance leading to anaemia .. 138
— lesions in pernicious anaemia .. 93
— lymphoma 154
— surgery, anaemia following .. 26, 138
— — pernicious anaemia following .. 104
— symptoms of Hodgkin's disease .. 151
Gastrotest for gastric acid secretion .. 91
General diseases causing risk of anaemia 138
Giant-cell arteritis 50
— granuloma 50
Glanzman's disease 230
Globulin levels 12
Glossitis due to vitamin-B_{12} and folate deficiency 98, 106
Granulocytopenia, drugs causing .. 267
Granuloma, giant-cell 50
— Hodgkin's 149
Granulomatosis, Wegener's 50
di Guglielmo's disease 183, 213

HAEMATEST tablet 70
Haematinic factors, serum levels of .. 140
Haematological complications of aplastic anaemia 266

Haematological conditions causing thrombocytopenia 228
Haemochromatosis 35
Haemoglobin catabolism (*Fig.* 30) 242
— in iron deficiency .. (*Fig.* 12) 63
— level(s), clinical assessment of .. 135
— — in relation to age and sex (*Fig.* 12) 63
— serum, and blood-urea levels in renal disease anaemia 39
— — iron in relation to .. .. (*Fig.* 17) 66
— synthesis 61
— values 2
— — following trauma 28
— — in infection and in vascular disease 22
Haemoglobinuria, paroxysmal cold .. 253
— — nocturnal 254, 267
Haemolysis in Hodgkin's disease .. 151
— increased 15
— intravascular 242, 244
Haemolytic anaemia(s) 126, (*Figs.* 80–83) 242–255
— — acquired .. .. (*Fig.* 83) 248
— — — auto-immunity in 245
— — acute, in paroxysmal cold haemoglobinuria 253
— — associated with cancer 25
— — classification of 242
— — congenital 245
— — non-spherocytic 247
— — diagnosis from other macrocytic anaemias 107
— — — of type 245
— — haemopathic 251
— — laboratory findings 244
— — micro-angiopathic .. 228, 254
— — secondary acquired 250
Haemopathic haemolytic anaemia .. 251
Haemophilia 234
Haemopoiesis and ageing .. (*Fig.* 1) 5
Haemorrhagic thrombocythaemia .. 229
Haemosiderin 61
— assessment .. (*Figs.* 18, 19) 67, 68
Headache in iron-deficiency anaemia .. 75
Health check-ups, routine periodic, importance of 140
Heavy-chain disease 197
Heparin in prevention of thrombosis .. 239
Hepatic cirrhosis causing haemolytic anaemia 257
— — serum electrophoresis in detection of .. .. .. (*Fig.* 60) 191
— folate 113
Hepatocellular necrosis 32
Hess's test of capillary resistance .. 225
Hiatus hernia, bleeding due to, causing anaemia 41
— 'leukaemicus' 173

INDEX

Histamine test, augmented, for achlorhydria 91
Histidine-loading test .. (*Fig.* 26) 112
Histiocytic leukaemia, chronic 164
Hodgkin's disease .. (*Fig.* 34) 149
— — age incidence of, by histological type .. .. (*Fig.* 34) 150
— — causing haemolytic anaemia .. 250
— — classifications of .. 149, 150
— — clinical features 150
— — haematological and systemic manifestations .. (*Fig.* 36) 158
— — incidence of (*Figs.* 32, 33) 142, 143
— — infections associated with .. 161
— — male preponderance in 144
— — prognosis in .. (*Fig.* 35) 155, 157
— — treatment of 153
Hydroxocobalamin in pernicious anaemia 104
Hyperchromic anaemia, mortality due to 5
Hypercoagulability, tendency to, in elderly 31
Hyperglobulinaemic purpura 232
Hypersensitivity to drugs causing thrombocytopenia 227
Hypersplenism 255
Hyperthyroidism 54
— associated with lymphoid tissue tumours 161
Hyperviscosity syndrome 197
Hypochromic anaemia due to bacterial endocarditis 19
— — in elderly 63
— — investigation of 15
— — sex-linked 126
— — with secondary iron loading .. 126
Hypogammaglobulinaemia, hypersplenism with 255
— in lymphatic leukaemia 182
— lymphoid tissue tumours 160
Hypoplasia of bone-marrow 257
Hypothyroidism 54
— diagnosis of, from other macrocytic anaemias 107
— macrocytic anaemia in 125
— pernicious anaemia in .. 54, 104, 125

IDIOPATHIC neutropenia, chronic .. 269
— thrombocytopenic purpura (I.T.P.) .. 225
IgA globulin 190
IgG globulin 190
IgM globulin 190
Ileal absorption, deficient, causing low serum vitamin B_{12} 108
Imferon (iron-dextran), intramuscular .. 81
— — intravenous, total dose infusion of 82
Immune mechanism causing granulocytopenia 267
— reaction disease 205

Immunoelectrophoresis 191, 192
Immunoglobulins .. .. (*Fig.* 58) 189
Immunological deficiencies in lymphoid tissue tumours 160
Incompatibility leading to anaemia .. 138
Infection(s) associated with blood changes 18
— — — lymphoid tissue tumours .. 161
— causing haemolytic anaemia 253
— — thrombocytopenia 228
— chronic, associated with blood changes 21
— purpura associated with (*Figs.* 74–79) 231
Intestinal absorption of iron .. (*Fig.* 10) 58
— malabsorption associated with lymphoid tissue tumours 161
— operations, anaemia following 26, 27
Intramuscular iron therapy 80
Intravenous iron therapy 81
Intrinsic cell antibody in pernicious anaemia 93
— factor 87
Ionizing radiations causing aplastic anaemia 259
Iron absorption .. .. (*Fig.* 10) 58
— — factors controlling 60
— deficiency .. .. (*Figs.* 10–20) 58–85
— — associated with folate deficiency 117, 121
— — — pernicious anaemia .. 90
— — clinical features of (*Fig.* 20) 72
— — complicating pernicious anaemia, treatment of 106
— — due to phlebotomy in polycythaemia vera 222, 223
— — in elderly, causes of .. 63
— — incidence of, in elderly (*Fig.* 15) 67
— — investigation of 70
— — laboratory findings and diagnosis (*Figs.* 12–19) 63
— — structural changes in .. 69
— — suspected, routine investigation of 71
— — with anaemia, clinical features of (*Fig.* 20) 73
— — without anaemia .. (*Fig.* 17) 67, 78
— — — test for 70
— excretion 60
— malabsorption causing anaemia .. 8
— metabolism .. .. (*Fig.* 11) 61
— — inborn error of 35
— overloading in haemochromatosis 35, 36
— preparations, oral, side-effects of .. 80
— — for oral therapy 79
— — prolonged-release 79
— — proprietary 83
— saturation 66, 67
— serum, and blood-urea levels in renal disease anaemia 39
— — correlation between T.I.B.C. and M.C.H.C. and .. (*Fig.* 17) 66
— — estimation of .. (*Figs.* 12–15) 64, 66

INDEX

	PAGE
Iron serum levels in portal cirrhosis	34
— — pernicious anaemia	91
— — values following trauma	28
— — — in infection and in vascular disease	22
— storage	61
— therapy, adjuvant substances	80
— — duration of	82
— — effect of, in diagnosis of anaemia of chronic infection	22
— — intramuscular	80
— — intravenous	81
— — in iron-deficiency anaemia	78
— — masking cause of anaemia	72
— — oral	78
— — preventive	133, 135, 136, 137
— — in rheumatoid arthritis	45
— tissue	68
— utilization, failure of, due to pyridoxine deficiency	124
— vitamin B_{12}, folic acid, ascorbic acid, interrelation of	128
Iron-binding capacity (see T.I.B.C.)	
Iron-deficiency anaemia	13
— — associated with specific diseases	14
— — clinical features (*Fig.* 20)	73
— — diagnosis from anaemia of chronic infection	21
— — — of underlying cause	72
— — due to blood-loss	7, 16
— — histamine-fast achlorhydria in	131
— — investigation	16
— — mild, routine treatment of, and neoplastic disease	140
— — morbidity and mortality	4
— — postoperative	26
— — in relation to other deficiencies	129, 130, 131
— — rheumatoid arthritis	43
— — treatment	78
Iron-dependent enzyme systems	62
Irradiation in Hodgkin's disease	153
— precipitating leukaemia	169
Ischaemic heart disease, anticoagulant therapy in	238
JAUNDICE, acholuric, complicating haemolytic anaemia	243, 247
— and anaemia, recurrent crises in	246
— due to Hodgkin's disease	151
— obstructive, causing blood-cell anomalies (*Fig.* 3)	32
Jectofer	81
Jejunum, diverticula of, associated with folate deficiency	114
— — — — vitamin-B_{12} deficiency	101
— — — raised folate	111

	PAGE
KOILONYCHIA due to iron-deficiency anaemia	72
LATEX agglutination test	52
L.E. cell phenomenon	51
Leucocyte(s) in acute leukaemia	173
— alkaline phosphatase activity in myeloid leukaemia	178
— count in Hodgkin's disease	159
— — myeloid leukaemia (*Figs.* 51, 52)	177
— in iron deficiency	64
Leuco-encephalopathy, multifocal, in Hodgkin's disease	152
Leuco-erythroblastic anaemia, diagnosis from other macrocytic anaemias	107
— — in myelofibrosis	210
Leucopenia associated with drugs	268
Leucopoietic system, functional capacity of, in age	6
Leukaemia (*Figs.* 37–57)	164–188
— acute (*Figs.* 44–49)	171
— — age distribution in (*Figs.* 38–40)	166
— — causing haemolytic anaemia	250
— — clinical features of	171
— — course and prognosis of	175
— — diagnostic laboratory features of (*Figs.* 48, 49)	173
— — incidence of (*Fig.* 40)	164
— — lymphoblastic	164, 175
— — monocytic 164, (*Fig.* 50) 174,	175
— — myeloblastic	164
— — pathological changes of	184
— — promyelocytic	164, 175
— — treatment of	185
— aetiology of (*Figs.* 41–43)	167
— age distribution in (*Figs.* 38, 39)	165
— aleukaemic	183
— — diagnosis from other macrocytic anaemias	107
— basophilic	183
— chronic histiocytic	164
— — incidence of (*Fig.* 40)	164
— — lymphatic	164, 180
— — — age distribution in (*Figs.* 38–40)	166
— — — associated conditions of	182
— — — causing haemolytic anaemia	250
— — — course and prognosis in	182
— — — 'latent'	181, 187
— — — M-components in	204
— — — pathological changes in	185
— — — treatment of	187
— — myeloid 164, (*Figs.* 51–57)	176
— — — age distribution in (*Figs.* 38–40)	166
— — — causing haemolytic anaemia	250
— — — diagnosis of	178
— — — laboratory findings in (*Figs.* 51, 52)	177

INDEX

Leukaemia, chronic myeloid, pathological changes in 184
— — — prognosis in .. (*Figs.* 53–57) 180
— — — radiation and 170
— — — treatment of 187
— classification of 164
— complicating polycythaemia vera 220, 221, 223
— drugs used in treatment of 186
— eosinophilic 183
— incidence of .. (*Figs.* 37–40) 164, 166
— lymphatic, associated with lymphosarcoma 146, 147, 162
— — low serum folate in 114
— lymphoblastic, incidence by age of (*Fig.* 42) 168
— mast-cell 183
— megakaryocytic 164
— monocytic, associated with reticulum-cell sarcoma 162
— neutrophilic 183
— non-lymphoblastic, incidence by age of (*Fig.* 43) 168
— plasma-cell 164, 183, 198, 199
— thrombocytopenia in 228
Leukaemic reticulo-endotheliosis .. 162
Leukaemoid blood reactions in tuberculosis 20, 21
— reactions 184
Liver disease causing macrocytic anaemia 125
— — chronic, diagnosis from other macrocytic anaemias 107
— disorders associated with blood disorders .. .. .. (*Fig.* 3) 32
Loneliness leading to anaemia 138
Lupus erythematosus associated with rheumatoid arthritis .. (*Fig.* 4) 44
— — causing haemolytic anaemia .. 251
— — systemic .. .. (*Figs.* 5–9) 51
Lymphadenopathy, causes of, other than malignant tumour 162
Lymphatic leukaemia (*see* Leukaemia, Lymphatic *and* Leukaemia, Chronic Lymphatic)
Lymph-node biopsy in diagnosis of malignant lymphoid tumours 162
Lymphoblastic leukaemia, acute 164, 176
— lymphosarcoma 146
Lymphocyte depletion in Hodgkin's disease .. (*Fig.* 34) 150, (*Fig.* 35) 157
— predominance in Hodgkin's disease (*Fig.* 34) 150, (*Fig.* 35) 157
Lymphocytic lymphosarcoma 146
Lymphoid tissue tumours (*Figs.* 32–36) 142–163
— — — age distribution of (*Figs.* 32, 33) 143
— — — associated conditions of .. 161
— — — classification of 142

Lymphoid tissue tumours, general prognosis in .. .. (*Fig.* 35) 156
— — — haematological and systemic manifestations of (*Fig.* 36) 158
— — — incidence of 142
— — — sex incidence of 144
— tumours, malignant, diagnosis of .. 162
Lymphoma, follicular 148
— — age distribution in 144
— — of gastric intestinal tract .. 155, 156
— — lymphosarcoma arising in .. 146
— — megaloblastic anaemia due to .. 159
— — prognosis in 156
— of gastro-intestinal tract 154
— giant follicular, of spleen 148
— malignant 250
— — causing leucoerythroblastic anaemia 158
Lymphosarcoma 145
— anaemia of 158
— causing haemolytic anaemia .. 250
— clinical features of 146
— follicular lymphoma developing into 148
— gastro-intestinal 154
— incidence of .. .. (*Figs.* 32, 33) 143
— prognosis in 156, 158
— treatment of 147

MACROCYTIC anaemia(s) due to folate deficiency 116, 117
— — in elderly, differential diagnosis of 107
— or megaloblastic anaemia, deficiency states giving rise to (*Fig.* 31) 123
Macrocytosis due to anticonvulsant therapy in epilepsy 114
Macroglobulinaemia, Waldenström's .. 196
Malabsorption causing anaemia .. 8
— — vitamin-B_{12} deficiency (*Figs.* 23, 24) 101
— investigation of 71
Malignancy, anaemia of 250, 260
Malignant lymphoma 250
— myelosclerosis 212, 213
Malnutrition causing anaemia 8
Marrow abnormalities in cirrhosis .. 35
— activity, impaired, in chronic infection 22
— aplasia, classification of 256
— aspiration 67, 68
— biopsy in myelofibrosis 210
— cellularity of, in relation to age (*Fig.* 1) 6
— changes in folate deficiency 111
— disease causing aplastic anaemia .. 258
— failure .. .. (*Figs.* 84, 85) 256–271
— — relative 270
— findings in myeloid leukaemia .. 178
— — polycythaemia vera 217
— function, tests of 15

INDEX

Marrow inadequacy in anaemia of cancer 24
— iron assessment .. (*Figs*. 18, 19) 67
— in leukaemia, acute 173
— lymphoid tissue tumours 160
— myeloma cells in
    (*Figs*. 61, 62) 193, (*Fig*. 63) 200
— in pernicious anaemia (*Fig*. 22) 90, 93
— picture in aplastic anaemia 262
— response, inadequate, to haematinic
    therapy 257
— smears, examination of 16
— toxicity causing granulocytopenia .. 267
— toxins, direct-acting, causing thrombo-
    cytopenia 227, 228
Mast-cell leukaemia 183
M-components in lymphatic leukaemia.. 204
— serum in multiple myelomatosis 200, 201
M.C.H.C. (mean corpuscular haemo-
    globin concentration) .. (*Fig*. 12) 64
— correlation between serum iron and
    (*Fig*. 17) 66
M.C.V. (mean corpuscular volume), in-
    creased, in pernicious anaemia .. 89
Mediastinal tumour, Hodgkin's disease
    simulating 151
Megakaryocytic anaemia 164
Megaloblastic anaemia(s) (*Figs*. 21–24) 86–109
— — 'refractory' 125, 126
— — in rheumatoid arthritis 117
— — subacute combined degeneration 97
— erythropoiesis 214
— or macrocytic anaemia, deficiency
    states giving rise to .. (*Fig*. 31) 123
Megaloblastosis in 'non-folate-deficient
    patients' 46, 47
Megaloblasts in marrow in pernicious
    anaemia .. .. .. (*Fig*. 22) 90
Melphalan in multiple myelomatosis .. 204
Memory loss in pernicious anaemia .. 94
Mental changes in pernicious anaemia 94, 106
— confusion in iron-deficiency anaemia
    74, 83
— — subacute combined degeneration 97
— disorder and anaemia 138
— disturbance due to vitamin-B_{12} defici-
    ency 95, 106
— symptoms due to folate deficiency .. 116
Mercaptopurine in acute leukaemia 185, 186
Mesenchymal stem cell, abnormal, dis-
    eases arising from .. (*Fig*. 73) 214
Methotrexate in acute leukaemia 185, 186
Methyldopa causing haemolytic anaemia 252
Micro-angiopathic haemolytic anaemia
    228, 254
Microbiological assays of serum vitamin
    B_{12} in pernicious anaemia 92
Mixed cellularity in Hodgkin's disease
    (*Fig*. 34) 150, (*Fig*. 35) 157

Mobility, decreased, leading to anaemia 138
Monoclonal gammopathy 196
— immunoglobulins 189
Monocytic leukaemia, acute
    164, (*Fig*. 50) 174, 175
Mononuclear 'blast cells' in acute leuk-
    aemia .. .. .. (*Figs*. 48, 49) 173
Morbidity and mortality 4
Mucous membrane, pallor of, in iron-
    deficiency anaemia 72
— — — value of, in assessment of
    haemoglobin level 135
Mustine hydrochloride in Hodgkin's dis-
    ease 153
Myeloblastic leukaemia, acute .. 164
— termination in chronic myeloid leuk-
    aemia .. .. (*Figs*. 53–57) 180
Myelofibrosis complicating polycythaemia
    vera 221
— course and prognosis in 213
— differential diagnosis of 213
— laboratory findings in 210
— and myelosclerosis 210
Myeloid leukaemia (*see* Leukaemia,
    Chronic Myeloid)
— metaplasia complicating polycyt-
    haemia 220
Myeloma, multiple, incidence of (*Fig*. 32) 143
— solitary 202
— — treatment of 203
Myelomatosis .. .. (*Figs*. 63, 64) 197
— age incidence of 195
— amyloidosis complicating .. 203, 204
— diffuse 201
— low serum folate in 114
— marrow in .. .. (*Figs*. 61, 62) 193
— multiple .. .. (*Figs*. 63, 64) 198
— — diagnosis of 200
— — prognosis in 201
— — treatment of 204
— serum electrophoresis in detection of
    (*Fig*. 59) 190
— treatment of 263
Myelopathy in pernicious anaemia .. 97
Myeloproliferative disorders (*Fig*. 73) 210–223
— syndrome .. .. (*Fig*. 73) 214
Myelosclerosis causing haemolytic
    anaemia 250
— low serum folate in 114
— malignant 212, 213
— myelofibrosis and 210
Myelosis, chronic erythraemic
    164, 183, 212, 213
Myelosuppressive therapy in polycyt-
    haemia vera 222, 223
Myoglobin 63
Myxoedema coma associated with haemor-
    rhages 233

INDEX

Neoplasm associated with paraproteinaemia .. .. .. (*Figs.* 65–72) 205
Neoplastic disease, folate deficiency associated with (*Figs.* 27–30) 118, 119
Nervous system, central, in pernicious anaemia 93, 94, 96
— — — symptoms of iron-deficiency anaemia in 73
Neuritis, peripheral, in pernicious anaemia 96
Neurological complications of pernicious anaemia 94, 106
— disease, anaemia associated with .. 139
— — and folate deficiency 116
Neutropenia, chronic idiopathic .. 269
Neutrophilic leukaemia 183
Nicotinic acid deficiency anaemia .. 124
Nitrogen mustard in polycythaemia vera 221
Nocturnal haemoglobinuria, paroxysmal 254, 267
Nodular sclerosing Hodgkin's disease (*Fig.* 34) 149, 150, (*Fig.* 35) 156
Non-thrombocytopenic purpura 225, 230
Normochromic anaemia due to folate deficiency 117
Normocytic anaemia, refractory 125, 126
— normochromic anaemia associated with cancer 21, 24
— — — postoperative 26
Nutritional folate deficiency 113
— megaloblastic anaemia, diagnosis from other macrocytic anaemias .. 107

Occult blood in faeces, tests for 70, 140
Occultest tablet 70
Optic neuritis in pernicious anaemia 97, 98
Oral lesions associated with iron deficiency 69
Organ-specific antibody to gastric parietal cells in pernicious and iron-deficiency anaemias 131
Orthotolidine test for occult blood .. 70
Osteo-arthritis 48
Osteolytic lesions in multiple myelomatosis 200, 201
Ovarian dermoids causing haemolytic anaemia 251

Pallor, mucosal, in iron-deficiency anaemia 72
— skin, in iron-deficiency anaemia .. 77
Palpitations in iron-deficiency anaemia 76
Pancytopenia, patterns of 257
Pantothenic acid deficiency 125
Paraesthesiae of hands and feet in iron-deficiency anaemia 75
Paragranuloma, Hodgkin's 149, 152, 156

Paraproteinaemia, age incidence of .. 195
— associated with neoplasm (*Figs.* 65–72) 205
— in lymphoid tissue tumours 160
— malignant causes of 194
Paraproteins .. .. (*Figs.* 58–62) 189
— classification of 194
— detection of .. .. (*Figs.* 59, 60) 190
— diagnostic implications of 195
— general features of 192
— production of .. .. (*Figs.* 61, 62) 193
— serum, in multiple myelomatosis 200, 201
Parietal cell antibody in pernicious anaemia 92
Paroxysmal cold haemoglobinuria .. 253
— nocturnal haemoglobinuria .. 254, 267
Paterson-Kelly syndrome 72
Pel-Ebstein fever in Hodgkin's disease .. 150
Penicillin allergy, spontaneous factor-VIII inhibitor associated with .. 235
— causing haemolytic anaemia 252
Pentagastrin test 91
Peptic ulceration, bleeding due to, causing anaemia 41, 42
— — leading to anaemia 138
Perls's technique .. .. (*Figs.* 18, 19) 68
Pernicious anaemia .. (*Fig.* 22) 89–101
— — aetiology of 100
— — associated with hyperthyroidism 54, 103
— — — — iron deficiency 69
— — — — other auto-immune disorders 103
— — biochemical changes in 91
— — clinical examination for 98
— — features of 94
— — in diabetes mellitus 55
— — diagnosis from other macrocytic anaemias 107
— — familial incidence of 100
— — in hypothyroidism 54, 154
— — laboratory and diagnostic features of .. .. (*Fig.* 22) 89
— — latent or early 98
— — morbidity and mortality of .. 14
— — pathology of 93
— — prevalence rate of 100
— — in relation to folate and iron deficiencies 128, 130
— — simulated by folate-deficiency anaemia 116
— — treatment of 104
— — — associated deficiencies .. 106
— — — with age 94
Peroxidases 62
Petechiae in idiopathic thrombocytopenic purpura 225
PGA (*see* Folic Acid)
Phenindione in prevention of thrombosis 238
Phenylbutazone precipitating leukaemia 168

INDEX

	PAGE
Philadelphia chromosome	178
Phlebotomy in polycythaemia vera	221, 222
Pigmentation, slaty, in haemochromatosis	36
Pituitary gland disease	55
Plasma cells, production of paraproteins in (Figs. 61, 62)	193, 195
— dried, in defibrination syndrome	237
— proteins	10
Plasma-cell leukaemia	164, 183, 198, 199
— proliferation in myelomatosis	197, 198
Plasma-iron clearance (P.I.C.) in myelofibrosis	211
Plasmacytoma, extramedullary	202, 203
Platelet abnormalities causing bleeding	224
— function, abnormal, in thrombasthenia	230
Polyarteritis nodosa	50
Polycythaemia	215
— in Cushing's syndrome	55
— erythropoietic	219
— in renal disease	37
— secondary	215
— 'stress'	219
— tumour-induced	219
— vera	216
— — complications in	220, 222
— — diagnosis of	218
— — — differential	219
— — treatment of	221
Portal cirrhosis	33
Postoperative anaemia	25
Prevention of anaemia	133–141
Primary atypical anaemia, cold agglutinins with	254
Primidone causing lymphadenopathy	162
Procarbazine hydrochloride in Hodgkin's disease	154
Promyelocytic leukaemia, acute	164
Prostate, carcinoma of, haemorrhage due to pathological fibrinolysis in	236
Protein(s) disorders (Figs. 58–72)	189–209
— — clinical classification of	196
— plasma	10
— serum, analyses at different ages	12
— — changes in carcinoma	25
— — — chronic infection	23
— — level in multiple myelomatosis	200
— — in lymphoid tissue tumours	160
Protoporphyrin, erythrocyte	70
'Pseudo-iron deficiency' in chronic bronchitis and chronic infection	21
Pseudolymphoma after anticonvulsant therapy	162
Pteroylglutamic acid (see Folic Acid)	
Pulmonary disease, chronic, leading to anaemia	139
— — polycythaemia secondary to	215
Purpura (Figs. 74–79)	224

	PAGE
Purpura, dysproteinaemia due to	232
— haemorrhagica in pernicious anaemia	98
— non-thrombocytopenic	225, 230
— senile	230
— thrombocytopenic	224, 225
— thrombotic thrombocytopenic	228
Pyelonephritis in myelomatosis	203
Pyridoxine deficiency	124
QUESTIONNAIRE, assessment of symptomatology by, in anaemia prevention	134
RADIATIONS, ionizing, causing aplastic anaemia	259
Radioassay of serum vitamin B_{12} in pernicious anaemia	92
Radio-isotope studies in haemolytic anaemia	242, 245
— — iron deficiency	69
— — myelofibrosis	211
Radiophosphorus in polycythaemia vera	216, 221
Radiotherapy in polycythaemia vera and leukaemia	220, 221, 223
Raynaud's syndrome, cold agglutinin haemoglobinuria and	254
Red-cell(s) aplasia	267
— count in pernicious anaemia	89
— destruction, evidence of	244
— folate content of	110, 112
— life, estimation of, by radio-isotopes	242
— regeneration, signs of	244
— volume determination in polycythaemia vera	216
Reed-Sternberg cells in Hodgkin's disease	149, 159
'Refractory' anaemias (see also Aplastic Anaemia)	257
— 'megaloblastic anaemia'	125, 126
Renal disease	37
— failure causing aplastic anaemia	259
— — — haemolytic anaemia	251, 254
— insufficiency, progress of, causing anaemia	37
— involvement in myelomatosis	203
— system, symptoms of iron-deficiency anaemia in	77
Respiratory system, symptoms of iron-deficiency anaemia in	77
Reticulocyte count in red-cell regeneration	244
Reticulosarcoma	147
— gastro-intestinal	154
— incidence of (Figs. 32, 33)	143
— prognosis in	156, 158
Reticulosarcoma causing haemolytic anaemia	250

INDEX

Reticuloses (see Lymphoid Tissue Tumours)
Reticulum-cell sarcoma (see also Reticulosarcoma) 147
— — associated with monocytic leukaemia 162
Rheumatoid arthritis .. .. (Fig. 4) 42
— — associated with folate deficiency 118
— — — — pernicious anaemia .. 104
— — leading to anaemia 139
Riboflavine deficiency anaemia .. 124
Rubidomycin in acute leukaemia .. 185

SARCOMA, anaplastic .. 147, 148, 156
— Hodgkin's 149
Saturation of transferrin 66, 67
Schilling test 92
Scurvy associated with anaemia 123
— haemorrhagic features of 231
Senile purpura 230
Septicaemia associated with purpura (Figs. 74–79) 231
— causing anaemia 26
— fulminating 20
Serum abnormalities causing bleeding .. 224
— electrophoresis in detection of paraproteins .. .. (Figs. 59, 60) 190
— levels, measurement of 140
— proteins (see Proteins, Serum)
— tests for paraproteins 191
Sex incidence of anaemia 2
— — lymphoid tissue tumours .. 144
Side effects of therapy with iron .. 80–82
— — — B_{12} 105
— — — folate 122
'Sidero-achrestic anaemia' .. 124, 126
Sideroblastic anaemia .. (Fig. 31) 126
— — in chronic alcoholism 119
— — following isoniazid and P.A.S. therapy 21
— — primary acquired 126
— — pyridoxine-sensitive 63
— — secondary 126, 127
Sideropenia (see also Iron Deficiency) 58
— in iron-deficiency anaemia 77
Skeletal involvement in Hodgkin's disease 152
Skin diseases associated with anaemia .. 130
— — — folate deficiency 120
— lesions in Hodgkin's disease .. 152
— reactions in chronic myeloid leukaemia 176
— symptoms of iron-deficiency anaemia 77
Smoking in causation of optic neuritis in pernicious anaemia 97
Social difficulties leading to anaemia .. 138
Spectroscopic tests for occult blood .. 71

Spherocytic anaemia, congenital (Figs. 81, 82) 245, 246
Spinal cord, subacute combined degeneration of 93, 97
Spleen in chronic myeloid leukaemia .. 185
Splenectomy in congenital spherocytic anaemia 246, 247
— haemolytic anaemia, acquired .. 249
— idiopathic thrombocytopenic purpura 226
— myeloproliferative syndrome .. 215
— polycythaemia vera 222
Splenic puncture in myelofibrosis .. 211
Splenomegaly associated with rheumatoid arthritis 44
— in follicular lymphoma .. 148, 149
— leukaemia, chronic myeloid 176
Spontaneous factor-VIII inhibitors .. 235
Sprue, folate deficiency in 120
Staphylococcal septicaemia associated with purpura .. (Figs. 74–79) 232
Steatorrhoea associated with folate deficiency 114
— — — vitamin-B_{12} deficiency .. 108
— in Hodgkin's disease 152
— idiopathic, associated with lymphoid tissue tumours 162
— in iron-deficiency anaemia 77
Steroid therapy in acquired haemolytic anaemia 249
— — contra-indicated in pernicious anaemia 106
Storage iron 61
Streptokinase for thrombolysis .. 239, 240
'Stress' polycythaemia 219
Subacute combined degeneration of cord in pernicious anaemia .. 93, 97
Succinic acid supplementary to iron therapy 80
Surgery associated with anaemia .. 25
— in Hodgkin's disease 153, 154
Systemic diseases causing macrocytic anaemia 125
Systolic murmur in iron-deficiency anaemia 76

TACHYCARDIA in iron-deficiency anaemia 76
Temporal arteritis 50
Thrombasthenia 230
Thrombocythaemia, haemorrhagic .. 229
Thrombocytopenia in pernicious anaemia 89
— secondary 227
Thrombocytopenic purpura 224
— — idiopathic (I.T.P.) 225
— — thrombotic 228
Thrombo-embolic disease, thrombolytic therapy in 238
Thrombolytic therapy 238, 239

INDEX

	PAGE
Thrombosis	31
— associated with atherosclerosis	49
Thrombotic thrombocytopenic purpura	228
Thyroid deficiency causing anaemia	54
— diseases	54
— disorders associated with pernicious anaemia	54, 103, 104
Thyroiditis, auto-immune	54
Thyrotoxicosis	54
T.I.B.C. in ageing (*Fig.* 12)	64, 65
— and blood-urea levels in renal disease anaemia	39
— estimation (*Figs.* 13, 14, 16)	65
Tissue iron	68
Tongue, sore, in pernicious anaemia	98
Torulosis associated with Hodgkin's disease	161
Transferrin	61
— iron saturation of	66
Trasylol in defibrination syndrome	237
Trauma associated with blood disorders	28
Tuberculosis associated with blood disorders	20
— — folate deficiency	118
— — Hodgkin's disease	161
— disseminated, giving leukaemoid reactions	184
— pulmonary, associated with acute leukaemia (*Figs.* 44–47)	171
Tumour-induced polycythaemia	219
Tumours, lymphoid tissue (*see* Lymphoid Tissue Tumours)	
URAEMIA associated with bleeding disorders	233
Urinary excretion of paraproteins	195
— — test in pernicious anaemia	92
Urine tests for paraproteins	191
VEGANS, low serum vitamin B_{12} level in	9
Venesection in polycythaemia vera	221, 222
Ventricular failure, left, in iron-deficiency anaemia	77, 83
— — — pernicious anaemia	96
Vertebral body collapse due to solitary myeloma	202
Vertigo in iron-deficiency anaemia	75
Vinblastine sulphate in Hodgkin's disease	154
Vitamin deficiency causing macrocytic or megaloblastic anaemia	123

	PAGE
Vitamin-B_6 deficiency	124
Vitamin-B_{12} absorption studies	92
— deficiency (*Figs.* 21–24)	86–109
— — abnormalities of ascorbate metabolism in	124
— — anaemia	13
— — associated with folate deficiency	116, 121
— — in chronic liver disease	125
— — due to malabsorption (*Figs.* 23, 24)	101
— — in myelofibrosis	211
— — pernicious anaemia	95
— — postoperative anaemia	26
— — relation to other deficiencies	128, 129, 130
— — side-effect of giving folate to patient with	122
— and folate deficiency, mixed	86
— injections in pernicious anaemia	104
— — preventive	133, 136
— intake and absorption	87
— iron, folic acid, ascorbic acid, inter-relation of	128
— malabsorption causing anaemia	8
— metabolism (*Fig.* 21)	86
— — in polycythaemia vera	218
— oral therapy	105
— serum, levels in disease categories	103
— — — low, comparison with haemoglobin levels	99
— — — — due to causes other than pernicious anaemia	106
— — — in portal cirrhosis	34
— — — renal disease	40
— — — rheumatoid arthritis	47
— — in pernicious anaemia	92
— — values, in acute hepatitis	32
— — — following trauma	28, 30
Vitamin-C deficiency associated with anaemia	123
— — — — folate deficiency	114, 123
— — causing purpura	231
Von Willebrand's disease, coagulation defect in	234
WALDENSTRÖM'S macroglobulinaemia	196
Weakness, general, in iron-deficiency anaemia	75
Wegener's granulomatosis	50
ZIEVE'S syndrome	252